Drugs in Pregnancy

Editor

CATHERINE S. STIKA

OBSTETRICS AND GYNECOLOGY CLINICS OF NORTH AMERICA

www.obgyn.theclinics.com

Consulting Editor
WILLIAM F. RAYBURN

March 2023 • Volume 50 • Number 1

ELSEVIER

1600 John F. Kennedy Boulevard • Suite 1800 • Philadelphia, Pennsylvania, 19103-2899

http://www.theclinics.com

OBSTETRICS AND GYNECOLOGY CLINICS OF NORTH AMERICA Volume 50 Number 1
March 2023 ISSN 0889-8545, ISBN-13: 978-0-323-93989-8

Editor: Kerry Holland
Developmental Editor: Hannah Almira Lopez

Obstetrics and Gynecology Clinics (ISSN 0889-8545) is published quarterly by Elsevier Inc., 360 Park Avenue South, New York, NY 10010-1710. Months of issue are March, June, September, and December. Periodicals postage paid at New York, NY, and additional mailing offices. Subscription price per year is $355.00 (US individuals), $757.00 (US institutions), $100.00 (US students), $428.00 (Canadian individuals), $956.00 (Canadian institutions), $100.00 (Canadian students), $487.00 (international individuals), $956.00 (international institutions), and $225.00 (international students). To receive student/resident rate, orders must be accompanied by name of affiliated institution, date of term, and the signature of program/residency coordinator on institution letterhead. Orders will be billed at individual rate until proof of status is received. Foreign air speed delivery is included in all *Clinics* subscription prices. All prices are subject to change without notice. POSTMASTER: Send address changes to *Obstetrics and Gynecology Clinics*, Elsevier Health Sciences Division, Subscription Customer Service, 3251 Riverport Lane, Maryland Heights, MO 63043. **Customer Service: Telephone: 1-800-654-2452 (U.S. and Canada); 314-447-8871 (outside U.S. and Canada). Fax: 314-447-8029. E-mail: journalscustomerservice-usa@elsevier.com (for print support); journalsonlinesupport-usa@elsevier. com (for online support).**

Reprints. For copies of 100 or more of articles in this publication, please contact the Commercial Reprints Department, Elsevier Inc., 360 Park Avenue South, New York, New York 10010-1710. Tel.: 212-633-3874; Fax: 212-633-3820; E-mail: reprints@elsevier.com.

Obstetrics and Gynecology Clinics of North America is also published in Spanish by McGraw-Hill Interamericana Editores S.A., P.O. Box 5-237, 06500, Mexico; in Portuguese by Reichmann and Affonso Editores, Rio de Janeiro, Brazil; and in Greek by Paschalidis Medical Publications, Athens, Greece.

Obstetrics and Gynecology Clinics of North America is covered in MEDLINE/PubMed (Index Medicus), Excerpta Medica, Current Concepts/Clinical Medicine, Science Citation Index, BIOSIS, CINAHL, and ISI/BIOMED.

Contributors

CONSULTING EDITOR

WILLIAM F. RAYBURN, MD, MBA
Affiliate Professor, Department of Obstetrics and Gynecology, College of Graduate Studies, Medical University of South Carolina, Charleston, South Carolina, USA; Emeritus Distinguished Professor, Department of Obstetrics and Gynecology, University of New Mexico School of Medicine, Albuquerque, New Mexico, USA

EDITOR

CATHERINE S. STIKA, MD
Clinical Professor of Obstetrics and Gynecology, Department of Obstetrics and Gynecology, Northwestern University Feinberg School of Medicine, Chicago, Illinois, USA

AUTHORS

MARTINA L. BADELL, MD
Division of Maternal Fetal Medicine, Department of Gynecology and Obstetrics, Emory University School of Medicine, Atlanta, Georgia, USA

JASPREET BANGA, MD, MPH
Division of Infectious Disease, Department of Medicine, Beth Israel Deaconess Medical Center, Harvard Medical School, Boston, Massachusetts, USA

LUCY C. BARKER, MD, FRCPC
Postdoctoral Fellow, Department of Psychiatry, Women's College Hospital and Research Institute, University of Toronto, Toronto, Ontario, Canada

BRANDON Z. BELL, DO
Department of Obstetrics and Gynecology, Indiana University School of Medicine, Indianapolis, Indiana, USA

RUPSA C. BOELIG, MD, MS
Assistant Professor, Director of Research, Division of Maternal Fetal Medicine, Department of Obstetrics and Gynecology, Department of Clinical Pharmacology and Therapeutics, Sidney Kimmel Medical College, Thomas Jefferson University, Philadelphia, Pennsylvania, USA

KATHLEEN F. BROOKFIELD, MD, PhD, MPH
Department of Obstetrics and Gynecology, Adjunct Associate Professor, Oregon Health & Science University, Legacy Medical Group, Maternal Fetal Medicine, Legacy Health System, Portland, Oregon, USA

KRISTINA M. BROOKS, PharmD
Department of Pharmaceutical Sciences, University of Colorado Anschutz Medical Campus, Aurora, Colorado, USA

AARON B. CAUGHEY, MD, MPH, PhD
Division of Maternal-Fetal Medicine, Department of Obstetrics and Gynecology, School of Medicine, Oregon Health & Science University, Portland, Oregon, USA

AI-RIS Y. COLLIER, MD
Division of Maternal Fetal Medicine, Department of Obstetrics and Gynecology, Beth Israel Deaconess Medical Center, Department of Obstetrics, Gynecology and Reproductive Biology, Harvard Medical School, Boston, Massachusetts, USA

MAGED M. COSTANTINE, MD
Division of Maternal Fetal Medicine, Department of Obstetrics and Gynecology, The Ohio State University Wexner Medical Center, Columbus, Ohio, USA

ANNA E. DENOBLE, MD, MSc
Assistant Professor of Obstetrics, Gynecology and Reproductive Sciences, Section of Maternal-Fetal Medicine, Yale School of Medicine, New Haven, Connecticut, USA

JOE EID, MD
Division of Maternal Fetal Medicine, Department of Obstetrics and Gynecology, The Ohio State University Wexner Medical Center, Columbus, Ohio, USA

ELIZABETH E. GERARD, MD
Associate Professor of Neurology, Feinberg School of Medicine, Northwestern University, Chicago, Illinois, USA

SARAH A. GOLDSTEIN, MD
Assistant Professor of Internal Medicine, Section of Cardiovascular Medicine, Yale School of Medicine, New Haven, Connecticut, USA

CYNTHIA GYAMFI-BANNERMAN, MD, MS
Samuel SC Yen Endowed Chair, Department of Obstetrics, Gynecology, and Reproductive Sciences, Professor, Maternal-Fetal Medicine, Obstetrics and Gynecology, University of California, San Diego, La Jolla, California, USA

DAVID M. HAAS, MD, MS
Department of Obstetrics and Gynecology, Indiana University School of Medicine, Indianapolis, Indiana, USA

JOANNA M. IZEWSKI, MD
Department of Obstetrics and Gynecology, Indiana University School of Medicine, Indianapolis, Indiana, USA

NAIMA T. JOSEPH, MD, MPH
Division of Maternal Fetal Medicine, Department of Obstetrics and Gynecology, Beth Israel Deaconess Medical Center, Department of Obstetrics, Gynecology and Reproductive Biology, Harvard Medical School, Boston, Massachusetts, USA

ELIZABETH E. KRANS, MD, MSc
Associate Professor, Department of Obstetrics, Gynecology and Reproductive Sciences, University of Pittsburgh School of Medicine, Magee-Womens Research Institute, Pittsburgh, Pennsylvania, USA

GRACE LIM, MD, MS
Associate Professor, Department of Anesthesiology and Perioperative Medicine, Division of Obstetric and Women's Anesthesiology, Department of Obstetrics Gynecology and Reproductive Sciences, University of Pittsburgh School of Medicine, Pittsburgh, Pennsylvania, USA

SHAKKED LUBOTZKY-GETE, PhD
Postdoctoral Fellow, Women's College Hospital and Research Institute, Toronto, Ontario, Canada

LESLIE MATTHEWS, MD, PharmD
Department of Anesthesiology and Perioperative Medicine, Division of Obstetric and Women's Anesthesiology, University of Pittsburgh School of Medicine, Pittsburgh, Pennsylvania, USA

OSINAKACHUKWU MBATA, MD
Department of Obstetrics and Gynecology, Oregon Health & Science University, Portland, Oregon, USA

MARK MIROCHNICK, MD
Boston University School of Medicine, Boston, Massachusetts, USA

ALEXANDRA C. MOISE, MD
Feinberg School of Medicine, Northwestern University, Chicago, Illinois, USA

CHRISTIAN M. PETTKER, MD
Professor of Obstetrics, Gynecology and Reproductive Sciences, Section of Maternal-Fetal Medicine, Yale School of Medicine, New Haven, Connecticut, USA

KELSEY PINSON, MD
Maternal Fetal Medicine Fellow, University of California, San Diego, La Jolla, California, USA

WILLIAM F. RAYBURN, MD, MBA
Affiliate Professor, Department of Obstetrics and Gynecology, College of Graduate Studies, Medical University of South Carolina, Charleston, South Carolina, USA; Emeritus Distinguished Professor, Department of Obstetrics and Gynecology, University of New Mexico School of Medicine, Albuquerque, New Mexico, USA

MICHAELA RICKERT, PA-C, RDN, CDCES
Division of Maternal-Fetal Medicine, Department of Obstetrics and Gynecology, School of Medicine, Oregon Health & Science University, Portland, Oregon, USA

KARA M. ROOD, MD
Division of Maternal Fetal Medicine, Department of Obstetrics and Gynecology, The Ohio State University Wexner Medical Center, Columbus, Ohio, USA

ANTONIO SAAD, MD
Associate Professor, Division of Maternal-Fetal Medicine, Department of Obstetrics and Gynecology, The University of Texas Medical Branch at Galveston, Galveston, Texas, USA

MELODY SAFARZADEH, MD, MS
Fellow, Division of Maternal-Fetal Medicine, Department of Obstetrics and Gynecology, The University of Texas Medical Branch at Galveston, Galveston, Texas, USA

AALOK R. SANJANWALA, MD
Fellow, Division of Maternal-Fetal Medicine, Department of Obstetrics, Gynecology and Reproductive Sciences, University of Pittsburgh School of Medicine, Pittsburgh, Pennsylvania, USA

KIMBERLY K. SCARSI, PharmD, MS
Department of Pharmacy Practice and Science, University of Nebraska Medical Center, Omaha, Nebraska, USA

MEGAN SHEPHERD, MD
Assistant Instructor, Division of Maternal-Fetal Medicine, Department of Obstetrics and Gynecology, The University of Texas Medical Branch at Galveston, Galveston, Texas, USA

CATHERINE Y. SPONG, MD
Department of Obstetrics and Gynecology, The University of Texas Southwestern Medical Center, Parkland Health, Dallas, Texas, USA

CATHERINE S. STIKA, MD
Clinical Professor of Obstetrics and Gynecology, Department of Obstetrics and Gynecology, Northwestern University Feinberg School of Medicine, Chicago, Illinois, USA

LISA R. THIELE, BS
Department of Obstetrics and Gynecology, The University of Texas Southwestern Medical Center, Dallas, Texas, USA

AMY M. VALENT, DO, MCR
Division of Maternal-Fetal Medicine, Department of Obstetrics and Gynecology, School of Medicine, Oregon Health & Science University, Portland, Oregon, USA

SIMONE N. VIGOD, MD, MSC, FRCPC
Professor, Department of Psychiatry, Women's College Hospital and Research Institute, University of Toronto, Toronto, Ontario, Canada

Contents

> Since the recognition of pregnancy as a special pharmacokinetic population in the late 1990s, investigations have expanded our understanding of obstetric pharmacology. Many of the basic physiologic changes that occur during pregnancy impact on drug absorption, distribution, or clearance. Activities of hepatic metabolizing enzymes are variably altered by pregnancy, resulting in concentrations sufficiently different for some drugs that efficacy or toxicity may be affected. Understanding these unique pharmacologic changes will better inform our use of medications for our pregnant patients.

> Pregnant and lactating individuals historically have been excluded from research studies because of the ethical concerns surrounding potential harm to the fetus. Several National Institutes of Health and Food and Drug Administration initiatives have attempted to improve inclusion; however, clinical trials continue to exclude pregnant and lactating people. Drug labeling for safety and efficacy in pregnancy has thus been forced to rely on data from animal studies or limited case reports. Recent changes have sought to improve prescriber understanding of risks, benefits, and limitations of safety information on medications; however, confusion persists.

> The obstetric provider should ask about over-the-counter drugs, although most are low dose, used only briefly, and any harm is unlikely and more theoretic than real.

Hypertensive disorders of pregnancy (HDP) can result in significant maternal morbidity and even mortality. Available data suggest that many antihypertensives can be safely used in pregnant patients, albeit with close supervision of parameters like fetal growth and amniotic fluid volume. This article summarizes current guidelines on the diagnosis and treatment of hypertension in pregnancy and provides an in-depth guide to the available safety and efficacy data for antihypertensives during pregnancy and postpartum.

Preeclampsia is a hypertensive disorder of pregnancy affecting up to 8% of pregnancies. It is associated with significant neonatal and maternal morbidities and mortality. Although its pathogenesis is not completely understood, abnormal placentation resulting in imbalance in angiogenic factors, increased inflammation, and endothelial dysfunction are thought to be key pathways in the development of the disease. Administration of low-dose aspirin is recommended by professional societies for the prevention of preeclampsia in high-risk individuals. In this review, we summarize the evidence behind the use of low-dose aspirin and pravastatin in pregnant individuals at high risk of preeclampsia.

Magnesium sulfate is one of the most commonly used medications in obstetrics, most notably for the prevention of eclamptic seizures and fetal neuroprotection of the extremely preterm neonate. Pharmacokinetic and pharmacodynamic studies have demonstrated a variety of IV and IM regimens are effective for these indications. Existing models and data can be used to tailor treatment regimens to increase coverage in poor resource areas, maximize efficacy and minimize toxicity for patients of different weights and renal function.

Specifically, meta-analyses of randomized trials demonstrate that vaginal progesterone reduces the risk of preterm birth in selected high-risk singleton pregnancies. 17-OHPC may also reduce the risk of recurrent preterm birth in singletons. Finally, one trial suggests that vaginal progesterone may also be beneficial in improving live birth rates in singletons with prior miscarriages and early pregnancy bleeding.

Preterm birth, typically defined as birth between 20 0/7 weeks and 36 6/7 weeks of gestation, is a major cause of neonatal morbidity, and rates of preterm birth continue to rise. Antenatal corticosteroids have demonstrated benefit for reduction of morbidities and mortality associated with preterm birth, with few observed maternal risks. As such, antenatal corticosteroids have become the standard of care for treating pregnant people at risk of preterm birth. Tocolytics may be beneficial in temporarily slowing uterine contractions to prolong pregnancy long enough for the administration of corticosteroids or stabilization and transfer of a parturient in preterm labor.

Persons with gestational and pregestational diabetes during pregnancy may require pharmacologic agents to achieve pregnancy glycemic targets, and the available medications for use in pregnancy are limited. Insulin is the only FDA-approved medication for use in pregnancy and has the greatest evidence for safety and efficacy. Metformin and glyburide are the most commonly used oral agents in pregnancy. Understanding each medication's unique pharmacokinetics, potential side effects, fetal or childhood risks, gestational age of medication initiation and patient's diabetes care barriers are important aspects of shared decision-making and choosing a regimen that will achieve glycemic and pregnancy goals.

Infections are common in obstetric care and often require specific antibiotics, depending on the infection site and prevailing organisms. Summaries of antibiotic recommendations and treatment algorithms are provided for the following conditions: routine labor, group B streptococcus prophylaxis, preterm prelabor rupture of membranes, operative vaginal delivery, cesarean delivery, obstetric anal sphincter lacerations, chorioamnionitis, postpartum endometritis, infections of the urinary tract, and bacterial endocarditis prophylaxis.

Pain management during labor and delivery is complex and must balance efficacy and toxicity to both the pregnant person and the fetus. There are numerous ways to achieve safe and effective analgesia and anesthesia during labor and delivery, including neuraxial and nonneuraxial techniques. This review describes important anesthetic considerations that should be made when formulating a pain management plan and an overview of common anesthesia-related complications encountered in the obstetric population.

psychological and pharmacological treatments for mental illness around the time of pregnancy. Rather, the focus is on therapeutic considerations for general obstetrical providers.

Overdose is a leading cause of pregnancy-associated morbidity and mortality in the United States. As such, all obstetric providers have a responsibility to provide evidence-based care for patients with opioid use disorder to mitigate adverse outcomes associated with substance use during pregnancy.

This article explores current recommendations for anticoagulation therapy in pregnancy, including antepartum, intrapartum, and postpartum guidelines. The authors review various screening strategies used to assess whether a patient is an appropriate candidate for anticoagulation during pregnancy and the postpartum period. The article includes dosing regimens, optimal surveillance, and medication reversal. The authors also address the challenges of transitioning between low-molecular-weight heparin and unfractionated heparin. Finally, there is a discussion of intrapartum anticoagulation management, especially as it relates to the administration of regional anesthesia, and the indications for and timing of thromboprophylaxis following delivery.

Globally, epilepsy affects up to 15 million of people assigned female at birth who are of childbearing age. Up to 65% of these people with epilepsy and gestational capacity (PWEGC) have an unplanned pregnancy. Seizure control during pregnancy is important for ths safety of both the childbearervand fetus. There are multiple antiseizure medications (ASMs) that can be used to control seizures; however, each medication has its own teratogenic risk profile, which must be considered. The majority of these ASMs will require frequent plasma concentration monitoring during pregnancy with corresponding dosage adjustments. Dosages should be reduced towards prepregnancy levels in the first 3 weeks postpartum. Breastfeeding is typically recommended as benefits of breastmilk outweigh risks of seizure medication exposure.

OBSTETRICS AND GYNECOLOGY CLINICS

SERIES OF RELATED INTEREST

Clinics in Perinatology
www.perinatology.theclinics.com
Pediatric Clinics of North America
https://www.pediatrics.theclinics.com

THE CLINICS ARE AVAILABLE ONLINE!
Access your subscription at:
www.theclinics.com

Introduction

Celebrating the 50-year Anniversary of *Obstetrics and Gynecology Clinics*

It is my pleasure to recognize and reflect on the 50-year anniversary of the "birth" of the *Obstetrics and Gynecology Clinics of North America* by W.B. Saunders Company. Known to most physicians as simply *"The Clinics,"* our periodical remains an essential addition of the successful *Clinics of North America* publishing program. The series was acquired by Elsevier, the world's largest medical publisher, which provided worldwide distribution to now more than 70 countries. For this reason, the title has changed to simply the *Obstetrics and Gynecology Clinics*.

Our issues provide clinical updates to readers, ensuring timely and relevant content. As a resident in training, I recall viewing brown hardbound copies of *The Clinics* in our department library beside hardbound volumes of our standard specialty journals. It served as a resource for me as a resident, fellow, and faculty member for systematic reviews by experts in a strong portfolio of topics relevant to my on-the-job educational needs.

Topics in this series were chosen to be clinically relevant to all practicing obstetricians and gynecologists. This 50-year period has marked the beginning and maturation of our subspecialties: gynecologic oncology, reproductive endocrinology and infertility, maternal-fetal medicine, female pelvic medicine and restorative surgery, complex family planning, pediatric and adolescent gynecology, and minimally invasive gynecologic surgery. We emphasize that each clinical review use systematic and explicit methods to identify, select, and critically appraise relevant primary research. Readily accessible information is available for acquiring new knowledge, enhancing health system team-based care, and incorporating preventative and public health while treating individual patients.

Shortly before I became the first consulting editor in 2004, the issues began to be published electronically, while print editions have continued since its inception. *The Clinics* eventually became covered in MEDLINE/PubMed (Index Medicus), Excerpta Medica, Current Concepts/Clinical Medicine, Science Citation Index, BIOSIS, CINAHL, and ISI/BIOMED. In 2021, there were over 115,000 page views on these platforms, and the impact factor has increased by 66% since 2018. Article utility remains high; of those articles viewed, 87% were downloaded in 2021. Likewise, the series' impact was seen in social media, with 64,000 citations and 175,000 engagements in 2022.

My approach has always been to choose a contemporary topic in which no current book is being marketed for obstetricians and gynecologists. I select topics that are highlighted at our prominent national specialty meetings or articles from our finest

Obstet Gynecol Clin N Am 50 (2023) xiii–xv
https://doi.org/10.1016/j.ogc.2023.01.001
0889-8545/23/© 2023 Published by Elsevier Inc.

obgyn.theclinics.com

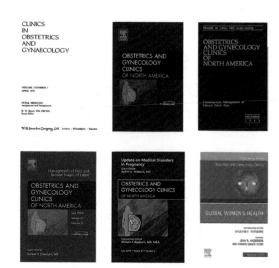

Fig. 1. The first-ever edition of *Obstetrics and Gynecology Clinics* is represented by the first image, the title page. Several images follow, showing the evolution of the cover designs over the years.

peer-reviewed journals in obstetrics and gynecology. Two editors now customarily undertake each *Obstetrics and Gynecology Clinics* issue, so that a junior faculty member can be mentored by a senior who is skilled in selecting topics of greatest interest and written by experts on the subject. We provide the possibility of each issue to be updated in 4 to 6 years depending on changes in the field and new topics of interest.

As consulting editor, I am pleased to provide career-building opportunities for fellows and junior faculty to gain publishing experience under the immediate direction of a senior author. The proportion of authors who are female faculty has risen considerably. All authors are delighted that their clinical reviews are discoverable on PubMed. Clinicians, students, and educators can access the content for free through subscriptions at their academic institution or hospital using the Science Direct and ClinicalKey platforms.

This acknowledgment of *Obstetrics and Gynecology Clinics'* 50th year in print would be incomplete without recognizing invaluable assistance from the outstanding Elsevier editorial staff. Those assigned to each issue work diligently and collaboratively with authors and editors on enforcing timelines and editing with proper grammar, formality, clarity, and consistency. In her longstanding leadership role as the senior manager of the entire series and global content, Kerry Holland has gained notoriety at Elsevier for her expertise, balanced approaches, and enthusiasm in overseeing our success.

The accompanying Fig. 1 displays the different cover designs of *Obstetrics and Gynecology Clinics* since 1974. Please peruse current and past issues at www. obgyn.theclinics.com. You will be impressed with the titles, key points and clinics care points, color illustrations, and videos in procedure-directed issues. On behalf of all issue editors and authors, I hope that you enjoy reading these articles as much as we appreciated working to bring them to you. As we begin the next 50 years, we welcome your feedback!

William F. Rayburn, MD, MBA
Departments of Obstetrics and Gynecology
University of New Mexico School of Medicine
Albuquerque, NM 87106, USA

Medical University of South Carolina
Charleston, SC 29425, USA

E-mail address:
wrayburnmd@gmail.com

Foreword

Drugs in Pregnancy: Common Use Despite Limited Information

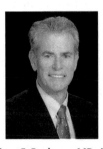

William F. Rayburn, MD, MBA
Consulting Editor

Basic science and clinical investigations continue to provide new information pertaining to drug therapy for disorders encountered during pregnancy, whether unique or preexisting. This information is now incorporated in a new *Obstetrics and Gynecology Clinics of North America* issue, "Drugs in Pregnancy," led by the Guest Editor, Catherine Stika, MD.

Guidelines for obstetric providers are provided for using common medications. Attention is balanced between safety to the fetus and maternal effectiveness and safety. For the student and practitioner of medicine, drugs of interest are generally confined to those of therapeutic value. In addition to iron, folic acid, or vitamin preparations, nearly all patients take one or more medications at some time during pregnancy. The most prescribed medications during pregnancy remain antibiotics, antiemetics, mild analgesics, and drugs for gastroesophageal reflux. The issue is well divided into subjects pertaining to medications for medical disorders (eg, diabetes, seizures, coagulation disorders, hypertension), antivirals, prevention or minimizing preeclampsia, and preparing for possible preterm delivery.

The issue begins with an overview of principles of obstetric pharmacology, including newer information about hepatic metabolism changes. Lessons learned and opportunities are then described about the inclusion of pregnant women and lactating women in clinical research. Medicines should be used during gestation only if the anticipated benefit is reasonable and considered to outweigh any known, suspected, or theoretic risk to the fetus. Conversely, drugs used to treat mothers-to-be with serious medical or mental health disorders may be intentionally discontinued before seeking advice from her obstetric provider. Special attention is devoted to opioid use, analgesia needs, and common psychiatric medications.

Obstet Gynecol Clin N Am 50 (2023) xvii–xviii
https://doi.org/10.1016/j.ogc.2022.11.002
0889-8545/23/© 2022 Published by Elsevier Inc.

obgyn.theclinics.com

Conclusions from case reports, epidemiologic studies, and animal investigations have definite limitations. Effects of a drug or its metabolites on the fetus require consideration of the dose, route of administration, duration, and fetal developmental stage of exposure. Drugs taken in high doses and near delivery may cause more immediate and sustained neonatal effects. Limited research has addressed the question of chronic exposure to therapeutic doses and subtle yet long-term consequences.

Relief of symptoms and the medical welfare of the pregnant patient must not be ignored. Drugs intended to improve maternal physical and mental health may benefit the fetus indirectly. To minimize any additional risks to the fetus or adverse side effects to the mother, a prescribed medication should be chosen properly and monitored closely, using the presumed most therapeutic dose for the shortest duration. Likewise, over-the-counter drugs for relief of symptoms should be used sparingly in the smallest dose for the shortest period. Despite this, individual variation in patient metabolism or clearance of certain drug must be appreciated, since recommended doses for nonpregnant women may be inadequate.

Careful attention was placed in this issue on the planning and writing of guidelines. Efforts were undertaken by 42 contributors specializing in general obstetrics, maternal-fetal medicine, internal medicine, and psychiatry. Their writings in the 18 articles describe not only new therapies that became available but also advances in both basic pharmacology and its application to obstetrics practice. Development of this large issue was successful due, in part, to the thoroughness and collaboration of the Elsevier publishing staff. I concur with Dr Stika's hope that this issue will provide readers with a broader understanding in caring better for our patients while inspiring investigators to pursue research in the growing field of obstetrics pharmacology.

William F. Rayburn, MD, MBA
Department of Obstetrics and Gynecology
Medical University South Carolina
1721 Atlantic Avenue
Sullivan's Island, SC 294482, USA

E-mail address:
wrayburnmd@gmail.com

Preface

Drugs in Pregnancy: Optimizing Care for our Pregnant Patients

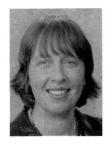

Catherine S. Stika, MD
Editor

Welcome to the most recent issue of *Obstetrics and Gynecology Clinics of North America* entitled, "Drugs in Pregnancy." Because pregnant people become sick and people with medical problems become pregnant, much of the care we provide to our pregnant patients involves the administration of drugs. Excluding vitamins and other supplements, a remarkable number of people take both prescribed and over-the-counter medications during their pregnancy. A cross-sectional, multinational, Web-based study,[1] which surveyed 9459 pregnant people in 2011 to 2012, found that 81.2% respondents reported use of at least one prescribed or over-the-counter medication during pregnancy. The percentage was even higher for participants in Canada and the United States: 84.8% reported any medication use in pregnancy, with 75.6% taking drugs for a short-term illness and 64.2% reporting use of over-the-counter medications.

Historically, many publications about drug use in pregnancy have focused on fetal safety. While still cognizant of fetal safety, this issue places the emphasis on maternal efficacy. Only nine drugs have undergone the extensive safety and efficacy evaluation required by the Food and Drug Administration (FDA) to achieve approval for an obstetric indication.[2] Of these, seven are currently still marketed, and four are uterotonics. All other drugs we prescribe to our pregnant patients are used off-label, supported by evidence in the literature but without formal FDA approval for use during pregnancy. Some drugs are prescribed for the same indication in both pregnant and nonpregnant people, like oseltamivir for influenza, but we also use medications for conditions other than their approved indications, such as the antihypertensive nifedipine prescribed for tocolysis. Because pregnant people are physiologically and pharmacologically different than nonpregnant people, we cannot assume that the same dosing strategies will work in both groups. For example, evidence from research performed in pregnant

Obstet Gynecol Clin N Am 50 (2023) xix–xx
https://doi.org/10.1016/j.ogc.2022.11.001
0889-8545/23/© 2022 Published by Elsevier Inc.

obgyn.theclinics.com

people has informed the creation of pregnancy-specific dosing guidelines for group B streptococci and cesarean antibiotic prophylaxis. But despite two decades of efforts by the FDA and National Institutes of Health as well as the 2018 recommendations of the 21st Century Cures Act Task Force on Research Specific to Pregnant Women and Lactating Women regarding gaps in knowledge and research on safe and effective therapies for pregnant and lactating women, timely research in this arena is woefully lagging, as witnessed by the recent delay in studying COVID-19 drugs and vaccinations in pregnant people. Our hope is that this issue of *Obstetrics and Gynecology Clinics of North America* will inspire investigators to pursue research in this exciting and growing field of obstetrics pharmacology.

However, the primary goal of "Drugs in Pregnancy" is to provide readers with a consolidated resource to aid in prescribing medications to treat common conditions that affect our pregnant patients. I am grateful to the many experts in their fields who have contributed to this publication. Topics they have addressed include the use of antihypertensive and antihyperglycemic medications, as well as antenatal steroids, tocolytics, and progestin therapy. You will find information about preeclampsia prophylaxis as well as guidelines for magnesium sulfate use in both high-income and low-/middle-income countries. Additional articles provide an overview of antiretroviral medications in pregnancy, COVID-19 therapies, and several other problematic viral infections. For our patients with chronic preexisting medical problems that require maintenance drugs while pregnant, we have included discussions of therapies for psychiatric conditions, opioid use disorder, epilepsy, and thromboembolic disease. Although we did not address uterotonics because that class of drugs has easily accessible FDA-approved guidance, we have included other labor-related topics, such as antibiotics for prophylaxis and treatment and analgesics prescribed during labor or postpartum. In addition, we start the issue with an overview of the changes in obstetric physiology and hepatic metabolism that impact drug use during pregnancy, a history of federal efforts to include pregnant and lactating people in drug research, and a discussion of common over-the-counter medications used by our patients.

We believe this first-of-its-kind resource will provide readers with a broader understanding of drug use in pregnancy and ultimately help us to better care for our pregnant patients.

Catherine S. Stika, MD
Department of Obstetrics and Gynecology
Northwestern University Feinberg School of Medicine
Chicago, IL 60611, USA

E-mail address:
c-stika@northwestern.edu

REFERENCES

1. Lupattelli A, Spigset O, Twigg MJ, et al. Medication use in pregnancy: a cross-sectional, multinational web-based study. BMJ Open 2014;4(2):e004365.
2. Wesley BD, Sewell CA, Chang CY, et al. Prescription medications for use in pregnancy-perspective from the US Food and Drug Administration. Am J Obstet Gynecol 2021;225(1):21–32.

Principles of Obstetric Pharmacology
Maternal Physiologic and Hepatic Metabolism Changes

Catherine S. Stika, MD*

KEYWORDS

- Pregnancy • Pharmacokinetics • Renal clearance • Renal secretion
- Drug metabolizing enzymes • Enzyme induction • Enzyme inhibition
- Pharmacogenetics

KEY POINTS

- Pregnancy is a pharmacologic special population, where changes in absorption, distribution, metabolism, and elimination of drugs can impact concentrations sufficiently that different dosing may be required.
- Normal physiologic changes in pregnancy (increases in plasma volume, total body water, glomerular filtration rate, and renal secretion and decreases in plasma proteins) can impact drug concentrations and clearance.
- Hormonal changes in pregnancy alter drug-metabolizing enzymes; activities of cytochrome P450 (CYP) 2D6, CYP2C9, CYP3A4, and uridine 5'-diphosphate glucuronosyltransferase (UGT) 1A1 and UGT1A4 increase, whereas CYP1A2 and CYP2C19 decrease.

The changes in pregnancy that affect drug absorption, distribution, metabolism, and elimination can be broken down into two categories: (1) physiologic changes in pregnancy that make intuitive sense to us as obstetricians and (2) changes that occur in hepatic metabolism, which for many of us are a confusing "black box." Although knowledge of obstetric physiology has evolved fairly commensurate with general medical knowledge, the first paper describing the failure of a standard drug dose to achieve therapeutic concentrations in pregnancy was not published until 1977.[1] Since then, and especially since the turn of the millennium with expansion of the United States Food and Drug Administration (FDA) and the National Institutes of Health (NIH) support, our understanding of pregnancy as a special pharmacologic population has significantly advanced.

Department of Obstetrics and Gynecology, Northwestern University Feinberg School of Medicine, 250 East Superior Street, Suite 03-2303, Chicago, IL 60611, USA
* Corresponding author.
E-mail address: c-stika@northwestern.edu

Obstet Gynecol Clin N Am 50 (2023) 1–15
https://doi.org/10.1016/j.ogc.2022.10.012
0889-8545/23/© 2022 Elsevier Inc. All rights reserved.

Although we often categorize these pharmacologic changes as pregnant versus nonpregnant, pregnancy is not uniform: pregnant people in the third trimester handle drugs differently than in the second or first trimester. Each pharmacokinetic parameter evolves across pregnancy on its own trajectory (**Table 1**). In addition, some of the hepatic enzymes have important pharmacogenetic differences, which further add to variability in pregnancy response.

Changes in pharmacokinetics do not always require changes in dosing regimens. If maximum or minimum concentrations and total drug exposures are different but still within therapeutic range, dosing guidelines may stay the same. However, optimal obstetric care requires that when we prescribe medications to this special maternal-fetal dyad, we understand each drug's unique pharmacokinetics during pregnancy so that its administration is both safe and effective.

IMPACT OF PHYSIOLOGIC CHANGES IN PREGNANCY ON PHARMACOLOGY
Case #1

A pregnant woman with a URI caused by ampicillin-sensitive *Haemophilus influenzae* was treated with oral ampicillin 500 mg every 6 hours. She failed to respond, and an ampicillin level was reported as "undetectable."[1] Why was the ampicillin concentration so low?

Increase in blood volume and total body water
Fundamental to many of the changes that occur in pregnancy is the 40% to 45% increase in blood volume. This expansion begins by 6 to 8 weeks and progressively

Table 1
Changes in maternal physiology and hepatic metabolism across pregnancy and postpartum

PK Parameter	Early First T	Late First T	Early Second T	Late Second T	Early Third T	Late Third T	<8 wk PP	>12 wk PP
Renal: CrCL	↑	↑↑	↑↑	↑↑↑	↑↑↑	↑↑	↑	=
Plasma volume/TBW	↑	↑	↑↑	↑↑	↑↑↑	↑↑↑	↑	=
Albumin	↓	↓	↓↓	↓↓	↓↓↓	↓↓↓	?	=
α1-acid glycoprotein	↓	↓	↓↓	↓↓	↓↓↓	↓↓	=	=
Hepatic arterial blood flow	?	=	=	=	=	=	?	=
Hepatic portal blood flow	?	↑	↑	↑	↑↑	↑↑	?	=
UGT1A1	?	↑	↑↑	↑↑	↑↑↑	↑↑↑	?	=
UGT1A4	↑	↑	↑↑	↑↑↑	↑↑↑↑	↑↑↑↑	=	=
CYP1A2	?	↓	↓↓	↓↓	↓↓	↓↓↓	↓	=
CYP2B6	?	?	?	=	=	=	?	=
CYP2C9	?	↑	↑	↑	↑↑	↑↑	?	=
CYP2C19 EM/RM/UM	?	?	?	?	↓↓↓	↓↓↓	?	=
CYP2D6 EM/RM	?	?	↑	↑↑	↑↑↑	↑↑↑	?	=
CYP3A4/5	?	↑↑↑	↑↑↑	↑↑↑	↑↑↑	↑↑↑	↑↑↑ ?	=

Abbreviations: =, no different from nonpregnant state; ?, parameter change is unknown; CrCL, creatinine, clearance; CYP, cytochrome P450; EM, extensive metabolizer; PK, pharmacokinetic; PP, postpartum; RM, rapid metabolizer; T, trimester; TBW, total body water; UGT, uridine 5'-diphosphate glucuronosyltransferase; UM, ultrarapid metabolizer.

adds 1200 to 1300 mL of blood, peaking at 32 to 34 weeks.[2,3] In twin gestations, the increase is approximately 20% greater.[3] Multiple factors contribute to these dramatic changes, including increases in steroid hormone concentrations and nitric oxide. Estrogen stimulates both production of hepatic angiotensinogen and renal renin, which increases aldosterone and subsequent sodium and fluid retention.[4] Extracellular fluid and total body water also increase proportional to patient weight.[5] In a nonpregnant woman, extracellular fluid space is approximately 0.156 L/kg versus approximately 0.255 L/kg in singleton pregnancies.[6]

This expansion of plasma volume and total body water increases the volumes of distribution (Vd) and reduces the concentrations of hydrophilic medications. Vd is the theoretic volume that would be necessary to contain the administered dose at the same concentration as measured in plasma: Vd = dose/concentration. An example of this effect, Casele and colleagues[7] reported that following the same dose of enoxaparin, whose Vd is essentially plasma volume, the anti-factor Xa activity at 4 hours was significant lower ($P < .05$) in the first and third trimester (19% and 29%, respectively) compared with 6 to 8 weeks postpartum.[7]

Because body fat has an extensive capacity to absorb lipophilic drugs, the Vd for these drugs greatly exceeds the actual volume of body fat. Although pregnant people gain body fat, the impact on Vd is less significant for lipophilic medications because this change only minimally increases the already large Vd.

Decreased protein binding

Plasma protein concentrations change during pregnancy. The best known is the decrease in plasma albumin from 4.2 g/dL in nonpregnancy to 3.6 g/dL in the midtrimester of pregnancy.[8] The plasma concentration of α_1-acid glycoprotein, which binds many basic drugs, is reduced by almost 50% during the third trimester of pregnancy.[9] These reductions in plasma protein concentrations increase the free fraction, Vd, and clearance of many drugs. For highly protein bound medications with a narrow therapeutic range (little difference between the minimal therapeutic and toxic concentrations), monitoring of free drug, rather than total drug, is often recommended in pregnancy, for example, digoxin and phenytoin.

Increase in cardiac output

Beginning early in the first trimester and peaking at 32 weeks, the 30%–50% increase in cardiac output follows the expansion of plasma volume,[10] with increases in both stroke volume and heart rate.[11] These cardiovascular changes do not fully return to normal until after 12 weeks postpartum.[12]

Changes in regional blood flow

The increased cardiac output in pregnancy is differentially distributed to the body. At term, the placenta with its low-pressure, arteriovenous shunt pulls 20%–25% of cardiac output and the kidney claims 20%.[13] Blood flow increases to the skin to dissipate heat generated by fetal metabolism[14] and to the developing mammary glands.[15] Arterial blood flow to the liver is unchanged but represents a smaller percentage of cardiac output. However, beginning at 28 weeks, portal venous blood flow increases to 150%–160% over nonpregnant levels.[16] This increase in portal blood flow enhances first-pass hepatic clearance of high-extraction ratio drugs. Because of these hemodynamic changes, less cardiac output is available for skeletal muscle and other vascular beds, and absorption of intramuscular administration of medications may be unpredictable.

Renal clearance

Renal elimination is composed of two components: (1) glomerular filtration (GFR) based on renal blood flow and (2) reabsorption and secretion within the tubule. Both processes change with pregnancy. The increase in GFR begins by 6 weeks, peaks late second to early third trimester, and then plateaus or decreases slightly until birth, followed by normalization by 6 to 8 weeks postpartum.[17] Creatinine clearance, which roughly parallels GFR, increases by 45% at 9 weeks, peaks 150% to 160% over nonpregnant values in mid-second trimester, and drifts down during late third trimester.[17]

Renal transporters

GFR is supplemented by the net effects of tubular reabsorption and secretion. Straddling membrane surfaces, drug transporters control movement of drugs and other compounds into and out of cells. In the kidney, specific transporters are found on tubular cell membranes facing either the afferent blood vessels or urine where they move compounds from the blood across the tubular cell and into urine (secretion) or from the urine back into the blood (reabsorption) (**Fig. 1**). Pregnancy increases the activity of some of these transporters, increasing renal clearance of their substrates.

Amoxicillin is primarily excreted unchanged through renal filtration plus the net effects of secretion via the organic anion transporter 1 (OAT1) and reabsorption by peptide transporter (PEPT1). Compared with postpartum, amoxicillin renal clearance, and secretion are increased by 50% in both second and third trimesters of pregnancy ($P < .001$).[18] Net amoxicillin secretion increases in pregnancy through a combination of upregulation of OAT1 secretion and progesterone inhibition of PEPT1 reabsorption.[18] With lower amoxicillin maximum concentrations plus the potential for subtherapeutic concentrations at the end of the dosing interval, pregnant people may require larger and more frequent dosing.

Metformin is eliminated unchanged by the kidneys with the assistance of another transporter, organic cation transporter 2 (OCT2). Compared with postpartum, renal clearance of metformin increases by 49% in the second and 29% in the third trimester ($P < .01$) and renal secretion increases by 45% and 38%, respectively ($P < .01$).[19]

Activity of a third transporter, P-glycoprotein (P-gp), also increases during pregnancy. With its long list of substrates, the efflux transporter, P-gp plays a protective role, controlling drug movement out of cells in the intestines, liver, kidney, blood brain

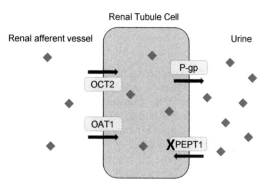

Fig. 1. Proximal renal tubule with selected drug transporters. OAT, organic anion transporter; OCT, organic cation transporter; PEPT, peptide transporter; P-gp, P-glycoprotein; X, progesterone decreases transcription of PEPT1 mRNA18.

barrier and, importantly, the placenta. Digoxin is a probe substrate for P-gp activity, for both placental fetal protection and renal secretion. Located on the apical, maternal-facing surface of syncytiotrophoblastic cells, P-gp transports digoxin back into maternal circulation. On the apical, urine-facing surface of renal tubular cells, P-gp moves digoxin into urine against its concentration gradient. Compared with post-partum, unbound digoxin renal clearance was 52% higher and unbound digoxin renal secretion clearance 107% higher during early third trimester.[20] The investigators hypothesized that this increase in digoxin secretion resulted from upregulation of either one or both, P-gp and OAT polypeptide (OATP), another digoxin transporter located on the basolateral surface of the tubules which moves digoxin from blood into the renal cell.[20]

Case #1: Discussion

This "undetectable" ampicillin concentration in a pregnant woman prompted the first pharmacokinetic drug study in pregnancy which found that compared with post-partum, the maximum ampicillin concentration following a 500 mg oral dose in pregnancy was 41% lower (2.2 ± 1.0 vs 3.7 ± 1.5 μ/mL, $P < .001$) and its clearance from plasma was 55% greater ($P < .001$).[1] Because hydrophilic ampicillin is only 15% to 25% protein bound and readily distributes to approximately total body water, its volume of distribution increases in pregnancy and concentrations for the same dose are lower. Ampicillin is renally cleared and is a substrate for the same renal transporters as amoxicillin, OAT1, and PEPT1. Ampicillin renal filtration and renal secretion both increase in pregnancy. As a result, pregnant people require higher and more frequent ampicillin dosing to achieve therapeutic concentrations. In nonpregnant patients, intravenous ampicillin 250 to 500 mg every 6 hours is sufficient to treat soft tissue infections. In pregnancy, ampicillin dosing is increased to 2 g initially followed by 1 g every 4 hours for Group B *Streptococcus* prophylaxis.

HEPATIC METABOLISM OVERVIEW

Metabolic enzymes evolved to detoxify potentially dangerous environmental chemicals (xenobiotics) and control concentrations of endogenous compounds. Phase II enzymes developed first. They facilitate simple biotransformations: the addition of readily available moieties (glucuronic acid, glutathione, amino acids glycine, taurine, glutamic acid, and methyl, acetyl and sulfate groups), making the toxic chemical more water soluble before renal clearance. Phase I enzymes catalyze chemical modifications, for example, oxidation-reduction reactions that in general, make drugs less toxic. The most important Phase I enzymes are the 12 cytochrome P450 (CYP) families, of which families 1, 2, and 3 are involved in drug metabolism. Although drug metabolizing enzymes can be found throughout the body, they are importantly located in the liver and small intestine, where they control xenobiotic (and drug) exposure through first-pass metabolism.[21] Some drugs are metabolized primarily by one enzyme; however, most medications are metabolized by multiple Phase I and II enzymes, sometimes sequentially, sometimes facilitating the same reaction. Redundancy helps to ensure successful elimination.[22]

PHASE I DRUG METABOLIZING ENZYMES AND PREGNANCY
Case #2

An African American patient at 32 weeks gestation was receiving immediate release nifedipine tocolysis (20 mg orally every 6 hours) for preterm labor. Contractions initially spaced but 5 hours after the first dose they recurred. Why?

CYP3A4/5

The CYP3A subfamily, composed of CYP3A4, CYP3A5, and fetal/neonatal CYP3A7, is the most abundant of the cytochrome enzymes in humans and contributes to the metabolism of many endogenous compounds and between 30% and 50% of drugs used today.[22] It is probably best known as the enzyme responsible for increased metabolism of contraceptive hormones by enzyme-inducing antiseizure medications. Enzyme-inducing drugs increase CYP3A4 activity through stimulation of the xenobiotic sensing system—a mechanism which ramps up drug metabolism when exposed to potentially toxic environmental chemicals (xenobiotics). The xenobiotic compound binds to pregnane-X-receptor (PXR) and/or constitutive androstane receptor (CAR), both of which evolved from a primitive estrogen receptor. This complex binds to the hormone responsive element within DNA, initiating transcription of the target gene and subsequent production of their proteins. For at least some of the hepatic enzymes, this is the mechanism responsible for changes in their activity in pregnancy. Cultured hepatocyte studies suggest that the primary stimulus for pregnancy induction of CYP3A4 is increasing cortisol, operating through PXR.[23]

Two studies with "probe" drugs demonstrate an approximate doubling in CYP3A4 activity during pregnancy.[20,24] A probe medication is uniquely metabolized by one CYP enzyme—changes in its metabolism reflect changes in that enzyme's activity. Midazolam hydroxylation is a CYP3A4 probe. After a pediatric dose of oral midazolam, the apparent oral clearance of midazolam in the third trimester was 108 ± 62% ($P = .002$) greater than postpartum.[20] Using N-demethylation of the cough suppressant, dextromethorphan, another probe for CYP3A, Tracy and colleagues[24] showed that CYP3A activity had already increased by early second trimester and remained elevated throughout pregnancy, 35% to 38% above its postpartum baseline. Obstetric therapeutics includes numerous drugs metabolized predominantly, or in part, by CYP3A. Multiple studies in pregnant people show increased clearance and reduced maximum concentrations of these medications, requiring dosing modifications to maintain efficacy[20,24–33] **(Table 2)**.

Case #2: Discussion

Metabolized by CYP3A, clearance of nifedipine increases 4-fold in pregnancy.[34] Because nifedipine can be metabolized by both CYP3A4 and CYP3A5, people who have CYP3A4 and functional CYP3A5 metabolize nifedipine faster than people without active CYP3A5. There are marked ethnic differences in the distribution of the major *inactive* CYP3A5*3 allele. This inactive variant is present in 92% to 94% of Europeans, 71% to 75% of East Asians, 55% to 65% of South Asians, 60% to 66% of Hispanics, but only 29% to 35% of people with African descent.[35] This means that the 65% to 71% of African Americans who have *active* CYP3A5 metabolize CYP3A drugs faster than other ethnic groups. Guidelines for tacrolimus, another CYP3A4/5 drug, advise increased dosing for African American transplant recipients. In a study of 14 people receiving nifedipine tocolysis, participants with active CYP3A5 (1 Hispanic and 3 African American patients) had lower average plasma concentrations and 2.7-fold greater nifedipine clearances than those with inactive CYP3A5.[25] Contractions recurred in our African American patient in Case #2 because the nifedipine concentrations became subtherapeutic before the next dose.

CYP2D6

CYP2D6 is the next most important of the CYP enzymes, contributing to the metabolism of about 20% of medications.[22] However, CYP2D6 has pharmacogenetic variants that are associated with almost 1000-fold differences in activity. Phenotypic

Table 2
Representative CYP3A medications studied in pregnancy

Medication	Key Findings
Midazolam (probe)[20]	Compared with PP, 72% increase in apparent oral clearance in 3T.
Dextromethorphan N-demethylation (probe)[24]	Compared with PP, clearance increases 35%–38% at 14–18, 24–28, and 36–40 wk.
Nifedipine (probe)[25,34]	Compared with historic nonpregnant controls, nifedipine clearance is 4-fold greater during 3T.[34] In patients treated for preterm labor, nifedipine clearance is 2.7-fold greater in people with one or two CYP3A5*1 alleles—active CYP3A5.[25]
Cholesterol (probe)[66,67] (endogenous)	Metabolic ratio 4βOHC/C is 26% greater in 3T compared with PP or nonpregnant control women.[68] 4βOHC/C ratios are similar in late 1T, 2T, and 3T but all are approximately 50% greater than ratio in nonpregnant women.[69]
Cortisol[26]	Compared with PP, CYP3A metabolic ratio before delivery is 4.9 times greater.
Betamethasone[27]	Compared with nonpregnancy, clearance increases 1.2–1.6-fold during 2T and 3T.
Darunavir[28]	Compared with PP, 2T and 3T darunavir AUCs are 38%–39% lower with once daily dosing and 26% lower with twice daily dosing.
Indinavir[29]	Compared with 6 wk PP, AUC is 68% lower at 30–32 wk
Atazanavir/ritonavir[30]	Coadministration of atazanavir/ritonavir with tenofovir decreases atazanavir AUCs by 31% both during pregnancy and PP. Compared with PP, 3T AUC of atazanavir is reduced by 27% both with and without tenofovir; 33% of women not receiving tenofovir and 55% receiving tenofovir fell below the atazanavir target AUC during pregnancy.
Lopinavir/ritonavir[31]	The geometric mean ratio of 3T and PP lopinavir AUCs is 0.72 (90%CI, 0.54–0.96) and 82% of the pregnant women do not meet target lopinavir AUC.
Carbamazepine[68]	Compared with nonpregnant baselines, no significant changes in clearances of free or total carbamazepine or free or total carbamazepine-epoxide occur in pregnancy. Changes in seizure frequency are not associated with decreased total or free carbamazepine concentrations.
Cyclosporine[69]	In patients with renal allographs, cyclosporine concentrations decline in five of six people during pregnancy.

(continued on next page)

Table 2 (continued)	
Medication	**Key Findings**
Lumefantrine[32]	Day 7 mean plasma concentrations are significantly lower in pregnant people: geometric mean ratio = 1.40; 95%CI (1.119–1.1745), P < .003, placing more women at risk for malaria treatment failure. The presence of active CYP3A5*1/*1 genotype is associated with lower concentrations in pregnancy.
Quetiapine[33]	Compared with nonpregnant baseline, 3T serum concentrations are 75% lower (95% CI, −83%, −66%, P < .001).
Tacrolimus[70]	Compared with PP, 39% increase in clearance during 3T.

Abbreviations: AP, antepartum; AUC, area under the concentration time curve; CYP, cytochrome P450; PP, postpartum; T, trimester.

extensive metabolizers have two "normally active" alleles; poor metabolizers have two alleles with the loss of function; intermediate metabolizers have one active and one loss of function alleles, and ultrarapid CYP2D6 metabolizers have multiple copies of a normal allele. Typically, CYP2D6 is not induced by PXR/CAR and the xenobiotic sensing system; however, studies of CYP2D6 substrates show enhanced metabolism during pregnancy[24,36–40] (**Table 3**). The exact mechanism by which this occurs is not known. The increase in CYP2D6 activity is progressive, with a 25% increase in early second trimester, progressing to 48% in late third trimester.[24] However, this increase in activity is restricted to the extensive and rapid metabolizers, with less change seen in the intermediate metabolizers, and no change in the poor metabolizers.[38,39]

CYP1A2
The CYP1 family of enzymes is composed of three enzymes: CYP1A1, CYP1A2, and CYP1B1. CYP1A2 is found only in the liver and the other two, only in extrahepatic tissues. CYP1A2 contributes to the metabolism of approximately 10% of our medications, including, caffeine, theophylline, tricyclic antidepressants, acetaminophen, and estrogens.[41] Among the compounds that inhibit CYP1A2, estradiol downregulates its transcription and decreases its activity.[42] Using caffeine metabolism as a probe, compared with postpartum, CYP1A2 activity progressively decreases across pregnancy with a 32.8 ± 22.8% reduction at 14 to 18 weeks, a 48.1 ± 27% reduction at 24 to 28 weeks, and a 65.2 ± 15.3% reduction at 36 to 40 weeks.[24] As a result, caffeine concentrations remain higher for a longer time, giving credence to pregnant peoples' avoidance of caffeinated beverages!

CYP2B6
Although estradiol induces transcription of CYP2B6 RNA in cultured hepatocytes,[43] studies in pregnancy with medications metabolized by CYP2B6 are less definitive. Part of the difficulty in assessing changes in CYP2B6 activity occurs because CYP2B6 contributes to the metabolism of approximately 25% to 30% of the drugs metabolized by CYP3A4, and few drugs are uniquely metabolized by CYP2B6.[44] The elimination clearance of efavirenz, a probe drug for CYP2B6, is unaffected by pregnancy.[45] Methadone concentration to dose ratios decrease and its clearance

Table 3
Representative CYP2D6 medications studied in pregnancy

Medication	Key Findings
Metoprolol[37]	Compared with PP, apparent oral clearance is 2–13 times greater in 3T. Peak plasma concentrations in 3T are only 12% to 55% of those after delivery.
Metoprolol[40]	In CYP2D6 EMs, compared with PP, apparent oral clearance is 1.8-fold higher in midpregnancy ($P < .05$) and 3-fold higher in late pregnancy ($P < .05$). IMs had a similar pattern of increased clearance in pregnancy, but their AP and PP clearances are lower than the EMs.
Dextromethorphan O-demethylation[24]	Compared with PP, CYP2D6 activity is 26 ± 58% greater at 14–18 wk, 35 ± 41% greater at 24–28 wk and 48 ± 25% greater at 36–40 wk.
Dextromethorphan O-demethylation[39]	Compared with PP, metabolism of dextromethorphan is significantly increased during pregnancy in EMs and IMs but decreased in PMs.
Clonidine[36]	Apparent oral clearance is two-fold greater in 2T and 3T compared with historic nonpregnant controls (440 ± 168 mL/min vs 245 ± 72; [$P < .0001$]) without change in clonidine renal clearance.
Paroxetine[38]	In 74 women with depression, paroxetine concentrations in CYP2D6 EMs progressively decrease across pregnancy, whereas concentrations in IMs and PMs increase.

Abbreviations: AP, antepartum; CYP, cytochrome P450; EM, CYP2D6 extensive metabolizers; IM, CYP2D6 intermediate metabolizers; PM, CYP2D6 poor metabolizers; PP, postpartum; T, trimester.

increases during pregnancy, but it is unclear if increased activity of CYP3A4 or CYP2B6 is responsible for these changes.[46]

CYP2C9

Estradiol increases CYP2C9 activity in cultured hepatocytes by unknown mechanisms, but unlike other enzymes, it does not involve increased mRNA transcription.[47] CYP2C9 activity increases during pregnancy based on studies with phenytoin, indomethacin, and glyburide.[48–51] Compared with historic controls, the apparent oral clearance of indomethacin in the second trimester was greater (14.5 ± 5.5 L/h vs 6.5–9.8 L/h), and the mean plasma concentration after a 25-mg oral dose was 37% lower.[49] Glyburide clearance was two-fold higher during the third trimester compared with nonpregnant women with type 2 diabetes.[48] Using modeling simulations, the investigators predicted that, compared with the usual twice daily dose of 1.25 to 10.0 mg, glyburide would have to be increased in pregnancy to as much as 23.75 mg twice daily for optimal glucose control.[48]

CYP2C19

CYP2C19 has common pharmacogenetic phenotypes with dramatically different activity: poor (two loss-of-function or no function alleles), intermediate (one loss-of-function and one normal function allele), extensive (two normal function alleles), rapid (one normal and one gain-of-function allele), and ultrarapid metabolizers (two gain-of-function alleles).[52] CYP2C19 converts the prodrug, proguanil, to the active antimalarial drug, cycloguanil. Both estrogen-containing contraceptives and pregnancy inhibit CYP2C19 conversion of proguanil to cycloguanil in extensive, rapid, and ultrarapid metabolizers.[53] Hepatocyte studies confirm downregulation of CYP2C19 expression by estrogens.[54]

PHASE II DRUG METABOLIZING ENZYMES AND PREGNANCY
Case #3

A 36-year-old pregnant woman at $25^{0/7}$ weeks of gestation with chronic hypertension previously stable on labetalol 200 mg bid (7 AM and 7 PM) reports the following blood pressures: 7 AM 165/98, 10 AM 125/82, 3 PM 134/88, and 6 PM 164/102. Preeclampsia evaluation was unremarkable, and the labetalol was increased to 300 mg twice daily. Two days later, she reports that she was feeling mildly orthostatic several hours after her morning dose. Why is this happening? What would be a better approach to manage her blood pressure?

UGT1A1

UGT1A1 metabolizes labetalol and bilirubin, as well as several of the antiretroviral integrase inhibitors, and it contributes to the metabolism of acetaminophen. In hepatocyte studies, progesterone increases the transcription of UGT1A1.[55] In pregnancy, glucuronidation of labetalol progressively increases.[56,57] In 57 women taking labetalol for chronic hypertension, compared with postpartum, the apparent oral clearance of labetalol in late first trimester was 1.4-fold greater and by term, 1.6-fold greater.[56] In an earlier study, the elimination half-life of labetalol in the third trimester was significantly shorter than in nonpregnant controls (1.7 vs 6–8 hours).[57]

Case #3: Discussion

The labetalol 200 mg orally twice daily is not controlling her blood pressure. Close examination of the readings reveals control at the time of maximum labetalol concentration but elevated pressures at the end of the dosing interval. UGT1A1 clearance of labetalol progressively increases across pregnancy, and her labetalol concentrations have become subtherapeutic before the next dose. However, increasing the dose to 300 mg twice daily causes orthostasis from hypotension when the concentration peaks at 2 to 4 hours post-dose. A better approach would be to increase the 24-h labetalol exposure to 600 mg but administer it as 200 mg every 8 hours.

UGT1A4

Of all the metabolic enzymes studied in pregnancy, none changes as dramatically as glucuronidation by UGT1A4. The anticonvulsant and mood-stabilizing drug, lamotrigine, is primarily metabolized by the Phase II enzyme, uridine 5'-diphosphate glucuronosyltransferase 1A4 (UGT1A4).[58] Using oral contraceptive pills, lamotrigine clearance did not change with progestin-only pills, whereas clearance increased and breakthrough seizures occurred in women on estrogen and progestin contraceptives.[59] The role of estrogen in inducing UGT1A4 mRNA was confirmed with cultured hepatocytes.[60] Multiple investigations since have shown that enhanced lamotrigine clearance begins as early as 5 weeks' gestation and progressively increases until it peaks in the third trimester at 248% to 330% over baseline.[61–63] However, Polepally and colleagues[64] identified two subpopulations; in 77% of 64 pregnancies, third trimester lamotrigine clearance had increased 219% over baseline, whereas, in 23%, clearance rose by only 21%. Factors that differentiated these populations have not been identified.

Because of the marked increase in lamotrigine clearance, serial dose increases are often necessary to maintain stable therapeutic lamotrigine concentrations.[61] After delivery, clearance of lamotrigine falls rapidly and returns to nonpregnant levels by 3 weeks postpartum. So, tapering the dose should begin within the first week after delivery to prevent possible lamotrigine toxicity.[61]

Not all UGT enzymes are upregulated during pregnancy. Based on pharmacokinetic studies with zidovudine in pregnant people, UGT2B7 activity does not change.[65]

SUMMARY

The changes in maternal physiology and hepatic metabolism that accompany pregnancy profoundly alter how drugs are distributed, metabolized, and eliminated. Because medical therapies play a major role in the care we provide to our pregnant patients, it is important to understand the pharmacokinetic evidence that informs the medication guidelines unique to pregnancy.

CLINICAL CARE POINTS

- Because of the changes that occur in pregnancy: decreased protein binding, increased volume of distribution and increased renal clearance, the recommended obstetric dosing regimens for penicillin and cephalosporin prophylaxis and treatment employ higher doses and shorter administration intervals, compared to recommendations for nonpregnant adults.

- To compensate for the increase in UGT1A1 metabolism of labetalol, changing the dosing frequency to every 8 hours may improve hypertensive control.

- Because of the increase in CYP3A metabolism, extended release nifedipine may need to be dosed every 12 hours to achieve control of blood pressures.

- The caffeine effects from coffee last much longer during pregnancy because caffeine metabolism by CYP1A2 is decreased.

- Because estradiol induction of UGT1A4 becomes clinically apparent early in pregnancy and abruptly falls after delivery of the placenta, to maintain therapeutic lamotrigine concentrations, monitoring with appropriate dosing adjustments should begin by 5-6 weeks in the first trimester and dose tapering should start 2-3 days after delivery with return to the pre-pregnancy regimen by 3 weeks post-birth.

DISCLOSURE

C.S. Stika has no conflicts of interest to disclose.

REFERENCES

1. Philipson A. Pharmacokinetics of ampicillin during pregnancy. J Infect Dis 1977; 136(3):370–6.
2. Lund CJ, Donovan JC. Blood volume during pregnancy. Significance of plasma and red cell volumes. Am J Obstet Gynecol 1967;98(3):394–403.
3. Hytten F. Blood volume changes in normal pregnancy. Clin Haematol 1985;14(3): 601–12.
4. Ouzounian JG, Elkayam U. Physiologic changes during normal pregnancy and delivery. Cardiol Clin 2012;30(3):317–29.
5. Petersen VP. Body composition and fluid compartments in normal, obese and underweight human subjects. Acta Med Scand 1957;158(2):103–11.

6. Frederiksen MC, Ruo TI, Chow MJ, et al. Theophylline pharmacokinetics in pregnancy. Clin Pharmacol Ther 1986;40(3):321–8.
7. Casele HL, Laifer SA, Woelkers DA, et al. Changes in the pharmacokinetics of the low-molecular-weight heparin enoxaparin sodium during pregnancy. Am J Obstet Gynecol 1999;181(5 Pt 1):1113–7.
8. Mendenhall HW. Serum protein concentrations in pregnancy. I. concentrations in maternal serum. Am J Obstet Gynecol 1970;106(3):388–99.
9. Bardy AH, Hiilesmaa VK, Teramo K, et al. Protein binding of antiepileptic drugs during pregnancy, labor, and puerperium. Ther Drug Monit 1990;12(1):40–6.
10. Lees MM, Taylor SH, Scott DB, et al. A study of cardiac output at rest throughout pregnancy. J Obstet Gynaecol Br Commonw 1967;74(3):319–28.
11. Robson SC, Hunter S, Boys RJ, et al. Serial study of factors influencing changes in cardiac output during human pregnancy. Am J Physiol 1989;256(4 Pt 2): H1060–5.
12. Capeless EL, Clapp JF. When do cardiovascular parameters return to their preconception values? Am J Obstet Gynecol 1991;165(4 Pt 1):883–6.
13. Metcalfe J, Romney SL, Ramsey LH, et al. Estimation of uterine blood flow in normal human pregnancy at term. J Clin Invest 1955;34(11):1632–8.
14. Ginsburg J, Duncan SL. Peripheral blood flow in normal pregnancy. Cardiovasc Res 1967;1(2):132–7.
15. Thoresen M, Wesche J. Doppler measurements of changes in human mammary and uterine blood flow during pregnancy and lactation. Acta Obstet Gynecol Scand 1988;67(8):741–5.
16. Nakai A, Sekiya I, Oya A, et al. Assessment of the hepatic arterial and portal venous blood flows during pregnancy with Doppler ultrasonography. Arch Gynecol Obstet 2002;266(1):25–9.
17. Odutayo A, Hladunewich M. Obstetric nephrology: renal hemodynamic and metabolic physiology in normal pregnancy. Clin J Am Soc Nephrol 2012;7(12): 2073–80.
18. Andrew MA, Easterling TR, Carr DB, et al. Amoxicillin pharmacokinetics in pregnant women: modeling and simulations of dosage strategies. Clin Pharmacol Ther 2007;81(4):547–56.
19. Eyal S, Easterling TR, Carr D, et al. Pharmacokinetics of metformin during pregnancy. Drug Metab Dispos 2010;38(5):833–40.
20. Hebert MF, Easterling TR, Kirby B, et al. Effects of pregnancy on CYP3A and P-glycoprotein activities as measured by disposition of midazolam and digoxin: a University of Washington specialized center of research study. Clin Pharmacol Ther 2008;84(2):248–53.
21. Lin JH, Chiba M, Baillie TA. Is the role of the small intestine in first-pass metabolism overemphasized? Pharmacol Rev 1999;51(2):135–58.
22. Zhao M, Ma J, Li M, et al. Cytochrome P450 enzymes and drug metabolism in humans. Int J Mol Sci 2021;22(23):12808.
23. Sachar M, Kelly EJ, Unadkat JD. Mechanisms of CYP3A induction during pregnancy: studies in HepaRG cells. AAPS J 2019;21(3):45.
24. Tracy TS, Venkataramanan R, Glover DD, et al. Human development network of maternal-fetal-medicine U. Temporal changes in drug metabolism (CYP1A2, CYP2D6 and CYP3A Activity) during pregnancy. Am J Obstet Gynecol 2005; 192(2):633–9.
25. Haas DM, Quinney SK, Clay JM, et al. Nifedipine pharmacokinetics are influenced by CYP3A5 genotype when used as a preterm labor tocolytic. Am J Perinatol 2013;30(4):275–81.

26. Ohkita C, Goto M. Increased 6-hydroxycortisol excretion in pregnant women: implication of drug-metabolizing enzyme induction. DICP 1990;24(9):814–6.
27. Della Torre M, Hibbard JU, Jeong H, et al. Betamethasone in pregnancy: influence of maternal body weight and multiple gestation on pharmacokinetics. Am J Obstet Gynecol 2010;203(3):254 e251–212.
28. Stek A, Best BM, Wang J, et al. Pharmacokinetics of once versus twice daily darunavir in pregnant HIV-infected women. J Acquir Immune Defic Syndr 2015; 70(1):33–41.
29. Unadkat JD, Wara DW, Hughes MD, et al. Pharmacokinetics and safety of indinavir in human immunodeficiency virus-infected pregnant women. Antimicrob Agents Chemother 2007;51(2):783–6.
30. Mirochnick M, Best BM, Stek AM, et al. Atazanavir pharmacokinetics with and without tenofovir during pregnancy. J Acquir Immune Defic Syndr 2011;56(5): 412–9.
31. Stek AM, Mirochnick M, Capparelli E, et al. Reduced lopinavir exposure during pregnancy. AIDS 2006;20(15):1931–9.
32. Mutagonda RF, Minzi OMS, Massawe SN, et al. Pregnancy and CYP3A5 genotype affect day 7 plasma lumefantrine concentrations. Drug Metab Dispos 2019;47(12):1415–24.
33. Westin AA, Brekke M, Molden E, et al. Treatment with antipsychotics in pregnancy: changes in drug disposition. Clin Pharmacol Ther 2018;103(3):477–84.
34. Prevost RR, Akl SA, Whybrew WD, et al. Oral nifedipine pharmacokinetics in pregnancy-induced hypertension. Pharmacotherapy 1992;12(3):174–7.
35. Xie HG, Wood AJ, Kim RB, et al. Genetic variability in CYP3A5 and its possible consequences. Pharmacogenomics 2004;5(3):243–72.
36. Buchanan ML, Easterling TR, Carr DB, et al. Clonidine pharmacokinetics in pregnancy. Drug Metab Dispos 2009;37(4):702–5.
37. Hogstedt S, Lindberg B, Peng DR, et al. Pregnancy-induced increase in metoprolol metabolism. Clin Pharmacol Ther 1985;37(6):688–92.
38. Ververs FF, Voorbij HA, Zwarts P, et al. Effect of cytochrome P450 2D6 genotype on maternal paroxetine plasma concentrations during pregnancy. Clin Pharmacokinet 2009;48(10):677–83.
39. Wadelius M, Darj E, Frenne G, et al. Induction of CYP2D6 in pregnancy. Clin Pharmacol Ther 1997;62(4):400–7.
40. Ryu RJ, Eyal S, Easterling TR, et al. Pharmacokinetics of metoprolol during pregnancy and lactation. J Clin Pharmacol 2016;56(5):581–9.
41. Kwon YJ, Shin S, Chun YJ. Biological roles of cytochrome P450 1A1, 1A2, and 1B1 enzymes. Arch Pharm Res 2021;44(1):63–83.
42. Xie C, Pogribna M, Word B, et al. In vitro analysis of factors influencing CYP1A2 expression as potential determinants of interindividual variation. Pharmacol Res Perspect 2017;5(2):e00299.
43. Koh KH, Jurkovic S, Yang K, et al. Estradiol induces cytochrome P450 2B6 expression at high concentrations: implication in estrogen-mediated gene regulation in pregnancy. Biochem Pharmacol 2012;84(1):93–103.
44. Walsky RL, Astuccio AV, Obach RS. Evaluation of 227 drugs for in vitro inhibition of cytochrome P450 2B6. J Clin Pharmacol 2006;46(12):1426–38.
45. Cressey TR, Stek A, Capparelli E, et al. Efavirenz pharmacokinetics during the third trimester of pregnancy and postpartum. J Acquir Immune Defic Syndr 2012;59(3):245–52.

46. Bogen DL, Perel JM, Helsel JC, et al. Pharmacologic evidence to support clinical decision making for peripartum methadone treatment. Psychopharmacology (Berl) 2013;225(2):441–51.
47. Choi SY, Koh KH, Jeong H. Isoform-specific regulation of cytochromes P450 expression by estradiol and progesterone. Drug Metab Dispos 2013;41(2):263–9.
48. Hebert MF, Ma X, Naraharisetti SB, et al. Are we optimizing gestational diabetes treatment with glyburide? The pharmacologic basis for better clinical practice. Clin Pharmacol Ther 2009;85(6):607–14.
49. Rytting E, Nanovskaya TN, Wang X, et al. Pharmacokinetics of indomethacin in pregnancy. Clin Pharmacokinet 2014;53(6):545–51.
50. Tomson T, Lindbom U, Ekqvist B, et al. Disposition of carbamazepine and phenytoin in pregnancy. Epilepsia 1994;35(1):131–5.
51. Yerby MS, Friel PN, McCormick K, et al. Pharmacokinetics of anticonvulsants in pregnancy: alterations in plasma protein binding. Epilepsy Res 1990;5(3):223–8.
52. Tornio A, Backman JT. Cytochrome P450 in Pharmacogenetics: An Update. Adv Pharmacol 2018;83:3–32.
53. McGready R, Stepniewska K, Seaton E, et al. Pregnancy and use of oral contraceptives reduces the biotransformation of proguanil to cycloguanil. Eur J Clin Pharmacol 2003;59(7):553–7.
54. Mwinyi J, Cavaco I, Pedersen RS, et al. Regulation of CYP2C19 expression by estrogen receptor alpha: implications for estrogen-dependent inhibition of drug metabolism. Mol Pharmacol 2010;78(5):886–94.
55. Jeong H, Choi S, Song JW, et al. Regulation of UDP-glucuronosyltransferase (UGT) 1A1 by progesterone and its impact on labetalol elimination. Xenobiotica 2008;38(1):62–75.
56. Fischer JH, Sarto GE, Hardman J, et al. Influence of gestational age and body weight on the pharmacokinetics of labetalol in pregnancy. Clin Pharmacokinet 2014;53(4):373–83.
57. Rogers RC, Sibai BM, Whybrew WD. Labetalol pharmacokinetics in pregnancy-induced hypertension. Am J Obstet Gynecol 1990;162(2):362–6.
58. Tomson T, Ohman I, Vitols S. Lamotrigine in pregnancy and lactation: a case report. Epilepsia 1997;38(9):1039–41.
59. Reimers A, Helde G, Brodtkorb E. Ethinyl estradiol, not progestogens, reduces lamotrigine serum concentrations. Epilepsia 2005;46(9):1414–7.
60. Chen H, Yang K, Choi S, et al. Up-regulation of UDP-glucuronosyltransferase (UGT) 1A4 by 17beta-estradiol: a potential mechanism of increased lamotrigine elimination in pregnancy. Drug Metab Dispos 2009;37(9):1841–7.
61. Fotopoulou C, Kretz R, Bauer S, et al. Prospectively assessed changes in lamotrigine-concentration in women with epilepsy during pregnancy, lactation and the neonatal period. Epilepsy Res 2009;85(1):60–4.
62. Karanam A, Pennell PB, French JA, et al. Lamotrigine clearance increases by 5 weeks gestational age: Relationship to estradiol concentrations and gestational age. Ann Neurol 2018;84(4):556–63.
63. Ohman I, Beck O, Vitols S, et al. Plasma concentrations of lamotrigine and its 2-N-glucuronide metabolite during pregnancy in women with epilepsy. Epilepsia 2008;49(6):1075–80.
64. Polepally AR, Pennell PB, Brundage RC, et al. Model-based lamotrigine clearance changes during pregnancy: clinical implication. Ann Clin Transl Neurol 2014;1(2):99–106.
65. O'Sullivan MJ, Boyer PJ, Scott GB, et al. The pharmacokinetics and safety of zidovudine in the third trimester of pregnancy for women infected with human

immunodeficiency virus and their infants: phase I acquired immunodeficiency syndrome clinical trials group study (protocol 082). Zidovudine Collaborative Working Group. Am J Obstet Gynecol 1993;168(5):1510–6.

66. Nylen H, Sergel S, Forsberg L, et al. Cytochrome P450 3A activity in mothers and their neonates as determined by plasma 4beta-hydroxycholesterol. Eur J Clin Pharmacol 2011;67(7):715–22.

67. Kim AH, Kim B, Rhee SJ, et al. Assessment of induced CYP3A activity in pregnant women using 4beta-hydroxycholesterol: Cholesterol ratio as an appropriate metabolic marker. Drug Metab Pharmacokinet 2018;33(3):173–8.

68. Johnson EL, Stowe ZN, Ritchie JC, et al. Carbamazepine clearance and seizure stability during pregnancy. Epilepsy Behav 2014;33:49–53.

69. Thomas AG, Burrows L, Knight R, et al. The effect of pregnancy on cyclosporine levels in renal allograft patients. Obstet Gynecol 1997;90(6):916–9.

70. Zheng S, Easterling TR, Umans JG, et al. Pharmacokinetics of tacrolimus during pregnancy. Ther Drug Monit 2012;34(6):660–70.

Inclusion of Pregnant and Lactating People in Clinical Research: Lessons Learned and Opportunities

Lisa R. Thiele, BS[a], Catherine Y. Spong, MD[a,b,*]

KEYWORDS

• Research inclusion • Pregnancy • Lactation • Medical ethics

KEY POINTS

- Pregnant and lactating individuals continue to be excluded from vital research under the guise of protection and expediency, leaving these populations vulnerable—as clearly demonstrated by their exclusion during a global pandemic.
- Lack of evidence for safety and efficacy of prescription and over-the-counter medications creates hesitancy among prescribers to treat pregnant patients or patients seeking pregnancy.
- New drug labeling is underutilized by prescribers due to lack of concise, straight forward data.

PREGNANT AND LACTATING PEOPLE AS A VULNERABLE POPULATION

Pregnant and lactating individuals historically have been excluded from clinical research trials under the guise of safety and protection for both mother and child. These exclusions however have led to limited data for these populations and thus a lack of evidence-based treatments for clinicians to use when counseling patients and families. Pregnant women were first identified as a vulnerable population in a 1975 Report from the National Commission for the Protection of Human Subjects of Biomedical and Behavioral Research.[1] The ethical debate of inclusion of a pregnant woman in clinical research has resulted in the overwhelming exclusion of pregnant and lactating patients from research—especially for studies and trials of general therapies. Numerous initiatives, groups, and reports have been published over the last several decades advocating for the inclusion of these groups in research.[2]

Financial Disclosures: none.
[a] Department of Obstetrics and Gynecology, University of Texas Southwestern Medical Center, 5323 Harry Hines Boulevard, Dallas, TX 75390-9032, USA; [b] Parkland Health, Dallas, TX 75390-9032, USA
* Corresponding author.
E-mail address: Catherine.spong@utsouthwestern.edu

Despite the lack of information available for drug safety and efficacy in pregnancy, more than 90% report taking at least one prescription or over-the-counter medication during pregnancy, with half reporting having taken 4 or more medications.[3] A 2002 study, examining the length of time required for newly approved medications to establish safety in pregnancy, found that 91% of agents approved in the prior 22 years had not yet been assessed for use in pregnancy.[4]

Despite this, the exclusion of pregnant and lactating people from observational as well as randomized controlled trials has persisted, forcing providers to rely on information from observational studies and expert opinion to counsel patients and in clinical decision-making.

FOOD AND DRUG ADMINISTRATION AND NATIONAL INSTITUTES OF HEALTH INITIATIVES

In the late 1950s and early 1960s, severe birth defects were found in children whose mothers who had been given thalidomide for nausea and vomiting in pregnancy.[5] Following this tragedy, Food and Drug Administration (FDA) guidelines released in 1977 essentially banned the inclusion of women of "childbearing potential," defined broadly as any woman capable of becoming pregnant, from early phase clinical trials. Under these guidelines, women of childbearing potential were only able to be included in studies where the medication would be used in life-threatening situations or in later phase trials after fertility trials and animal studies were completed.[6]

The near-complete exclusion of women from research led to widening gaps in knowledge on efficacy and safety of drugs in pregnant and nonpregnant women **(Fig. 1)**. In the 1980s, in the midst of shifts in public opinion, the US Public Health Service Task Force on Women's Health Issues Report recommended that long-term studies on women's health be conducted to better understand the effect of behavior, biology, and social factors on diseases prevalent or unique to women.[7] In 1989, the National Institutes of Health (NIH) created policy requiring that researchers justify exclusion of women and minorities from research.

In 1990 the US General Accounting Office found that little improvement in inclusion of women had been made and that implementation had been poorly communicated and inconsistently applied.[7,8] Governmental reports from the late 1980s and 1990s showed that women were represented significantly less in studies of diseases that affected both sexes, including human immunodeficiency virus (HIV)/AIDS and cardiovascular disease.[6]

Before 1993 inclusion of women in research trials was strongly recommended but not required by law. The NIH Revitalization Act of 1993 created a law requiring the

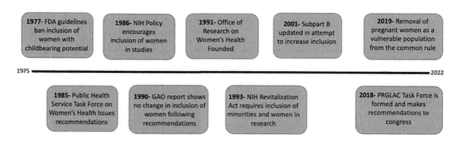

Fig. 1. Timeline of FDA and NIH initiatives to increase inclusion of pregnant and nonpregnant women in research.

inclusion of these groups in NIH-funded trials.[6,7] Under this act, trials must meet 4 criteria to obtain NIH funding: (1) that women and minorities be included in all clinical research; (2) that numbers in phase 3 clinical trials be sufficient to allow for valid analyses of potential differences by gender or race; (3) that these groups could not be excluded due to trial costs; and (4) that the NIH creates programs and supports outreach efforts to enroll and retain women and minorities in clinical trials.[6,7] Following implementation of the Revitalization Act, studies assessing the rates of inclusion for men and women in clinical trials showed mixed outcomes. Some found that men and women were overall included in trials at rates similar to the prevalence of the disease in the general population and that many trials included information on differences by sex.[9] Other studies reported that women continued to be excluded from trials studying HIV/AIDS.[8]

Although inclusion of nonpregnant, nonlactating, and minority populations increased in clinical research throughout the late 1990s and early 2000s, policies designed to increase inclusion of pregnant or lactating individuals were not passed. Pregnant women continued to be listed as a vulnerable population under the Common Rule.[10] In addition, requirements for inclusion of pregnant women were more stringent than other groups, as listed under Subpart B of 45 CFR 46. Although updated in 2001 as an attempt to increase inclusion, additional requirements are needed including that pregnant women or fetuses may be involved in research if all 10 criteria are met[10] (**Table 1**).

In 2004, the Eunice Kennedy Shriver National Institute of Child Health and Human Development (NICHD) created the Obstetric-Fetal Pharmacology Research Units Network (OPRU) in response to growing concern about the lack of information on drug use in pregnancy and the necessity of using off-label medications for patients.[11] The aims of OPRU were to improve the safety of medication use in pregnancy by conducting research on the pharmacokinetics and pharmacodynamics on common drugs. In the early 2000s, studies through these programs established changes in drug metabolism, absorption, distribution, and excretion in pregnant individuals.[11,12] Studies on glyburide found that glyburide was detected in cord blood at 70% of the maternal blood levels; this drastically differed from the understanding at the time that glyburide did not cross the placenta and was not in fetal blood. Developments from this work led to changes in national recommendations and practice standards.[12] These studies demonstrate the importance of studying therapeutics in pregnancy.

Despite major improvements in inclusion for women and minorities in the twenty-first century, pregnant patients continued to be generally excluded from research. In 2018, a study of actively recruiting NIH-funded phase III and IV clinical trials found 68% explicitly excluded pregnant women and 47% explicitly excluded lactating women.[13] Since this time, the FDA has signaled a "paradigm shift" in the inclusion of pregnant and lactating women in clinical research, including guidance expanding recognition of the obligation to include pregnant women.[14,15] Even with this guidance, however, there has been little movement in the inclusion of pregnant or lactating women in research.[14]

PRGLAC TASK FORCE RECOMMENDATIONS

Given the increasing concern regarding the lack of sound data on medication use in pregnant and lactating patients, the US Congress sought to understand the cause of the persistence of exclusion of women from clinical trials and the necessary steps to improve inclusion. In 2016, the 21st Century Cures Act established the Task Force on Research Specific to Pregnant Women and Lactating Women (PRGLAC) to provide recommendations to the Secretary of The Department of Health and Human Services

Table 1
Current wording of §46.204 subpart B

45 CFR46 Subpart B	Category	Explanation
§46.46.204	Pregnant women or fetuses may be involved in research if ALL of the following conditions are met	a. Where scientifically appropriate, preclinical studies, including studies on pregnant animals, and clinical studies, including studies on nonpregnant women, have been conducted and provide data for assessing potential risks to pregnant women and fetuses b. The risk to the fetus is caused solely by interventions or procedures that hold out the prospect of direct benefit for the woman or the fetus, or, if there is no such prospect of benefit, the risk to the fetus is not greater than minimal and the purpose of the research is the development of important biomedical knowledge that cannot be obtained by any other means c. Any risk is the least possible for achieving the objectives of the research d. If the research holds out the prospect of direct benefit to the pregnant woman, the prospect of a direct benefit both to the pregnant woman and the fetus, or no prospect of benefit for the woman nor the fetus when risk to the fetus is not greater than minimal and the purpose of the research is the development of important biomedical knowledge that cannot be obtained by any other means, her consent is obtained in accord with the informed consent provisions e. If the research holds out the prospect of direct benefit solely to the fetus then the consent of the pregnant woman and the father is obtained in accord with the informed consent provisions of subpart A of this part, except that the father's consent need not be obtained if he is unable to consent because of unavailability, incompetence, or temporary incapacity or the pregnancy resulted from rape or incest f. Each individual providing consent under paragraph (d) or (e) of this

(continued on next page)

Table 1 (continued)		
45 CFR46 Subpart B	**Category**	**Explanation**
		section is fully informed regarding the reasonably foreseeable impact of the research on the fetus or neonate g. For children as defined in Sec. 46.402(a) who are pregnant, assent and permission are obtained in accord with the provisions of the Protections for Children Involved as Subjects (subpart D) h. No inducements, monetary or otherwise, will be offered to terminate a pregnancy i. Individuals engaged in the research will have no part in any decisions as to the timing, method, or procedures used to terminate a pregnancy j. Individuals engaged in the research will have no part in determining the viability of a neonate.

and Congress on improvement of inclusion of pregnant and lactating individuals in research.[11] This task force was composed of representatives from federal agencies, medical societies, nonprofit organizations, and the pharmaceutical industry.[11] The report from this committee was submitted in September of 2018 and included 15 recommendations to help facilitate inclusion of pregnant women in trials.[16] The task force also subsequently provided a detailed plan for implementation of the recommendations in August of 2020.

The recommendations from PRGLAC centered on altering cultural assumptions regarding inclusion of pregnant and lactating women in research that have led to limited knowledge of therapeutic safety, effectiveness, and dosing of medications for these groups.[16] The recommendations included removal of pregnant women as a vulnerable population in the Common Rule as well as altering regulations that made inclusion of pregnant women more difficult for priniciple investigators (PIs) and reducing liability for researchers who included these populations in studies.[16] The task force also focused on increasing funding and resources to increase research on medications in pregnancy, expanding the workforce of clinicians studying these populations, and increasing public awareness on importance of inclusion.[16] In 2020, the task force provided an implementation plan to Congress to facilitate the adoption of the previous recommendations. The report offers detailed proposed implementation plans for all recommendations.[17]

Following the PRGLAC recommendations, in 2019 pregnant individuals were removed as an example of a vulnerable population in the Common Rule. However, as of the time of this writing, further policy has not been enacted to require justification of exclusion in study design for pregnant or lactating women.

Since 2018, there have been ample opportunities to enact many of the PRGLAC recommendations. As one example, the COVID pandemic provided a clear opportunity to include pregnant and lactating women in vaccination and therapeutic research.

Importantly, a study conducted more than 3 years after the PGRLAC recommendations found there was no change in exclusion rates of pregnant and lactating individuals in NIH-funded research trials compared with the findings in 2018[18] **(Fig. 2)**. Despite removal of pregnant women as a vulnerable population, lack of official policy has left the burden of increasing inclusion of pregnant and lactating women to individual principal investigators and as such, changes have not been implemented.

PREGNANCY LABELING

The FDA's alphabetic risk stratification system was used in the United States from the late 1970s until 2015 to inform clinicians on the availability of data on drug use and safety in pregnancy.[19] The system categorized drugs as A, B, C, D, or X, with category A representing medications with adequate and well-controlled studies proving safety in pregnancy and category X drugs with evidence in animal or human studies demonstrating teratogenicity or fetal risk. The intention of this system was to inform clinicians of the amount of available data on the use of a drug in pregnancy; however, this system led to clinicians misusing the categorization as an assessment of absolute risk in pregnancy.[19,20] The use of a letter system was misinterpreted that class B therapies were "safer" and "better" than class C, which was not true.

Concerns about the potential for misinterpretation of the alphabetical system were first raised in the early 1990s. Critics reported that clinicians would wrongly assume that 2 drugs had equal safety when in actuality, the drugs only had similar levels of evidence for or against their usage in pregnancy.[21] In response to concerns about misuse of the alphabetical system, the FDA established the Pregnancy Labeling Task Force to evaluate more effective systems characterizing the information about therapies.[21] The Pregnancy Labeling Task Force, along with increasing public frustration with the categorization system led to an FDA publication in 1999 that outlined potential changes to drug labeling in pregnancy and lactation.[19,21] Nearly a decade later, the FDA introduced a new labeling requirement, eliminating the alphabetical system and replacing it with a more structured approach that attempts to provide clinicians with a better understanding of the data on safety in pregnancy.[19,21]

In June of 2015, the FDA implemented this new system of categorization of drugs and biologic agents known as the Pregnancy and Lactation Labeling Rule (PLLR). The new system includes summaries of data on safety as well as the strength of the data and covers information for pregnancy and lactation in reproductive-aged men and women.[22] The FDA mandated that newly submitted drugs and biologics begin using the new system immediately with a slow rollout for previously approved medications.[22] The new

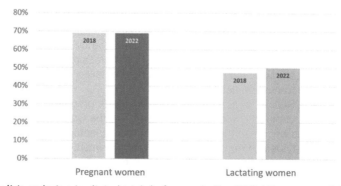

Fig. 2. Explicit exclusion in clinical trials before and after PRGLAC recommendations.

mandate required that the alphabetic classification be removed from all labeling by June of 2018 and that all drugs approved after 2001 use the new system by June of 2020.[21] This new system improved the presentation of pregnancy-related information in prescription drug labeling; however, it also highlighted the need to improve the quality and quantity of human data for prescription therapies in pregnancy.[23]

A study in 2020 by Byrne and colleagues[19] found that although newly approved medications complied with the PLLR labeling system, one-third of older medications had not converted their labels to comply with the new regulation. Furthermore, they found most of the information on labels was from animal studies rather than human trials, demonstrating again the lack of well-controlled, sound data available for pregnant and lactating individuals.[19] Other studies found that although drug companies were required to update labels and remove the alphabetical categorization by June of 2018, several online drug information resources commonly used by prescribers continued to list previous categorizations.[24]

A study from 2020 found that among providers in the Academy of Allergy, Asthma, and Immunology who saw an average of 2 pregnant patients a month, less than half were aware of changes to drug labeling in 2015. After being shown examples of the new labeling information, 95% of respondents reported that they would continue to use the alphabetical categorization system when making decisions regarding prescribing.[25] Despite changes to drug labeling for pregnant and lactating women, providers continue to rely on the older system of categorization, which has been shown to lead to incorrect conclusions regarding safety of use in pregnancy. The benefits of changing the labeling system are limited by the lack of strong, well-controlled clinical evidence of safety and efficacy and resistance from providers to using a less concise system. Furthermore, pharmacists and physicians have limited understanding of the PLLR labeling system.[26] A large deficit in well-controlled data on drug use in pregnancy creates complex and often confusing information that cannot be easily reduced to a letter classification system. At the same time, provider workload demands push physicians to use concise and overly simplified models in making clinical judgements for prescribing medications.

Labeling of drugs with safety information in pregnancy and lactation is key for aiding providers in making decisions on whether to initiate or continue therapy in patients while pregnant or nursing. Although obstetricians are practiced in navigating medication uses during pregnancy, providers in other specialties may not feel as confident prescribing medications to these patients. It is critical that information on dosing and safety is easily accessible and understandable for these providers when encountering patients in pregnancy. Despite decades of concern, FDA initiatives, and drastic changes in drug labeling, issues persist, including the continued lack of sound, well-controlled data available to guide medical decision-making.

SUMMARY

Despite decades of concern surrounding the inclusion of pregnant and lactating individuals in clinical trials, there has been limited movement forward. During the COVID-19 pandemic, pregnant and lactating women were again excluded from the initial trials that led to emergency authorization of the COVID-19 vaccinations.[27] The COVID-19 pandemic presented a ripe opportunity for pregnant and lactating women to be included in clinical trials. Although the pandemic occurred after PRGLAC recommendations, the vaccination trials once again excluded pregnant and lactating patients, resulting in delayed evidence regarding vaccination for these groups. Interestingly, despite NIH and FDA actively leading the PRGLAC recommendations and implementation, at each opportunity to include pregnant women in the vaccine trials, the decision was made—under the guise of expediency—to exclude pregnant women; this increased vaccine hesitancy and fear among patients and left clinicians without sound data to make recommendations to expectant mothers who were at increased risk of severe COVID-19 complications. Lack of controlled trial data also led to pregnant health care workers being excluded from vaccine mandates and in some institutions prevented pregnant and breastfeeding employees from accessing the vaccine.[28]

Four years after PRGLAC recommendations, there remains a lack of policy requiring justification for exclusion of pregnant and lactating individuals from research trials. Currently, the NIH requires justification for the exclusion of nonpregnant and nonlactating women or children from research; however, with no policy requiring justification for exclusion for pregnant or lactating individuals, the responsibility to include these groups falls to individual investigators. Although not all clinical trials may be suitable for inclusion of these groups, exclusion remains the default for many researchers. This exclusion results in a severe lack of information of drug safety and efficacy in this population; although intended to protect this "vulnerable" population, the ultimate effect is to provide care without adequate evidence.

CLINICS CARE POINTS

- Exclusion of pregnant and lactating women in research limits evidence for management.
- Requiring a justification for exclusion of pregnant and lactating women from research may increase inclusion.
- The new drug labeling system provides information on safety and strength of the data however the utility is hindered by limited human data

REFERENCES

1. Research, N.C.f.t.P.o.H.S.o.B.a.B. Research on the fetus. U.S Department of Health, Education, and Welfare; 1975.
2. Byrne JJ, Saucedo AM, Spong CY. Task force on research specific to pregnant and lactating women. Semin Perinatol 2020;44(3):151226.
3. Mitchell AA, Gilboa SM, Werler MM, et al. Medication use during pregnancy, with particular focus on prescription drugs: 1976-2008. Am J Obstet Gynecol 2011; 205(1):51.e1–8.
4. Lo WY, Friedman JM. Teratogenicity of recently introduced medications in human pregnancy. Obstet Gynecol 2002;100(3):465–73.
5. Kim JH, Scialli AR. Thalidomide: the tragedy of birth defects and the effective treatment of disease. Toxicol Sci 2011;122(1):1–6.
6. Liu KA, Mager NA. Women's involvement in clinical trials: historical perspective and future implications. Pharm Pract (Granada) 2016;14(1):708.
7. Health, N.I.o. History of Women's Participation in Clinical Research. NIH Inclusion Outreach Toolkit: How to Engage, Recruit, and Retain Women in Clinical Research 2022. 2022. https://orwh.od.nih.gov/toolkit/recruitment/history. [Accessed 12 July 2022].
8. Merkatz RB. Inclusion of women in clinical trials: a historical overview of scientific, ethical, and legal issues. J Obstet Gynecol Neonatal Nurs 1998;27(1):78–84.

9. Evelyn B, Toigo T, Banks D, et al. Participation of racial/ethnic groups in clinical trials and race-related labeling: a review of new molecular entities approved 1995-1999. J Natl Med Assoc 2001;93(12 Suppl):18s–24s.
10. Blehar MC, Spong C, Grady C, et al. Enrolling pregnant women: issues in clinical research. Womens Health Issues 2013;23(1):e39–45.
11. Ren Z, Bremer AA, Pawlyk AC. Drug development research in pregnant and lactating women. Am J Obstet Gynecol 2021;225(1):33–42.
12. Parisi MA, Spong CY, Zajicek A, et al. We don't know what we don't study: the case for research on medication effects in pregnancy. Am J Med Genet C Semin Med Genet 2011;157c(3):247–50.
13. Spong CY, Bianchi DW. Improving public health requires inclusion of underrepresented populations in research. JAMA 2018;319(4):337–8.
14. Nooney J, Thor S, de Vries C, et al. Assuring access to safe medicines in pregnancy and breastfeeding. Clin Pharmacol Ther 2021;110(4):941–5.
15. Waggoner MR, Lyerly AD. Clinical trials in pregnancy and the "shadows of thalidomide": revisiting the legacy of Frances Kelsey. Contemp Clin Trials 2022;119:106806.
16. Health NIo. Task force on research specific to pregnant women and lactating women. PRGLAC; 2018.
17. Health NIo. TASK force on research specific to pregnant women and lactating women- report implementation plan. PRGLAC; 2020.
18. Thiele L, Thompson J, Pruszynski J, et al. Gaps in evidence-based medicine: underrepresented populations still excluded from research trials following 2018 recommendations from the Health and Human Services Task Force on Research Specific to Pregnant Women and Lactating Women. Am J Obstet Gynecol 2022. https://doi.org/10.1016/j.ajog.2022.07.009.
19. Byrne JJ, Saucedo AM, Spong CY. Evaluation of Drug Labels Following the 2015 Pregnancy and Lactation Labeling Rule. JAMA Netw Open 2020;3(8):e2015094.
20. Brucker MC, King TL. The 2015 US food and drug administration pregnancy and lactation labeling rule. J Midwifery Women's Health 2017;62(3):308–16.
21. Freeman MP, Farchione T, Yao L, et al. Psychiatric medications and reproductive safety: scientific and clinical perspectives pertaining to the US FDA pregnancy and lactation labeling rule. J Clin Psychiatry 2018;79(4).
22. Content and format of labeling for human prescription drug and biological products; requirements for pregnancy and lactation labeling. Final rule. Fed Regist 2014;79(233):72063–103.
23. Dinatale M, Roca C, Sahin L, et al. The importance of clinical research in pregnant women to inform prescription drug labeling. J Clin Pharmacol 2020; 60(Suppl 2):S18–25.
24. Harris JB, Holmes AP, Eiland LS. The Influence of the food and drug administration pregnancy and lactation labeling rule on drug information resources. Ann Pharmacother 2021;55(4):459–65.
25. Namazy J, Chambers C, Sahin L, et al. Clinicians' perspective of the new pregnancy and lactation labeling rule (PLLR): results from an AAAAI/FDA survey. J Allergy Clin Immunol Pract 2020;8(6):1947–52.
26. Alem G, Awuonda M, Haastrup D, et al. Evaluation of knowledge of the new Pregnancy and Lactation Labeling Rule among pharmacists and physicians. J Am Pharm Assoc (2003) 2022;62(2):427–31.
27. Rubin R. Pregnant people's paradox—excluded from vaccine trials despite having a higher risk of COVID-19 complications. JAMA 2021;325(11):1027–8.
28. Adhikari EH, Spong CY. Pregnancy is not a disability: including pregnant healthcare workers in COVID-19 vaccine mandates. Am J Obstet Gynecol 2022;226(5):757–9.

Over-The-Counter Drugs and Pregnancy

William F. Rayburn, MD, MBA[a,b,*]

KEYWORDS

- Common conditions • Drugs • Medications • Nonprescription • Over-the-counter
- Pregnancy

KEY POINTS

- Over-the-counter (OTC) medication use is common in pregnancy. However, information about potential maternal or fetal adverse reactions is often limited or unavailable regarding human exposure.
- Avoid drug exposure during the first trimester, as it is the period of organogenesis. Continued fetal exposure to some medications later in gestation can result in subtle morphologic abnormalities, functional problems, and growth impairment.
- When an OTC drug must be taken, discuss the risks and benefits of taking versus not taking the drug.
- Most OTC drugs are low dose and used only briefly, so any harm is unlikely and more theoretic than real.
- OTC drugs have ingredients that have been used for years, which is the reason for confidence about safety.

INTRODUCTION

Despite growing patient awareness of avoiding exposures, most women take several medications during pregnancy. Drug ingestion is most common during the first and third trimesters, exposing the fetus during the critical period of organogenesis and shortly before labor and delivery.[1] Nonprescription or over-the-counter (OTC) medicines are taken more often than prescribed drugs during pregnancy[1,2]; this is particularly worrisome, as many OTC medications are used without physician awareness and are occasionally not recognized by the patient as being potentially harmful.

Dilemmas exist when studying any drug, whether prescribed or OTC. Most OTC drugs taken during human pregnancy are not discussed in standard obstetrics textbooks or lay books. Although published research can be valuable, findings from

[a] Department of Obstetrics and Gynecology and College of Graduate Studies, Medical University of South Carolina, Charleston, SC, USA; [b] Department of Obstetrics and Gynecology, University of New Mexico School of Medicine, Albuquerque, NM, USA
* 1721 Atlantic Avenue, Mt. Pleasant, SC 29482.
E-mail address: wrayburnmd@gmail.com

Obstet Gynecol Clin N Am 50 (2023) 27–37
https://doi.org/10.1016/j.ogc.2022.10.002
0889-8545/23/© 2022 Elsevier Inc. All rights reserved.
obgyn.theclinics.com

most studies about OTC drugs are not always conclusive. Data may be biased or reflect the patients' background risk for birth defects regardless of exposure.[1,2] In many cases, the only data come from animal studies, which involve administration of doses high enough to cause maternal morbidity or fetal toxicity. Therefore, in many situations where the only reported human experience involves case reports or small series, the medication is often avoided during pregnancy unless the benefits clearly outweigh the risks.[1,2]

Although information about prescription medications can be scant or limited and difficult to interpret, assessing the risks associated with OTC medications is even more difficult. A review of the *Physician' Desk Reference for Non-Prescription Drugs* reveals little or no information about reproductive toxicity in humans for most OTC medications. Many agents contain multiple ingredients, both active and inactive, making it more difficult to determine whether the combined effect of these ingredients might potentiate teratogenic effect.

Doses may not be included in the labeling of the drug, although the lowest effective dose is customarily used to relieve symptoms in most persons. Patients may misinterpret dosage instructions and take either larger amounts or more frequently than recommended, resulting in an increased exposure to the fetus. This manuscript attempts to summarize principles of educating pregnant patients and address points in counseling about specific ingredients in OTC drugs for common pregnancy-related conditions.

PRINCIPLES OF EDUCATING PREGNANT PATIENTS

The initial prenatal visit should include a review of all medications taken around the time of conception and early in gestation. People commonly use OTC medicine to treat nutritional needs, pain or discomfort, cold and cough, allergies, skin rashes or hives, diarrhea or constipation, heartburn, and insomnia. Most OTC medicines relieve the symptoms for a brief time but do not correct the condition causing the symptoms.

OTC medicines contain low doses and, with a few exceptions such as nonsteroidal antiinflammatory drugs (NSAIDs), are presumably safe during pregnancy. The same dose is taken despite physiologic change due to pregnancy and the postpartum. However, experts do not know for sure about the safety of many medications, as studies in humans have not been conducted, especially in a controlled manner. Whether an OTC medicine taken infrequently increases the risk of any fetal harm is believed to be unlikely.

Birth defects happen in the first few months of pregnancy. Sufficient information to determine the additional risk is available for less than 168 of all medications approved by the US Food and Drug Administration.[3] The background risk that a fetus will have a major birth defect is 2% to 4%. A study would require 2000 pregnancies exposed to a drug during the first trimester to provide sufficient power (80% at 5% significance level) to exclude a 3-fold higher overall risk and 700 for a 2-fold higher risk.[4]

Patients are encouraged that the best way to know if an OTC medicine is safe is to ask her obstetrics clinician. Locating information about drug safety online is often difficult for patients, and any reported effects may be inexact or misleading. Calling the no-cost MotherToBaby hotline (1–866–626–6847), which is a service of the Organization of Teratology Information Services, may be beneficial. Other evidence-based resources about specific drugs in pregnancy are shown in **Box 1**.

The prenatal period is an opportune time for counseling patients about OTC drug use during lactation. Most active ingredients in OTC drugs are transferred into human

---

Box 1
Standard resources for evidence-based information about specific drugs during pregnancy and lactation

Briggs Drugs in Pregnancy and Lactation: A Reference Guide to Fetal and Neonatal Risk
    Wolters Kluwer, 12th ed.
    ISBN-13: 978-1975162375

Drugs during Pregnancy and Lactation: Treatment Options and Risk Assessment
    Academic Press, 3rd ed.
    ISBN-13: 978 to 0,124,080,782

Shepard's Catalog of Teratogenic Agents
    Johns Hopkins University Press, 13th ed.
    ISBN-13 978 to 0,801,897,849

MotherToBaby, Organization of Teratology Information Specialists (OTIS)
    www.OTISpregnancy.org
    866-626-6847; 877-311-8972

Reproductive Toxicology Center (REPROTOX)
    Washington, Columbia Hospital for Women Medical Center, Washington, DC
    www.reprotox.com
    202-293-5137

Teratogen Information System (TERIS)
    School of Public Health, University of Washington, Seattle, WA
    206-543-2465

UpToDate drug database
    Software system for point-of-care, Wolters Kluwer Health
    www.uptodate.com

Cochrane Database of Systematic Reviews, Cochrane Library
    John Wiley & Sons
    www.cochrane.org

---

milk in insignificant amounts. Unless the mother consumes copious quantities, the calculated infant dose via breastfeeding is very small. Limited information on drugs in breastmilk is also found in those resources in **Box 1**.

A trip to the chain store pharmacy will reveal hundreds of different OTC drugs. Furthermore, there are often several OTC medications for treating each of the common conditions. This review focuses on active ingredients in OTC products for specific conditions and does not encourage a particular branded product.

ADVICE ABOUT OVER-THE-COUNTER DRUGS FOR SPECIFIC CONDITIONS

Conditions encountered during prenatal care that are amenable to use of commonly used drugs are described by Lockwood and Magriples in UpToDate.[5] Specific OTC drugs for specific conditions are summarized later. The primary active ingredient in each drug is shown in italics. Examples of OTC brands and their active ingredients are shown for each condition in **Table 1**.

"Quick takes" about OTC drugs during pregnancy come primarily from searching for the active ingredient of each drug in the REPROTOX system (www.reprotox.org). REPROTOX contains summaries of maternal and fetal effects from medications and chemicals on pregnancy, reproduction, and development. The system was developed as an adjunct information source for clinicians, scientists, and government agencies. References in this manuscript are provided selectively only for further reading;

Table 1
Common conditions during pregnancy and active ingredients in examples of brands of over-the-counter drugs

Condition	Active Ingredient	Examples of OTC Brands
Nausea	Pyridoxine/doxylamine	Diclegis, Unisom
Localized pain	Acetaminophen	Tylenol
	NSAIDs	Advil, Motrin, Bayer, Aleve, aspirin
Nasal congestion	Oxymetazoline	Afrin, Sinex, Zicam
	Triamcinolone acetonide	Nasacort
	Phenylephrine	Sudafed, Mucinex, Dayquil
Cold remedy	Zinc	Zicam
Allergy relief	Antihistamines	Claritin, Allegra
Heartburn/reflux	Antacids	Tums, Mylanta, Rolaids
	Sucralfate	Carafate
	H2RAs	Pepcid, Zantac 360
	PPIs	Prilosec, Nexium, Peracid
Flatulence	Alpha galactosidase	Beano
Diarrhea	Loperamide	Imodium, Diamode
	Bismuth subsalicylate	Pepto Bismol, Kaopectate
	Kaolin	Kaopectalin
Constipation	Bisacodyl, docusate	Dulcolax, Colace
Hemorrhoids	Phenylephrine, pramoxine	Preparation H max strength
Acne	Benzoyl peroxide	Clearasil, Neutrogena acne
Dandruff	Zinc pyrithione	Head & Shoulders, Dove, Selsun
	Coal tar	DHS shampoo, Tarsum shampoo
Cuts/Abrasions	Bacitracin, polymyxin	Neosporin, Polysporin
Skin itching	Hydrocortisone	Cortizone-10
	Diphenhydramine	Benadryl spray
	Zinc oxide	Desitin, Calamine
Insomnia	Melatonin	Nature Made, Nature's Bounty
	Diphenhydramine	Benadryl
	Doxylamine	Sleep Aid, Unisom
Insecticide repellents	DEET	OFF!, Murphy's
Sunscreens	Oxybenzone	Coppertone, Neutrogena, Sun Bum
Nicotine replacement	Nicotine	Nicorette gum and lozenges

Note: many comparable generic brands with the same ingredients are available, often at a lower cost.

otherwise, the reference list would be too exhaustive and is available from standard resources shown in **Box 1**.

Prenatal Vitamins/Mineral Supplements

Most *prenatal multivitamins* contain the same amounts of vitamins, iron, and folic acid to satisfy the daily requirements of most pregnant patients. Vitamin use may not improve maternal and neonatal outcomes, as most persons are adequately nourished, and food is vitamin fortified. Nevertheless, it seems reasonable to ingest one prenatal multivitamin daily. In addition, prenatal vitamins contain *omega-3 fatty acids* (docosahexaenoic acid and eicosapentaenoic acid) from fish oil. These normal components of the diet are essential for brain and retinal function. Any benefit to the fetus is questionable, but adverse pregnancy outcomes from exposure to these agents seem unlikely.

Iron supplantation at the recommended dose of 27 mg daily is not harmful during pregnancy. Similar to any medication, intoxication with iron (eg, intentional overdose) can lead to adverse maternal and fetal effects. Prenatal multivitamins typically contain 27 mg of elemental iron to reduce pregnancy-induced iron deficiency. The Centers for Disease Control and Prevention recommends 30 mg daily to achieve the Recommended Daily Allowance (RDA) for pregnant patients.[6] If a daily multivitamin with iron is not well tolerated, iron supplementation (1 to 3 times per week) seems to be as effective and better tolerated.[7] Many OTC iron products contain different amounts of iron, and any intake of 45 mg or more can lead to gastrointestinal discomfort (usually constipation).

Prenatal multivitamins typically contain 800 mcg of *folic acid*. A 400 to 800 mcg daily dose may aid in reducing the risk of open neural tube defects during the period of neural tube closure. Supplementing folic acid beyond what is in prenatal multivitamins may have additional benefits, but available data are insufficient to support a clear benefit of a higher dose (ie, 4.0 mg) given before or after conception. Additional information is provided in the antiseizure medications paper in this issue. An adverse effect of excessive folic acid includes masking maternal vitamin B12 deficiency.

Vitamin D is an essential nutrient. High doses of vitamin D (eg, 2000–4000 international units/day) have not been associated with a syndrome of congenital anomalies. Serum concentrations of vitamin D3 are not routinely measured during pregnancy.

Calcium is an essential mineral. Intestinal absorption of calcium increases in pregnancy and enables accumulation for fetal skeletal development. Supplements are available as salts and found in some antacids. When consumed in excessive amounts, calcium may pose a greater risk of neonatal hypoparathyroidism and hypocalcemia.

Nausea/Heartburn/Reflux

All pregnant patients experience nausea. Behavioral changes, expectant management, and medication are most effective. *Pyridoxine*, or vitamin B6, is a normal component of the diet. Although the RDA is 1.9 mg/d, the recommended limits for pregnant and lactating women are 100 mg/d. Used as an antiemetic in early pregnancy either alone or combined with doxylamine (Unisom), pyridoxine is often recommended, although it has not been consistently documented as being effective in controlled studies.

Antacids are commonly taken for intermittent relief of dyspepsia by alkalinizing contents of the stomach. Antacids based on aluminum, calcium, or magnesium are believed not to increase the risk of congenital anomalies when used in appropriate doses. Unrestricted use of antacids containing sodium bicarbonate can produce metabolic alkalosis and fluid overload in mother and offspring.

No studies in humans have been conducted about the harmful effects of antacids during pregnancy. All antacids can cause diarrhea or constipation. Aluminum in certain antacids has been shown in animals to cross the placenta and accumulate in fetal tissues, leading to death or abnormal skeletal growth, impaired learning, and memory. However, no such toxic effects have been reported in human pregnancies. Limited use of calcium-containing antacids would seem to present no additional risk to the fetus or mother.

Gastroesophageal reflux affects half or more of pregnant patients. Similar to treatment of nausea, initial management consists of lifestyle and dietary modifications. Drug therapy should begin with antacids followed by *sucralfate*, an antiulcer agent composed of an alkaline aluminum complex. Sucralfate is not expected to increase risks during pregnancy. Those who fail to respond are encouraged to take OTC *histamine 2 receptor antagonists (H2RAs)* and then *proton pump inhibitors (PPIs)* to control symptoms. The brand Zantac had previously contained ranitidine, a probable carcinogen (N-nitrosodimethylamine), and now contains famotidine. None of those drugs is associated with a greater risk of congenital anomalies or adverse pregnancy outcomes. Any relation between maternal H2RAs and PPIs and later childhood asthma remains speculative.

Analgesia

Acetaminophen is the most taken medication during pregnancy outside of prenatal vitamins and iron. It is widely used for treatment of pain and fever, with no high-quality evidence in humans of increased risks of pregnancy loss, congenital anomalies, or neurodevelopmental delay in offspring.[8] Acetaminophen use during pregnancy does not increase adverse outcomes in most studies, although some studies suggested associations between prolonged acetaminophen with cryptorchidism, childhood wheezing/asthma, and neurodevelopmental problems in offspring (attention disorders, child autism).[9,10]

The extensive use of acetaminophen by pregnant people combined with the paucity of documented adverse effects has served to make this medication the pain reliever and antipyretic of choice when short-term drug therapy is indicated.[8] In addition, it is possible that fever reduction with acetaminophen reduces the risk of some congenital anomalies, but further study is needed.[9] Overuse may be more likely in pregnancy due to limitations on use of other medications and perceptions of its safety. Limited data suggest good fetal outcomes in cases of maternal overdose/overuse (more than 4 g daily), but the potential for maternal morbidity is high.

The risks and benefits of NSAIDs for treatment of pain, fever, or rheumatologic disease depend on the dose, gestational age, and duration of therapy.[11] An increased risk of miscarriage is weakly associated with use of ibuprofen or naproxen, particularly near the time of conception. After 20 weeks, NSAIDs can affect the fetal kidneys, leading to oligohydramnios, typically after at least 48 hours of therapy. As early as 24 weeks gestation, use of NSAIDs other than low-dose aspirin for more than 48 hours can cause in utero constriction of the ductus arteriosus.

Aspirin exposure in experimental animal studies reveals an increase in congenital anomalies. A consistent pattern of anomalies was not identified in human reports of typical exposures to aspirin. An increase in miscarriage risk around conception has been proposed. As other NSAIDs, aspirin is to be avoided later in gestation. Concerns about oligohydramnios, closure of the ductus arteriosus, and bleeding abnormalities do not apply to low doses (60–100 mg/d) used to reduce the risk of developing preeclampsia.[11] Repeated doses of aspirin are not recommended during breast feeding because of possible newborn accumulation of the drug and the theoretic risk of Reye syndrome.

Nasal Congestion

Many pregnant patients encounter symptomatic nasal congestion (rhinitis of pregnancy), which is hormonally mediated with no known allergic cause. It does not usually require therapy nor respond well to medications. Preexisting allergic rhinitis or "cold"-induced rhinitis is common during pregnancy and seem to last longer. Symptoms from allergies are often accompanied with sneezing, nausea, watery rhinorrhea, and conjunctival itching. Treatment is focused on maximizing allergen avoidance and rinsing the nose and sinuses with saline once or twice daily. The nasal passages can be rinsed with an OTC saline spray or the lower sinuses rinsed with larger volumes using a steam pot or squeeze bottle. External nasal dilator strips may be useful for nocturnal nasal congestion.

OTC drug sprays or pills for nasal congestion contain phenylephrine/pseudoephedrine, oxymetazoline, antihistamines, or glucocorticoids. *Phenylephrine* and *pseudoephedrine* are sympathomimetic drugs used as decongestants in nonprescription cold medicines. It is best to minimize or avoid during pregnancy because of their vasoconstrictive property. Any association with malformations in some studies has not been confirmed. Use in normotensive patients with upper respiratory congestions is likely safe when used sparingly beyond the first trimester. *Oxymetazoline* is an alpha-adrenergic agonist found in decongestant nasal sprays. It is not expected to cause any fetal harm including any additional risk of birth defects.

There are many H1 and H2 histamine receptor blocker agents to reduce nasal congestion. Several sedating (eg, chlorpheniramine) and nonsedating (eg, loratadine) *antihistamines* are often used without apparent harm. If sedation is desired, chlorpheniramine, often in a sustained release form, has a good safety record for residual itching and sneezing (although less effective for congestion and postnasal drip). If symptoms continue, multidosing of *cromolyn sodium* nasal sprays or once daily *glucocorticoid* nasal sprays has proved safety during pregnancy. Allergic rhinitis is often accompanied by conjunctivitis. Eye drops for allergic relief contain *pheniramine maleate*, which should be safe during pregnancy when used as directed.

Zinc, an essential nutrient, is the primary ingredient in cold remedies that are promoted to shorten the duration of symptoms. Adverse pregnancy outcomes have been associated with high concentrations of zinc in the blood and tissues. A role for excess zinc intake in the production of congenital anomalies has not been established, however.

Diarrhea/Flatulence

Diarrhea is not more common in pregnancy. The management of patients with acute diarrhea initially involves general supportive measures such as hydration and alteration of the diet. *Loperamide* was not teratogenic in animal studies, but human data are conflicting, and no malformation has been confirmed. It shares some of the opioid-binding properties of meperidine but very little loperamide enters the central nervous system and is unlikely to be abused.

Bismuth subsalicylate is frequently used for relief for indigestion, nausea and vomiting, and diarrhea. Any harm from bismuth salts during pregnancy is controversial and most likely theoretic. It is known that bismuth is concentrated in the placenta and readily transferred to the fetus where it may bind to numerous tissues including the bones. It is unknown whether this would result in fetal damage. There may also be concerns about the salicylate component of bismuth subsalicylate, as this may decrease platelet adhesiveness and aggregation as well as increase the risk of premature closure of the fetal ductus arteriosus.

Kaolin, a clay composed of hydrated aluminum silicate, is administered orally in treating diarrhea. Kaopectate, a mixture of kaolin, pectin, and bismuth subsalicylate, has not been studied for adverse pregnancy outcomes. The agent is not teratogenic in rats, but there are no epidemiologic studies in humans. Consumption of copious amounts of kaolin may be associated with maternal anemia. In addition, there are some indications that use of kaolin-containing agents may serve as a significant source of aluminum loading during pregnancy. Therefore, there seems to be little clinical basis to support the use of kaolin-containing medications for treating diarrhea during pregnancy.

Excess flatulence is treated with *alpha galactosidase*, one of the enzymes that hydrolyzes terminal galactosyl linkages from glycolipids. Its activity is normally present in the plasma of pregnant people. There are no known published studies of possible reproductive or lactation effects.

Constipation/Hemorrhoids

Constipation is more common during pregnancy due to hormonal (progesterone) and mechanical factors. Increasing dietary fiber and fluids or using bulk-forming laxatives (see **Table 1**) is preferred, as these agents are not absorbed. Occasional use of *magnesium hydroxide, lactulose, or bisacodyl* is not thought to be harmful. Magnesium salts have been used widely during pregnancy with good safety, whereas lactulose and bisacodyl are minimally absorbed. It is better to avoid *castor oil* during pregnancy, as it may stimulate uterine contractions and interfere with absorption of fat-soluble vitamins in excessive use.

Approximately one-third of pregnant or postpartum patients are affected by hemorrhoidal discomfort. An emphasis on dietary and lifestyle modification is often accompanied by recommending mild laxatives and stool softeners to avoid constipation. Antihemorrhoidal suppositories or creams contain *pramoxine, glycerin, phenylephrine* (see nasal congestion section), and often hydrocortisone. Pramoxine is a local anesthetic marketed in topical analgesic, antiitch, and hemorrhoidal preparations. The use of pramoxine in combinations with hydrocortisone during the third trimester was not associated with adverse effects on birthweight, prematurity, or gestational age at delivery.

Skin Conditions

Several topical OTC preparations are available for treating acne, dandruff, skin cuts and abrasions, and localized itching. These products are absorbed and could potentially lead to exposure to the fetus with excessive use.

Benzoyl peroxide is the active ingredient in many topical acne medications. There is no increase in congenital malformations in rats. Although any additional risk during human pregnancy is unknown, the low level of systemic absorption should provide protection. *Resorcinol* is an aromatic alcohol used in treating acne, seborrhea, eczema, and psoriasis. The agent is not teratogenic in animal studies and not associated with an increased frequency of congenital anomalies.

Oral *tretinoin* is expected to increase the risk of birth defects if the exposure level is sufficiently high. Low-dose topical preparations of tretinoin do not increase adverse pregnancy outcomes with minimal or intermittent use. There are case reports of birth defects after continued topical tretinoin that form the basis of topical tretinoin avoidance during pregnancy.

Zinc pyrithione is an antidandruff agent in medicated shampoos. There have been no studies in humans, perhaps because of the poor absorption and negative teratogenic studies in animals. A role of excessive zinc intake in the production of congenital anomalies has not been established. *Coal tar* is also used to treat dandruff. Although a small series of women who used coal tar products did not have an increase in congenital anomalies, no epidemiologic studies were found about human reproductive toxicity.

Bacitracin and *polymyxin B* are antimicrobials in topical antiseptics. No relation between their exposure and adverse pregnancy outcomes has been noted. Based on experimental animal studies and limited human experience, both topical therapies are not expected to increase the risk of congenital anomalies or any fetal harm.

The amount of *hydrocortisone* or *zinc oxide* in topical antiitch creams is believed to be too low to cause any additional concern during pregnancy.

Sleep Aids

Insomnia is characterized by complaints of difficulty initiating or maintaining sleep, early morning awakening, and nonrestful sleep. Sleep hygiene consists of a set of simple recommendations that include ensuring a comfortable sleep environment, regularity of sleep schedule, regular exercise, allowing time for the patient to unwind before bedtime, and relief of any stressors.[12,13] Cognitive behavioral therapy for insomnia is the first-line treatment of chronic insomnia.

In general, avoidance of common herbal or "natural" remedies touted as insomnia treatments, such a valerian, tryptophan, or melatonin receptor agonists (melatonin, ramelteon), is recommended due to both an absence of evidence for efficacy as well as safety.[13] Endogenous melatonin is present normally during pregnancy.[14] There is no evidence of adverse fetal outcomes with exogenous melatonin, although studies have been small.[15]

Diphenhydramine, a first-generation antihistamine, has convincing evidence for lack of clinical effect in many pregnant patients. Although there is no increased risk of congenital malformations, continued antihistamine use during lactation is associated with infant irritability and mild sedation.[13] *Doxylamine*, another first-generation antihistamine, is a reasonable OTC option to treat insomnia.[13] Based on experimental animal studies and human experience with the doxylamine/pyridoxine combination, use of doxylamine during pregnancy is not expected to increase the risk of congenital anomalies. As with diphenhydramine, continued use of doxylamine and other antihistamines during lactation is associated with infant irritability and mild sedation.

Insect Repellents/Sunscreens

Pregnant patients are advised to take precautions to reduce their risk of acquiring arboviral infections (eg, Zika virus, West Nile virus, malaria) by avoiding mosquito bites using protective clothing and *DEET* (N,N-diethy-3-methylbenzamide)-based repellents.[16] Topically applied DEET does not pose hazards to the fetus, regardless of gestational age. Despite this, it is likely better for pregnant women to limit their exposure to smaller amounts and apply it to protective clothing rather than on the skin.

Avoiding prolonged exposure to the sun is particularly desirable during pregnancy. Limited use of sunscreens is likely better than none. Sunscreens applied topically contain many ingredients: *oxybenzone*, homosalate, octisalate, and avobenzone. There is no reference on pregnancy or lactation effects of these agents.

Smoking and Other Tobacco Products

Nicotine in cigarette smoking, chewing tobacco, and other smokeless tobacco products are associated with a greater risk of restricted fetal growth. Some nicotine products are sold without a prescription to adults. Marketed as an aid for stopping smoking, nicotine in gum and lozenges is a vasoconstrictor with potential for elevations in blood pressures.

Use of nicotine replacement products is debatable. Nicotine replacement products by pregnant women might reduce fetal exposure to other agents in cigarette smoke. Nicotine replacement might have beneficial effects on total cigarette consumption, lengthening gestational age, and increasing birth weight in pregnant women who are trying to quit smoking. Use of the lowest dose is urged, as replacement products might lead to higher nicotine concentrations than those found in cigarettes. Monitoring for fetal growth would be a worthwhile consideration.

SUMMARY

Pregnancy is often accompanied with many symptoms for which nonprescription or OTC drugs are used or recommended. Most obstetric clinicians consider OTC medicines to be safe because of their low dose with very short-term use. However, studies of sufficient sample size in humans are often lacking about the safety of most OTC medicines during pregnancy and lactation. In general, products containing the lowest effective dose of only necessary ingredients are to be taken during the shortest period. Safety information about ingredients in most drugs can be found on the Reproductive Toxicology Center Web site (REPROTOX) and other resources provided in this overview.

CLINICS CARE POINTS

- Some patients may not perceive OTC drugs as being important to report. The initial and subsequent prenatal examinations should include questions and documentation about use of any specific OTC drugs.
- OTC medications should generally be avoided in pregnancy, especially during the first trimester, due to a lack of human data.
- Pregnant patients are encouraged to consult their obstetric clinician rather than rely on online summaries of drug effects.
- Limited information in experimental animals exists about most OTC drugs during pregnancy and lactation. Although generally considered to be safe, it is not prudent to assume that these products are without reproductive toxicity.
- The obstetrician should be aware of the ingredients in OTC preparations and recommend those products that contain the safest ingredients at the lowest possible dose to relieve symptoms.
- As gestation advances, conditions leading to the need for OTC drugs are more common.
- Patients should be instructed to follow the directions carefully and use the medications for the shortest period.
- Concern about maternal or fetal risks would be greatest when any OTC drug is taken continually or in amounts more than directed.
- OTC drugs taken in customary doses can be safe while lactating, as infant concentrations are very low. If taken regularly or continually, discussion with the clinician is to be encouraged beforehand.

ACKNOWLEDGMENTS

The authors acknowledge the review of references in **Box 1** and editorial assistance by Dr Gale G. Hannigan, a research professor and librarian, University of New Health Sciences Library and Informatics Center, University of New Mexico Health Sciences, Albuquerque, NM.

DISCLOSURE

The author of this review has no relevant commercial interests to disclose.

REFERENCES

1. Conover EA, Rayburn WF. Over the-the-counter drugs during pregnancy. In: Rayburn WF, Zuspan FP, editors. Drug therapy in obstetrics and gynecology. 3rd edition. St Louis: Mosby; 1992. p. 45–56.

2. Haas DM, Marsh DJ, Dang DT, et al. Prescription and other medication use in pregnancy. Obstet Gynecol 2018;131:789–96.
3. Adam MP, Polifka JE, Friedman JM. Evolving knowledge of the teratogenicity of medications in human pregnancy. Am J Med Genet C Semin Med Genet 2011; 157C:175.
4. Anderson JT, Futtrup TB. Drugs in pregnancy. Adverse Drug React Bull 2020; 321:1243.
5. Lockwood C, Magriples U. Prenatal care: patient education, health promotion, and safety of commonly used drugs. UpToDate July 29, 2022. Available at: www.uptodate.com/prenatal   -care-patient-education-health-promotion-and -safety-of-commonly -used-drug/print?. Accessed August 17, 2022.
6. Centers for Disease Control and Prevention. Recommendations to prevent and control iron deficiency in the United States. Available at: www.cdc.gov/mmwr/ preview/mmwrhtml/00051880.htm. Accessed July 30, 2022.
7. Peña-Rosas J, De-Regil L, Gomez Malave H, et al. Intermittent oral iron supplementation during pregnancy. Cochrane Database Syst Rev 2015;10:CD009997. https://doi.org/10.1002/14651858.CD009997.pub2.
8. Society for Maternal-Fetal Medicine (SMFM) Publications Committee. Prenatal acetaminophen use and outcomes in children. Am J Obstet Gynecol 2017;216: B14. Available at: pubs@smfm.org.
9. Feldkamp ML, Meyer RE, Krikov S, et al. Acetaminophen use in pregnancy and risk of birth defects: findings from the National Birth Defects Prevention Study. Obstet Gynecol 2010;115:109–16.
10. Bauer AZ, Swan SH, Kriebel D, et al. Paracetamol use during pregnancy — a call for precautionary action. Nat Rev Endocrinol 2021;17:757–66.
11. FDA drug safety communication. FDA has reviewed possible risks of pain medicine use during pregnancy. US Food and Drug Administration. Wolters Kluwer; 2015.
12. Facco FL, Chan M, Patel SR. Common sleep disorders in pregnancy. Obstet Gynecol 2022;140:321–39.
13. Okun ML, Ebert R, Saini B. A review of sleep-promoting medications used in pregnancy. Am J Obstet Gynecol 2015;212:428–35.
14. Reiter RJ, Tan DX, Korkmaz A, et al. Melatonin and stable circadian rhythms optimize maternal, placental and fetal physiology. Hum Reprod Update 2014;20: 293–8.
15. Tamura H, Nakamura Y, Terron MG, et al. Melatonin and pregnancy in the human. Reprod Toxicol 2008;25:291–7.
16. Centers for Disease Control and Prevention. Traveler's health: vaccines, medicines, advice. Available at: www.cdc.gov/travel/bugs.htm. Accessed August 19, 2022.

Antihypertensives in Pregnancy

Anna E. Denoble, MD, MSc[a],*, Sarah A. Goldstein, MD[b], Christian M. Pettker, MD[a]

KEYWORDS

- Antihypertensive • Chronic hypertension • Gestational hypertension • Preeclampsia
- Pharmacokinetics in pregnancy • American Heart Association
- American College of Cardiology
- American College of Obstetricians and Gynecologists

KEY POINTS

- Most antihypertensives can be safely used during pregnancy. Exceptions include angiotensin-converting enzyme inhibitors, angiotensin receptor blockers, and aldosterone antagonists.
- Physiologic changes may alter the pharmacokinetics of antihypertensives in pregnancy; however, pharmacokinetic data specific to pregnancy are limited.
- Antihypertensive therapy should be considered for chronic hypertension during pregnancy at a threshold blood pressure of greater than or equal to 140/90 mm Hg.
- Extended-release nifedipine and labetalol are first-line drugs for the treatment of nonsevere hypertension in pregnancy, but other antihypertensives may be safe and reasonable alternatives. Patients should be counseled about the uncertain risk of fetal growth restriction, particularly with use of beta-blocker therapy.
- Most antihypertensives are safe for lactating parents; therefore, postpartum antihypertensive selection should be based on the most effective therapy.

Hypertensive disorders of pregnancy (HDP) are estimated to occur in 77.8 per 1000 livebirths, while chronic hypertension is present in 1.5% of pregnancies.[1,2] HDP can result in significant maternal morbidity and even mortality. Treatment of chronic and acute hypertension in pregnancy improves maternal and fetal outcomes; however, the optimal antihypertensive regimen and approach in pregnancy remain elusive.[3] Available data suggest that many antihypertensives can be safely used, albeit with close supervision of parameters like fetal growth and amniotic fluid volume. This article

[a] Section of Maternal-Fetal Medicine, Department of Obstetrics, Gynecology & Reproductive Sciences, Yale University School of Medicine, New Haven, CT, USA; [b] Section of Cardiovascular Medicine, Department of Internal Medicine, Yale University School of Medicine, New Haven, CT, USA
* Corresponding author. Department of Obstetrics, Gynecology & Reproductive Sciences, 333 Cedar Street, PO Box 208063, New Haven, CT 06510.
E-mail address: anna.denoble@yale.edu

Obstet Gynecol Clin N Am 50 (2023) 39–78
https://doi.org/10.1016/j.ogc.2022.10.008
0889-8545/23/© 2022 Elsevier Inc. All rights reserved.

obgyn.theclinics.com

summarizes current guidelines on the diagnosis and treatment of hypertension in pregnancy and provides an in-depth guide to the available safety and efficacy data for antihypertensives during pregnancy and postpartum.

CASE

Jane is a 37-year-old nullipara who presents to her obstetrician/gynecologist for pre-conception counseling. She has chronic hypertension treated with lisinopril. She self-discontinued the lisinopril in anticipation of pregnancy. Her blood pressure at this visit is 145/95.

- Question 1: How is hypertension defined outside of pregnancy, and when is treatment recommended?

DIAGNOSIS AND TREATMENT OF HYPERTENSION OUTSIDE OF PREGNANCY

Diagnostic and treatment thresholds for hypertension differ during and outside of pregnancy. In 2017, the American College of Cardiology (ACC)/American Heart Association (AHA) Task Force on Clinical Practice Guidelines (referred to henceforth as the ACC/AHA guidelines) published new recommendations for the management of high blood pressure in adults.[4] The authors of the ACC/AHA guidelines concluded that there is progressively higher cardiovascular risk as blood pressure increases from normal to elevated to stage 1 hypertension and beyond. For this reason, the guidelines proposed new blood pressure categories, which differed from previous guidelines and are presented in **Table 1**. New to these guidelines was the characterization of stage 1 hypertension.[4] Although diagnostic thresholds for hypertension remain systolic blood pressure (SBP)/diastolic blood pressure (DBP) 140/90 mm Hg in pregnancy, according to the American College of Obstetricians and Gynecologists (ACOG), a growing body of evidence suggests a similar gradation of risk during pregnancy for those

Table 1
American College of Cardiology/American Heart Association categories of blood pressures in adults and recommendations for pharmacologic treatment for primary prevention of atherosclerotic cardiovascular disease

Blood Pressure Category	Definition (in mm Hg)	Pharmacologic Treatment Recommendations
Normal	SBP <120 and DBP <80	None
Elevated blood pressure	SBP 120–129 and DBP <80	None
Hypertension		
Stage 1	SBP 130–139 or DBP 80–89	Antihypertensive therapy recommended if: • Clinical cardiovascular disease present or, • 10-y , atherosclerotic cardiovascular disease risk is $\geq$ 10%
Stage 2	SBP $\geq$ 140 or DBP $\geq$ 90	Antihypertensive therapy recommended

Data from Whelton PK, Carey RM, Aronow WS, et al. 2017 ACC/AHA/AAPA/ABC/ACPM/AGS/APhA/ASH/ASPC/NMA/PCNA guideline for the prevention, detection, evaluation, and management of high blood pressure in adults: a report of the American College of Cardiology/American Heart Association Task Force on Clinical Practice Guidelines. Circulation. 2018;138(17):e484-e594.

meeting criteria for stage 1 hypertension. Therefore, patients with the diagnosis of hypertension established by these new criteria should retain a diagnosis of chronic hypertension.[5] The ACC/AHA recommendations for the treatment of hypertension to prevent future atherosclerotic cardiovascular disease outside of pregnancy are also presented in **Table 1** and should be considered when evaluating the need for postpartum antihypertensive therapy. Classes of antihypertensives identified by the ACC/AHA guidelines as first-line for the treatment of hypertension in adults are bolded and marked by an asterisk in **Table 3**.

CASE, CONTINUED

Jane meets criteria for stage 2 hypertension and warrants antihypertensive treatment. At her preconception visit, it was recommended that she discuss switching to a pregnancy-safe antihypertensive with her primary care physician (PCP) prior to conceiving. However, she presents 3 months later at 6 weeks' gestation before her scheduled follow-up with her PCP.

- Now that Jane is pregnant, how is hypertension defined, and what treatment thresholds should be used?
- What physiologic changes are anticipated during pregnancy that may impact hypertensive disorders of pregnancy and the pharmacokinetic properties of antihypertensive medications?

DIAGNOSTIC AND TREATMENT THRESHOLDS FOR HYPERTENSION IN PREGNANCY

The diagnosis of hypertension in pregnancy requires the presence of 2 blood pressure measurements $\geq$140 mm Hg systolic or $\geq$90 mm Hg diastolic on 2 occasions at least 4 hours apart.[5] Severe hypertension in pregnancy is defined as an SBP greater than or equal to 160 mm Hg or DBP greater than or equal to 110 mm Hg. Hypertension is considered chronic if diagnosis or onset occurs prior to pregnancy or before 20 weeks of gestation.[5] The hypertensive disorders of pregnancy (ie, gestational hypertension, preeclampsia, eclampsia, or hemolysis, elevated liver enzymes, and low platelets [HELLP] syndrome) should be suspected when new-onset hypertension occurs at greater than or equal to 20 weeks of gestation.[6]

Thresholds for the initiation of antihypertensive medications vary depending on the diagnosis, severity of hypertension, and comorbidities. Acute severe-range hypertension in pregnancy requires urgent treatment, generally within 30 to 60 minutes, to prevent complications, while treatment thresholds for nonsevere blood pressure ranges remain controversial.[6] Results from the recently published Chronic Hypertension and Pregnancy (CHAP) Study support the initiation of an antihypertensive agent in individuals with nonsevere chronic hypertension in pregnancy.[3] Subjects in this trial were randomized to initiation of an antihypertensive agent at a blood pressure threshold of 140/90 mm Hg or no treatment until severe hypertension (SBP $\geq$160 or DBP $\geq$105 mm Hg) developed. Initiation of antihypertensive therapy at a threshold of 140/90 mm Hg resulted in a reduced risk of the primary composite outcome (preeclampsia with severe features, medically indicated preterm birth at less than 35 weeks' gestation, placental abruption, or fetal or neonatal death). Importantly, the incidence of birthweight below the 10th percentile was similar between groups. Thus, there may be maternal and fetal/neonatal benefit from initiation of antihypertensive therapy at a blood pressure threshold of 140/90 mm Hg without an increase in accompanying fetal/neonatal risk. As a result, both ACOG and the Society for Maternal-Fetal Medicine now support initiating or titrating antihypertensive therapy in the setting of mild chronic hypertension at a threshold of 140/90 mm Hg.[7,8] The CHAP study did not specifically study a target goal for blood pressure treatment in patients on antihypertensive therapy, so it is unclear what an appropriate blood pressure target is in this population. To summarize, the recommendations provided in **Table 2** reflect current guidelines regarding initiation of antihypertensive therapy in pregnancy.

CASE, CONTINUED

Jane returns to clinic at 16 weeks' gestation. Her SBP/DBP is 138/92 mm Hg and she brings a record of her home blood pressure measurements, which are mostly greater than or equal to ≥140/90 mm Hg. After discussion, she agrees to initiate an antihypertensive agent.

- Which antihypertensive medications are safe in pregnancy? What risks should be discussed?
- Which antihypertensive medication(s) should be considered first-line for the treatment of nonsevere hypertension in pregnancy?

REVIEW OF ANTIHYPERTENSIVE SAFETY IN PREGNANCY

With respect to efficacy and safety, the optimal antihypertensive regimen for pregnancy and the postpartum period is not yet determined. Randomized-controlled trials to answer this question are unlikely to be feasible, requiring sample sizes estimated at 2,500 to 10,000 women necessary per arm.[9] Therefore, data to guide selection of antihypertensives will continue to be derived from cohort studies and meta-analyses and will continue to be influenced by individual patient factors. There is an accumulating body of evidence, reviewed here, to suggest that some antihypertensives are safe and effective in pregnancy. However, there are concerns regarding teratogenicity of certain classes (eg, angiotensin-converting enzyme [ACE] inhibitors) that preclude their use. The 3 medications most commonly used are labetalol (β-blocker, BB), nifedipine (calcium channel blocker, CCB), and methyldopa (α-agonist).[4,5] Patients with chronic hypertension often enter pregnancy on other antihypertensives, as the ACC/

Table 2
Hypertension in pregnancy: diagnosis, blood pressure criteria, and treatment thresholds and targets

Hypertension in Pregnancy Diagnosis	Reference Guideline	Blood Pressure Criteria on ≥2 Occasions ≥ 4 h Apart, mm Hg	Treatment Threshold, mm Hg	Treatment Target, mm Hg
Mild or severe chronic hypertension	5,7,8	140 ≤ SBP <160 or 90 ≤ DBP < 110	SBP 140 or DBP 90	120 ≤ SBP <160 and 80 ≤ DBP < 110
Gestational hypertension and preeclampsia without severe features	Not specified	140 ≤ SBP <160 or 90 ≤ DBP < 110	SBP 160 or DBP 110	Not specified
Acute severe hypertension[a]	6	SBP ≥ 160 or DBP ≥ 110	SBP 160 or DBP 110	SBP < 160 and DBP < 110

[a] Acute severe hypertension may include severe gestational hypertension, preeclampsia with severe features, or worsening chronic hypertension.

AHA guidelines state that thiazide diuretics, ACE inhibitors, angiotensin receptor blockers (ARBs), and CCBs should be used preferentially outside of pregnancy as they have been shown to reduce clinical adverse events.[4] It is a reasonable first step to consider whether to continue the antihypertensive medication used before pregnancy or to switch to an antihypertensive more commonly used in pregnant patients for the duration of pregnancy. Antihypertensive classes, their indications, contraindications, and pregnancy and lactation considerations are reviewed in **Table 3**. A more in-depth discussion of the antihypertensive medications commonly employed in pregnancy follows and may help guide patient counseling regarding the specific risks associated with each class.

β-blockers

There does not appear to be a significant increase in the risk of major congenital malfo90ormations with ß-blocker use in the first trimester.[10,11] As a class, however, ß-blockers have been associated with an increased risk for small-for-gestational (SGA), neonatal bradycardia, and hypoglycemia. The risk of neonatal SGA seems to be higher with second- and third-trimester ß-blocker use than first-trimester use and may vary depending on the ß-blocker selected.[10,12] A case-control study using the Quebec Pregnancy Registry found that cardioselective ß-blocker use carried the highest odds of SGA, followed by combined α- and β-receptor blockers and centrally acting adrenergic antihypertensives, although the sample size within each class was small.[10] Similar findings were noted in a recent meta-analysis comparing the efficacy and safety of oral antihypertensives in pregnancy. Concerns were raised regarding the neonatal safety of ß-blockers, with atenolol and labetalol noted to significantly increase the risk of SGA and cesarean delivery. It should be noted that not all BBs are created equal when it comes to SGA risk. A retrospective cohort study of 379,238 women with singleton pregnancies, of whom 4,847 were exposed to ß-blockers, demonstrated the lowest birthweights and percent low birthweight for labetalol (2926 ± 841g; 24%) and atenolol (3058 ± 748g; 18%), compared with metoprolol (3163 ± 725g; 13%), propranolol (3286 ± 651g; 7%) and nonexposed controls (3353 ± 702g; 5%), with a significantly increased odds of infants born SGA if exposed to atenolol and labetalol.[13] Reassuringly, labetalol use in the treatment of acute severe hypertension has not been shown to alter fetal Doppler studies.[14] In addition to the potential risk for SGA, ß-blockers may impart a risk of neonatal bradycardia (occurring in 1.6% of ß-blocker-exposed neonates vs 0.5% unexposed neonates) and hypoglycemia (4.3% of B ß-blocker-exposed neonates vs 1.2% unexposed neonates). Compared with other ß-blockers, labetalol appears to carry the highest risk of neonatal bradycardia (propensity-score matched odds ratio [OR 1.34, 95% confidence interval [CI] 1.08 to 1.67).

Despite these studies associating ß-blocker use with SGA, there are well-designed studies and meta-analyses that refute this finding. The most up-to-date Cochrane review examining the maternal and fetal effects of antihypertensive treatments for mild-to-moderate hypertension suggested that the various antihypertensives studied, including ß-blockers, have no significant effect on the risk of fetal death, fetal growth restriction, or premature birth, a finding also corroborated by the recent CHAP trial.[3,15] The retrospective nature of most of the studies of ß-blocker use in pregnancy – with a lack of data on the underlying pathology and disease severity – introduces the possibility of confounding by indication. A crucial question arises: is it the antihypertensive medication or the severity of the disease being treated that most appreciably contributes to restricted fetal growth in pregnancy? A retrospective cohort study using linked health care records for children born in Scotland from 2010 to 2014 demonstrated an

Table 3
Antihypertensive medications: mechanism of action, indications, contraindications, adverse effects, and use in pregnancy and lactation

Antihypertensive Class	Mechanism of Action	General Indications	Contraindications	Adverse Effects	Important Notes	Pregnancy	Lactation
β-blockers							
β-blockers – noncardioselective • Nadolol • Propranolol	Bind to β-1 (located primarily in the heart and kidneys) and β-2 (located in diverse locations, including smooth muscles) receptors and induce antagonizing effects β-2 blockade results in smooth muscle relaxation	Hypertension (second-line agent outside of pregnancy) Arrhythmias Congenital long QT syndrome Essential tremor Thyrotoxicosis Migraine prophylaxis Restless leg syndrome Performance anxiety β-blockers are not recommended as first-line agents for hypertension unless the patient has ischemic heart disease or heart failure	Asthma Chronic bradycardia Hypotension Raynaud's (risk of exacerbation)	Bradycardia Hypotension Fatigue Nausea Dizziness Constipation Sexual dysfunction Bronchospasm (particularly in patients with asthma) Hyperglycemia Insomnia Sleep changes Nightmares Worsens edema Risk of heart block	Avoid abrupt cessation Noncardioselective β-blockers should be avoided in patients with reactive airway disease May mask symptoms of hypoglycemia in patients with diabetes	Teratogenic: no Placenta permeable: unknown May cause hypoglycemia, bradycardia, and hypotension in neonate Other fetal effects: may be associated with increased risk of SGA newborn	Compatible: yes Transfer to breastmilk: minimal
β-blockers – cardio-selective • Atenolol • Betaxolol • Bisoprolol • Metoprolol tartrate • Metoprolol succinate • Nebivolol	Bind to β-1 receptors only with antagonizing effects β-1 blockade results in negative chronotropic, inotropic and dromotropic effects on the heart, slowing the heart rate	Hypertension (second-line agents outside of pregnancy) Heart failure (bisoprolol and metoprolol preferred) Arrhythmias Aortic dilatation Ischemic heart disease	Complete heart block Use with caution if second-degree heart block Use with caution if moderate-to-severe asthma or chronic obstructive pulmonary disease (COPD)	Bradycardia Decreased exercise capacity AV nodal block Heart failure Hypotension Fatigue Nausea Dizziness Dry mouth and eyes Constipation Sexual dysfunction	Avoid abrupt cessation These are the preferred β-blocker agents in patients with mild-to-moderate reactive airway disease May mask symptoms of hypoglycemia in patients with diabetes	Teratogenic: no, with exceptions Placenta permeable: yes (atenolol achieves doses in fetal circulation equivalent to maternal) Other fetal effects: may be associated with increased risk of SGA newborn, with atenolol imparting the highest risk of SGA Neonatal effects: may cause	Compatible: yes Transfer to breastmilk: minimal Atenolol and metoprolol concentrate in breastmilk and may result in higher neonatal concentrations; therefore, more protein-bound

Drug	Mechanism	Indications	Contraindications	Adverse effects	Clinical considerations	Pregnancy	Breastfeeding
• Esmolol (intravenous only)	and myocardial oxygen demand, and decreases renin release, resulting in lower blood pressure Nebivolol also induces nitric oxide-induced vasodilation	Migraine prophylaxis Tremor reduction Symptomatic treatment of anxiety disorders		Masking of hypoglycemia symptoms Insomnia Sleep changes Nightmares Worsens edema		hypoglycemia, bradycardia, and hypotension in neonates	β-blockers (eg. labetalol or carvedilol) may be preferred
β-blockers – combined α– and β-receptor • Carvedilol • Labetalol	Bind to α₁ adrenoreceptors, as well as β₁ and β₂ adrenoreceptors equally, resulting in α₁ and nonselective β blockade No intrinsic sympathomimetic activity β blockade is greater than α₁ blockade Results in reduction in systemic arterial pressure and total peripheral resistance, without significant effects on resting heart rate or cardiac output Heart rate and cardiac output response to exercise may be blunted Glomerular filtration rate and renal blood flow are preserved Carvedilol is more potent than	Carvedilol: Hypertension Heart failure (carvedilol preferred for heart failure with reduced ejection fraction) Dilated cardiomyopathy Impaired left ventricular function caused by myocardial infarction Gastroesophageal varices Labetalol: Hypertension (second-line agent outside of pregnancy)	Cardiogenic shock Decompensated heart failure Complete heart block Use with caution if second-degree heart block Severe bradycardia Use with caution if moderate-to-severe asthma or COPD Hypersensitivity	Bradycardia Decreased exercise capacity Hypotension Peripheral edema Headaches Abnormal weight gain Hyperglycemia Diarrhea and nausea Dizziness Fatigue AV nodal block Rare: Erythema multiforme, Stevens-Johnson syndrome, toxic epidermal necrolysis Aplastic anemia Acute severe exacerbation of asthma Hepatotoxicity	Avoid abrupt cessation Avoid in patients with reactive airway disease May mask symptoms of hypoglycemia in patients with diabetes	Teratogenic: no Placenta permeable: yes Other fetal effects: may be associated with increased risk of SGA newborn	Compatible: yes Transfer to breastmilk: minimal

(continued on next page)

Table 3
(continued)

Antihypertensive Class	Mechanism of Action	General Indications	Contraindications	Adverse Effects	Important Notes	Pregnancy	Lactation
	labetalol with regard to β and α_1 blockade and may prevent formation of oxidized low-density lipoproteins Of the β-blockers, carvedilol and labetalol are expected to have the greatest antihypertensive effect						
β-blockers – intrinsic sympathomimetic activity • Acebutolol • Penbutolol • Pindolol	Cardioselective β blockade with weak sympathomimetic properties, theoretically resulting in reduced systemic blood pressure and total peripheral resistance without significant changes in heart rate, cardiac output, and renal blood flow Can have antianginal, antiarrhythmic, and antihypertensive effects	Angina Hypertension (second-line agents outside of pregnancy) Hyperthyroidism	Asthma or COPD Cardiogenic shock or heart failure Hypersensitivity Complete heart block Use with caution if second-degree heart block Severe bradycardia	Dizziness Headache Fatigue Edema Insomnia Anxiety Arthralgias/myalgias Bradyarrhythmia Heart failure Rare: Hepatotoxicity Anaphylaxis Drug-induced lupus	Avoid abrupt cessation Avoid in patients with reactive airway disease May mask symptoms of hypoglycemia in patients with diabetes	Teratogenic: no Placenta permeable: yes Other fetal effects: may be associated with increased risk of SGA newborn	Compatible: • Acebutolol: avoid if possible because of relatively extensive excretion into breastmilk • Penbutolol: minimal excretion in breastmilk, but minimal data available • Pindolol: likely safe because of minimal excretion and short half-life

Central α_2-agonists

Drug	Mechanism	Indications	Contraindications	Adverse effects	Comments	Teratogenicity/Placenta	Breastmilk
• Methyldopa	Exerts effects through false neurotransmitter alpha-methyl-norepinephrine, which acts on central inhibitor α-adrenergic receptors, resulting in decreased central sympathetic outflow and lower plasma renin activity Results in reductions in heart rate, blood pressure, and total peripheral resistance without significant change in cardiac index	Hypertension (generally considered last-line agents because of significant central nervous system adverse effects)	Active hepatic disease Hemolytic anemia (direct Coombs positive) Significant drug history of monoamine oxidator inhibitor therapy Pheochromocytoma Known hypersensitivity to methyldopa in any form	Nausea Diarrhea Headache Dizziness Sedation Dry mouth Rash Rebound hypertension Weight gain Rare: Hemolytic anemia (usually appears within a few weeks of initiation) Lupus-like syndrome Myocarditis Pancreatitis Hepatotoxicity (weeks to years after initiation) Immune thrombocytopenia Reversible leukopenia	Methyldopa historically considered first-line for maternal hypertension because of fetal safety, but not always effective Monitor complete blood count and liver function while on therapy because of the risk of hemolytic anemia and abnormal liver function tests	Teratogenic: no Placenta permeable: yes Similar to β-blockers, methyldopa has been associated with ↑ ncreased SGA risk	Compatible: yes Transfer to breastmilk: minimal
• Clonidine	Stimulates α₂-adrenergic receptors in the central nervous system, resulting in reduced sympathomimetic outflow and decreased total peripheral resistance, renal vascular resistance, heart rate, and blood pressure	Hypertension Sedation in ICU setting Vasomotor symptoms of menopause Nicotine dependence Opioid withdrawal Attention-deficit hyperactivity disorder	Bradyarrhythmia, including sick sinus syndrome Galactosemia Hypersensitivity to clonidine Use with caution if chronic renal impairment, cerebrovascular disease, or severe coronary insufficiency	Withdrawal syndrome with rebound Dry mouth Sedation Bradycardia Hypotension Hypertension Abdominal pain Dizziness Headache Constipation Nausea Urinary incontinence Tremor	Avoid abrupt discontinuation of clonidine, which may induce rebound hypertension and hypertensive crisis	Teratogenic: no Placenta permeable: yes Sleep disturbances and hypotension in neonates exposed to clonidine in utero Clonidine may result in transient neonatal hypertension up to 3 d after birth	Compatible: yes Transfer to breastmilk: minimal
CCBs							
Nondihydropyridine CCBs[a] • Diltiazem	L-type (slow) calcium channel inhibitors	Cardiac arrhythmias (atrial fibrillation and sustained	Avoid in heart failure with reduced ejection fraction	Constipation (dose-dependent) Worsening cardiac	Significant drug interactions exist with diltiazem and	Teratogenic: • Verapamil: no	Compatible: yes Transfer to breastmilk: minimal

(continued on next page)

Table 3
(continued)

Antihypertensive Class	Mechanism of Action	General Indications	Contraindications	Adverse Effects	Important Notes	Pregnancy	Lactation
• Verapamil	Block calcium ion influx during depolarization of cardiac and vascular smooth muscle Decrease total peripheral vascular resistance, resulting in smooth muscle relaxation, thereby decreasing SBP and DBP Reduce cardiac workload through moderate bradycardic effect and decreased peripheral resistance Also cause moderate slowing in heart rate and slows AV conduction Diltiazem is a potent coronary vasodilator, but mild arterial vasodilator, and does not have negative inotropic effect Verapamil dilates coronary and peripheral arteries, slows conduction through the AV	ventricular tachycardia) Hypertension (dihydropyridines preferable) Chronic stable angina Proteinuria reduction in diabetes Heart failure with preserved ejection fraction	(because of negative inotropy and risk of worsening heart failure) Second- or third-degree atrioventricular block Sick sinus syndrome (can cause bradycardia and worsening cardiac output) Known hypersensitivity Caution with severe hepatic impairment	output Bradycardia Gingival hyperplasia Peripheral edema (although less than with dihydropyridines)	verapamil (CYP3A4 major substrate and moderate inhibitor) Avoid concomitant use of β-blocker therapy because of increased risk of bradycardia and heart block	• Diltiazem: association with skeletal abnormalities in animal studies not replicated in human studies at usual doses • Potential for fetal AV block and bradycardia cannot be excluded • Placenta permeable: yes	

	Mechanism	Indications	Contraindications/Cautions	Adverse Effects	Notes	Pregnancy/Lactation
Dihydropyridine CCBs[a] • Amlodipine • Felodipine • Isradipine • Nicardipine • Nifedipine • Nisoldipine	Block calcium ion influx during depolarization in cardiac and vascular smooth muscles, with greater vascular smooth muscle cell than cardiac activity. Act directly on smooth muscle to decrease intracellular calcium, resulting in reduced total peripheral resistance and blood pressure. Reduces coronary vasospasm. May result in increased heart rate and cardiac contractility, node, and has negative inotropic and chronotropic effects	Hypertension (preferred over non-dihydropyridines) Chronic stable angina Heart failure with preserved ejection fraction	Avoid in heart failure with reduced ejection fraction Severe aortic stenosis Known hypersensitivity Caution with severe hepatic impairment Severe hypotension Acute myocardial infarction Pulmonary congestion	Lightheadedness Flushing Headaches Gingival hyperplasia Dose-related pedal edema in 20%–30% Short-acting formulation: reflex tachycardia and increase in sympathetic tone (use with caution in heart failure and coronary artery disease)	Because of increased CYP3A4 activity, there is increased oral clearance and decreased peak plasma levels and half-life of CCBs in pregnancy; this may require increased doses in pregnancy Sublingual nifedipine should be avoided because of the risk of significant hypotension	Teratogenic: no Placenta permeable: yes Compatible: yes Transfer to breastmilk: minimal (No information available for felodipine or nisoldipine)
Diuretics						
Thiazide diuretics[a] • Chlorthalidone • Hydrochlorothiazide • Indapamide • Metolazone	Affect electrolyte reabsorption in the distal renal tubule, resulting in increased excretion of sodium and chloride and accompanying water Exact mechanism by which changes in electrolyte r	Hypertension (considered 1 st-line outside of pregnancy) Edema	Allergy to sulfonamides Anuria Use with caution if history of gout Hypersensitivity to medication	Hypokalemia Hyponatremia Metabolic alkalosis Hypercalcemia Hyperglycemia Hyperuricemia Hyperlipidemia	Chlorthalidone is preferred (long half-life and proven reduction in cardiovascular disease) Require monitoring for hyponatremia and hypocalcemia, as well as uric acid and calcium levels	Teratogenic: no Placenta permeable: yes May cause maternal volume depletion→use with caution in pregnancy, especially pregnancies affected by reduced uteroplacental perfusion (eg, preeclampsia and fetal growth Compatible: yes, higher doses may suppress lactation Transfer to breastmilk: low

(continued on next page)

**Table 3
(continued)**

Antihypertensive Class	Mechanism of Action	General Indications	Contraindications	Adverse Effects	Important Notes	Pregnancy	Lactation
	eabsorption result in antihypertensive effects is not known, but may result in alterations in peripheral vascular resistance Response to thiazide diuretics occurs in 2 phases: in the first, the hypotensive effect results directly from diuresis, and, in the second, plasma sodium and volume return to normal, but hypotensive effects persist, perhaps because of arteriolar vasodilation					restriction) Use with close fetal monitoring , as may result in fetal/neonatal electrolyte imbalance and oligohydramnios	
Loop diuretics • Bumetanide • Furosemide • Torsemide	Inhibit reabsorption of sodium and chloride in the proximal and distal tubules and loop of Henle, resulting in increased sodium and potassium secretion and decreased	Symptomatic heart failure Preferred over thiazides if moderate-to-severe chronic kidney disease	Anuria History of hypersensitivity to loop diuretics or sulfonamides (except for ethacrynic acid) Hepatic coma (consider potassium-sparing diuretics in patients with hepatotoxicity or cirrhosis) Severe electrolyte	Electrolyte imbalances – hyponatremia, hypokalemia, hypochloremia, hypomagnesemia, metabolic alkalosis, prerenal azotemia Dehydration Hypertriglyceridemia and hypercholesterolemia Hyperuricemia and gout Hyperglycemia in	Use with caution with nephrotoxic medications Monitor for electrolyte disturbances and correct pre-existing electrolyte imbalances before treatment	Teratogenic: no Placenta permeable: yes for furosemide (bumetanide and torsemide unknown) Use only if necessary and with close monitoring, as may result in fetal/neonatal electrolyte imbalance and oligohydramnios Neonatal effects:	Compatible: yes, at lower doses (furosemide doses of 20 mg daily do not suppress lactation, but higher doses might decrease lactation) Transfer to breastmilk: unknown Furosemide displaces bilirubin, can cause

	Mechanism	Contraindications / Precautions	Adverse Effects	Pregnancy	Lactation
	reabsorption, thus producing diuresis	depletion Use with caution in combination with digoxin	diabetes Restlessness Headache Dizziness, postural hypotension, syncope Vertigo Skin photosensitivity Interstitial nephritis Tinnitus and ototoxicity Myalgias and muscle soreness Rare: Erythema multiforme Stevens-Johnson syndrome Toxic epidermal necrolysis Cytopenias	kernicterus has been reported	unconjugated hyperbilirubinemia when used in neonates (uncertain transfer in breastmilk)
Potassium-sparing • Amiloride • Triamterene	Antikaliuretic activity with weak natriuretic, diuretic, and antihypertensive properties Block reabsorption of sodium at the distal convoluted tubule, cortical collecting tubule and collecting duct, leading to net negative potential of the tubular lumen and decreased secretion/excretion of hydrogen and potassium Does not inhibit aldosterone	Minimally effective antihypertensive agents, but can be considered in conjunction with thiazides in patients with hypokalemia Acute or chronic renal insufficiency Anuria Concomitant use of potassium-sparing agents (spironolactone, ACE inhibitors, and others) or potassium supplementation Diabetic nephropathy Hyperkalemia Hypersensitivity Use with caution if renal disease Use with caution if hyperuricemia or gout	Hyperkalemia Diarrhea Loss of appetite Nausea and vomiting Muscle cramps Dizziness Headache Cough Dyspnea Cardiac dysrhythmias Palpitations Hyperuricemia (triamterene) Rare: Aplastic anemia Neutropenia Thrombocytopenia (triamterene) Encephalopathy Increased intraocular pressure	Avoid in patients with significantly reduced renal function Teratogenic: likely not based on animal studies, but human data limited Placenta permeable: yes	Compatible: data limited; other agents preferred Transfer to breastmilk: yes
Aldosterone antagonists	Bind to the mineralocorticoid	Hypertension (as adjunct) Potassium-sparing diuretics	Hyperkalemia Electrolyte disturbances	Preferred agents in primary aldosteronism Teratogenic:	Compatible: yes, may reduce breastmilk

(continued on next page)

Table 3
(continued)

Antihypertensive Class	Mechanism of Action	General Indications	Contraindications	Adverse Effects	Important Notes	Pregnancy	Lactation
• Eplerenone • Spironolactone	receptor and competitively inhibit binding of aldosterone, resulting in blood pressure reduction. May have antifibrotic effects in the myocardium and vasculature. Spironolactone has greater affinity for aldosterone receptor, but also great affinity for other steroid receptors, which may increase its side effects (gynecomastia and menstrual irregularities). Both agents have similar aldosterone-mediated effects	Mild systolic heart failure Edema Hyperaldosteronism	Potassium-supplements Addison disease Significant renal dysfunction Hyperkalemia Avoid use with strong CYP3A inhibitors Type 2 diabetes with hypertension and microalbuminuria Serum creatinine >1.8 mg/dL	Metabolic acidosis Gynecomastia and menstrual irregularities (spironolactone only) Increased gamma-glutamyl transferase activity Dizziness Headache Worsening renal function Angina Myocardial infarction Hepatotoxicity Rare: Agranulocytosis Stevens-Johnson syndrome Toxic epidermal necrolysis Breast cancer Drug-induced systemic lupus erythematosus	and resistant hypertension	• Eplerenone likely safe, but data limited • Spironolactone is associated with antiandrogenic effects and oral clefts and is contraindicated in pregnancy Placenta permeable: yes	production Transfer to breastmilk: likely minimal, but limited data Data on spironolactone suggest it is compatible with breastfeeding Eplerenone data are more limited
Other vasodilators							
Nitrates • Isosorbide dinitrate • Nitroprusside • Nitroglycerin	Induce vascular smooth muscle relaxation resulting in dilation of peripheral veins and arteries (affects veins more than	Angina Myocardial infarction Congestive heart failure Hypertensive emergency Pulmonary edema	Allergy to nitrates Concomitant use of phosphodiesterase inhibitors Right ventricular infarction or poor right ventricular contractility (preload sensitive)	Headaches Hypotension Cutaneous flushing Syncope Reflex tachycardia Methemoglobinemia Tachyphylaxis/nitrate tolerance Monday disease	Typically reserved for acute treatment of hypertensive emergency May be used for afterload reduction in peripartum cardiomyopathy	Teratogenic: likely not, but data minimal Placenta permeable: unknown Nitroprusside carries risk of fetal cyanide poisoning and should	Compatible: • Nitroprusside: avoid because of risk of cyanide and thiocyanate in breastmilk

arteries) Venous dilatation reduces left ventricular end-diastolic pressure and pulmonary capillary wedge pressure. Arterial dilation reduces systemic vascular resistance, systolic arterial pressure, and mean arterial pressure (afterload)	Hypertrophic cardiomyopathy (decreased preload worsens outflow tract obstruction)	(tachycardia, headache, and dizziness during re-exposure)	not be used for a prolonged period	• Isosorbide dinitrate: unknown; Nitroglycerin: unknown • Transfer to breastmilk: unknown
Hydralazine	Unknown mechanism of action, although appears to interfere with calcium movement responsible for smooth muscle contraction, resulting in peripheral vasodilation through direct relaxation of vascular smooth muscle. This leads to a decrease in blood pressure. Must be metabolized after attachment to the vessel wall, resulting in slower onset of action Hypertensive emergency Hypertension Congestive heart failure	Coronary artery disease (because of stimulation of sympathetic nervous system, increased CO, and increased myocardial oxygen demand) Sodium and water retention Reflex tachycardia Headaches Nausea Flushing Hypotension Palpitations Dizziness Angina Rare: Drug-induced lupus erythematosus Drug-induced liver injury Toxic epidermal necrolysis Serum sickness Hemolytic anemia Vasculitis Glomerulonephritis	Consider using with a β-blocker and diuretic to avoid reflex tachycardia and sodium and water retention	Teratogenic: likely not, although hypospadias has been reported with first trimester use Placenta permeable: yes Neonatal effects: neonatal thrombocytopenia has been reported
				Compatible: yes Transfer to breastmilk: minimal
ACE inhibitors and angiotensin-receptor and renin blockers				
ACE inhibitors[a] • Benazepril	Prevent the conversion of Hypertension (first-line therapy)	History of angioedema or hereditary Dry, nonproductive paroxysmal cough	Increased risk of hyperkalemia in	Teratogenic: yes Placenta
				Compatible: yes Transfer to breastmilk:

(continued on next page)

Table 3
(continued)

Antihypertensive Class	Mechanism of Action	General Indications	Contraindications	Adverse Effects	Important Notes	Pregnancy	Lactation
• Captopril • Enalapril • Fosinopril • Lisinopril • Moexipril • Perindopril • Quinapril • Ramipril • Trandolapril	angiotensin I to angiotensin II, a potent vasoconstrictor Decreased angiotensin II leads to decreased vasopressor activity and decreased aldosterone Suppression of the renin-angiotensin-aldosterone system results in beneficial cardiac and renal effects Cardiac preload and afterload are reduced Renal blood perfusion is increased and renal vascular resistance is decreased as long as renal perfusion is normal (ie, absence of conditions like renal artery stenosis or aggressive diuresis)	Myocardial infarction Heart failure, including with reduced ejection fraction Hypertension in chronic kidney disease and diabetes Diabetic nephropathy Migraine prophylaxis	angioedema History of angioedema related to ACE-I treatment Concomitant treatment with direct renin-inhibitor (aliskiren) or neprilysin inhibitors (eg, sacubitril) Pregnancy Bilateral renal artery stenosis (risk of acute renal failure)	(1%–10%) Angioedema Life-threatening anaphylaxis Decline in renal function, especially if heart failure or renal insufficiency Hypotension Syncope Hyperkalemia Cholestatic jaundice or hepatitis (rare, but serious) Photosensitivity Rare: Pemphigus Psoriasis Stevens-Johnson syndrome Toxic epidural necrolysis Gynecomastia Pancreatitis Hemolytic anemia Thrombocytopenia Leukopenia Neutropenia/ pancytopenia	patients with renal dysfunction and in those on K^+ supplements or K^+-sparing diuretics	permeable: yes Possible increased risk of cardiovascular and central nervous system anomalies with first trimester use Second and third trimester use associated with oligohydramnios, neonatal and fetal renal failure, pulmonary hypoplasia, skull hypoplasia, fetal growth restriction, hypotension, and joint contractures	minimal Of the ACE inhibitors, enalapril and captopril may be considered first-line f or postpartum hypertension because of minimal excretion in breast milk

Angiotensin II receptor blockers[a]	Angiotensin receptor antagonists selectively block the binding of angiotensin II to the AT1 receptor subtype, resulting in blocking of the vasoconstrictor and aldosterone-secreting effects of angiotensin II	Hypertension (first-line therapy) Heart failure Myocardial infarction Hypertension in chronic kidney disease and diabetes Diabetic nephropathy Left ventricular hypertrophy	Heart failure with hypotension Bilateral renal artery stenosis (risk of acute renal failure) Pregnancy Do not use in combination with ACE-I or direct renin inhibitor History of angioedema with ARBs (can try 6 weeks after ACE-I discontinued for angioedema with ACE-I)	Angioedema Cough (rare; less than ACE-I) Hypotension Renal failure Hyperkalemia (in those with renal disease or on other agents that increase potassium) Abdominal pain Nausea Diarrhea Back ache Headache Rare: Urticaria Anaphylaxis Vasculitis Cytopenias Liver function test abnormalities Rash Anemia Neutropenia Thrombocytopenia	Increased risk of hyperkalemia in patients with renal dysfunction and in those on K+ supplements or K+-sparing diuretics	Teratogenic: yes Placenta permeable: unknown	Compatible: unknown, likely compatible, no published human evidence Transfer to breastmilk: unknown Theoretic risk of neonatal hypotension
• Azilsartan • Candesartan • Eprosartan • Irbesartan • **Losartan** • Olmesartan • Telmisartan • Valsartan							
Direct renin inhibitor	Directly inhibits renin, decreasing plasma renin activity and inhibiting conversion of angiotensinogen to angiotensin I	Hypertension Chronic kidney disease Diabetic nephropathy	Do not use in combination with ACE inhibitors or ARBs Bilateral renal artery stenosis (risk of acute renal failure) Pregnancy	Hypotension Hyperkalemia Diarrhea Dizziness Headache Increased serum creatinine and serum urea nitrogen Increased creatine kinase Seizure Renal impairment Rare: Angioedema	Very long acting Increased risk of hyperkalemia in patients with renal dysfunction and in those on K+ supplements or K+-sparing diuretics	Teratogenic: possible, no teratogenicity in animal studies Placenta permeable: unknown	Compatible: unknown Transfer to breastmilk: yes
• Aliskiren							

[a] First-line for treatment of essential hypertension outside of pregnancy.

increased, but similar risk for preterm birth, SGA, and low birthweight in pregnancies complicated by untreated hypertension, late-onset hypertension, and in utero antihypertensive exposure.[16] Hypertension may be the key risk factor for low birthweight, rather than the antihypertensive medication selected.[16–18] That said, enough evidence exists regarding a gradation in risk with different ß-blockers that consideration should be given to monitoring of fetal growth and mitigation of this risk by using the lowest effective doses necessary.

Calcium Channel Blockers

CCBs are considered first-line for the treatment of hypertension outside of pregnancy and appear to be safe and efficacious for the management of chronic and acute severe hypertension in pregnancy.[4,15] Of the CCBs, nifedipine is probably the most commonly used in pregnancy. CCBs do not appear to represent a major teratogenic risk in human studies.[19,20] Early animal studies found an increase in skeletal malformations with in utero exposure to diltiazem, although this finding was not replicated in later human studies.[21,22] Similarly, while early studies found an increased risk of neonatal seizures with in utero CCB exposure,[19] a more recent, large, population-based cohort study did not corroborate these findings, with 0.23% of infants born to mothers exposed to CCB experiencing neonatal seizures compared with 0.18% of infants unexposed (OR 0.95, 95% CI 0.70–1.30).[23]

There are no signals to suggest that CCBs are associated with an increased risk of SGA or preterm birth compared with placebo and other antihypertensives.[9,12,15] Although the potential to dangerously lower uteroplacental blood flow to the detriment of the fetus is a concern in the treatment of hypertension in pregnancy, oral nifedipine, like labetalol, produces minimal doppler changes in fetal and uteroplacental vessels, suggesting that this concern may be insignificant with the use of nifedipine.[24] Nifedipine has been associated with a decreased risk of placental abruption in pregnancies complicated by hypertension.[12]

Central α_2-Agonists

Most studies examining the α-blockers have focused on methyldopa; less data exists regarding clonidine use during pregnancy. Of all the antihypertensives, methyldopa has the most data (albeit limited by methodological concerns) regarding long-term postnatal effects, with safety data available up to 7.5 years following in utero exposure demonstrating minimal long-term effects.[25] There are no signals in the literature to suggest that methyldopa increases the risk of congenital malformations.[26] Results are mixed regarding the efficacy of methyldopa compared with other antihypertensives in the prevention of severe hypertension. The 2018 Cochrane Systematic Review found methyldopa to be less effective than ß-blockers and CCBs in the prevention of severe hypertension, while still carrying a risk of SGA.[15] Methyldopa has been associated with a decreased risk of placental abruption in pregnancies complicated by hypertension.[12] A recent population-based study found those treated with methyldopa had a higher risk of preeclampsia (adjusted odds ratio [aOR] 1.43, 95% CI 1.19 to 1.73), but lower odds of fetal growth restriction (aOR 0.66, 95% CI 0.48–0.90) than those prescribed ß-blockers.[27] Additionally, 1 limited study found an increased risk of postpartum depression among those taking methyldopa for hypertension in the postpartum period.[28] Given that methyldopa is considered last-line for the treatment of hypertension outside of pregnancy and given some studies suggesting lower efficacy compared with ß-blockers and CCBs in pregnancy, it is reasonable to consider methyldopa as a safe, but second-line antihypertensive choice. In the end, however, manufacturer availability of methyldopa may be the most important limiting factor for its use in the United States.

Direct Vasodilators

Hydralazine is the direct vasodilator most commonly used in pregnancy. Hydralazine is not considered first-line for the treatment of hypertension outside of pregnancy.[4] Most studies of hydralazine in pregnancy have focused on the intravenous treatment of acute severe hypertension, with few studies examining its chronic use in pregnancy. Data on oral hydralazine use in the first trimester are lacking, although there are no overt signals suggesting teratogenicity in available animal and human reports. Hydralazine does readily cross the placenta, with fetal concentrations equal to or greater than maternal.[29] Although not considered first-line for the treatment of chronic hypertension in pregnancy, hydralazine remains an important alternative to ACE inhibitors for afterload reduction in the treatment of heart failure.

Concerns regarding hydralazine in the treatment of acute severe hypertension center mainly around the unpredictability of the maternal blood pressure response to intravenous hydralazine with the potential for excessive hypotension. Significant maternal hypotension and tachycardia are possible with hydralazine administration, which may result in reduced uteroplacental perfusion.[30] However, this risk may be mitigated by ensuring correction of hypovolemia prior to hydralazine administration and fluid administration if hypotension is noted after administration. Intravenous hydralazine may be considered as an alternative regimen in the treatment of acute severe hypertension.[31]

Thiazide and Thiazide-Like Diuretics

Thiazide diuretics are among the first-line therapies for essential hypertension outside of pregnancy, as they have been demonstrated to reduce clinical adverse cardiovascular events.[4] Hydrochlorothiazide is considered by ACOG to be a second-line agent for the treatment of chronic hypertension in pregnancy.[5] In utero exposure to hydrochlorothiazide has not been associated with congenital malformations in animal or human studies.[32,33] Theoretic concerns exist about the prolonged use of diuretics in pregnancy because of potential restriction of normal volume expansion. Although reduced plasma volume expansion has been demonstrated in pregnant individuals using thiazide diuretics in a small study, this occurred without adverse fetal or neonatal effects.[34] A meta-analysis of 9 randomized trials and a systematic review of diuretics for the prevention of preeclampsia did not support an increased risk for fetal growth restriction or oligohydramnios with diuretic use.[32,35] Placental transfer of hydrochlorothiazide (HCTZ) does occur, with HCTZ demonstrated in amniotic fluid and umbilical cord blood.[36] For this reason, fetal and neonatal electrolyte imbalances and oligohydramnios are possible, and close fetal and neonatal monitoring is warranted.

Loop Diuretics

Loop diuretics are not indicated for single-agent therapy for hypertension but may be added as adjunctive therapy for women with heart failure in pregnancy. There are no large, randomized trials of loop diuretic use in pregnancy. However, a historical meta-analysis of 7000 neonates with in utero exposure to diuretics failed to show significant harm.[32] It is reasonable to avoid loop diuretics in settings in which intravascular volume depletion or reduced uteroplacental perfusion is suspected, such as cases of severe fetal growth restriction and preeclampsia with severe features, as the administration of diuretics may worsen volume depletion. Furosemide does cross the placenta. Animal studies have demonstrated an increased risk of skeletal abnormalities; however, this was reversed with adequate potassium supplementation.[37] Unlike the association in adults between high doses of furosemide and ototoxicity, the proportion of infants with prolonged in utero exposure to furosemide with an abnormal hearing screen is similar to controls.[38]

Renin-Angiotensin-Aldosterone System Blockers

The use of ACE inhibitors and angiotensin receptor blockers (ARBs) in pregnancy is contraindicated, although they represent a mainstay of hypertension treatment outside of pregnancy. Numerous studies have demonstrated increased risks of congenital malformations and adverse fetal effects with first-, second-, and third-trimester use of ACE inhibitors and ARBs. Historically, first-trimester ACE inhibitor use has been associated with an increased risk of cardiovascular and central nervous system anomalies compared with other antihypertensives.[39] Other studies suggested that this association may be confounded by indication (ie, hypertension or diabetes). Review of data from the ROPAC registry on cardiac medication use for cardiac disease in pregnancy found that 8% of those using an ACE inhibitor, even for a short time, had fetuses with congenital malformations.[40] More recently, Bateman and colleagues used Medicaid claims data to examine the association between first-trimester ACE inhibitor exposure and the risk for overall major, cardiac, and central nervous system malformations. The authors of this analysis, which was limited to the use of ACE inhibitors for chronic hypertension and was adjusted for other confounders, concluded that exposure to ACE inhibitors in the first trimester was not associated with an increased risk of major congenital malformations.[41] Controversy remains as to the absolute risk of congenital malformations with first-trimester exposure to ACE inhibitors and ARBs. Patients of reproductive age, particularly those not using a reliable contraceptive method, should be counseled about the potential risks and need to convert to an alternative agent if pregnancy is being considered. Although ACE inhibitors and ARBs should be avoided in pregnancy, patients with unwitting first-trimester exposure to ACE inhibitors or ARBs can be reasonably reassured that the overall risk of congenital malformations is low.

There may be a higher risk of fetopathy with ACE inhibitor and ARB use in the second and third trimesters. A systematic review of case reports and case series found that 48% of newborns exposed to ACE inhibitors and 87% of newborns exposed to ARBs exhibited fetal renin-angiotensin system blockade syndrome.[42] Given the limitations of the data included in this systematic review and risk for reporting bias, these results should be interpreted with caution. However, this review was able to summarize the features of the fetal renin-angiotensin system blockade syndrome from second- and third-trimester use: oligohydramnios, neonatal and fetal renal failure, pulmonary hypoplasia, skull hypoplasia, fetal growth restriction, hypotension, and joint contractures. Although controversy exists as to the magnitude of the increase in risk of fetopathy, these drugs should also be avoided in the second and third trimesters.

ANTIHYPERTENSIVE SELECTION FOR NONSEVERE HYPERTENSION IN PREGNANCY

Fig. 1 outlines a suggested clinical pathway for the evaluation and management of patients with nonsevere hypertension in pregnancy. New hypertension at greater than or equal to 20 weeks' gestation necessitates an immediate evaluation for hypertensive disorders of pregnancy (preeclampsia). At less than 20 weeks' gestation, or once hypertensive disorders of pregnancy have been evaluated, treatment should be initiated for nonsevere hypertension if the systolic blood pressure is greater than or equal to 140 mm Hg or the diastolic blood pressure is greater than or equal to 90 mm Hg on 2 or more occasions at least 4 hours apart.[3] In accordance with ACOG's recommendations, labetalol and nifedipine are considered first-line therapy. Options for

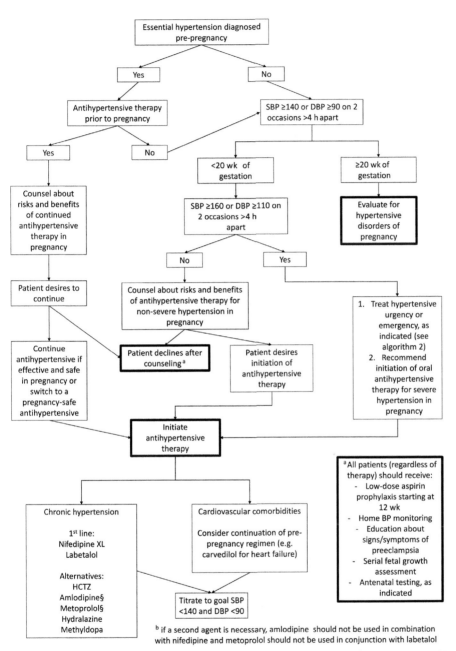

Fig. 1. Treatment of nonsevere hypertension in the outpatient setting in pregnancy. DBP, diastolic blood pressure; HCTZ, hydrochlorothiazide; SBP, systolic blood pressure.

second-line therapy include oral methyldopa (included as second-line as it is considered less effective than labetalol and nifedipine) if available, hydrochlorothiazide, amlodipine, and carvedilol. **Table 4** includes potential dosing regimens. Effective single-agent therapy is preferred over multiple agents when possible.

Table 4
Antihypertensive medications in pregnancy: indications in pregnancy, pharmacokinetics, dosing regimens for acute severe hypertension and nonsevere hypertension

Antihypertensive Class and Available Medications	Use in Pregnancy	Pharmacokinetic (PK) Characteristics[53,54]	Acute Severe Hypertension in Pregnancy		Nonsevere Hypertension in Pregnancy		Alternative Indications
			Indicated	Dose and Route of Administration	Indicated	Dose and Route of Administration	
β-blockers – combined alpha- and β-receptor antagonists							
Carvedilol	Use with caution (available evidence is limited, but without major concerns)	F: 25%–35% Onset: 1 h T_{max}: 1–1.5 h PPB: 95% V_d: 115 L Metabolism: CYP2D6 $T_{1/2}$: 6–10h Renal excretion: 16% Blood pressure response: 4-7h	No	–	Use only if potential benefit outweighs risk	Initial dose: 6.25 mg orally twice daily Dose titration: increase after 1–2 weeks to a maximum of 25 mg twice daily Maximum: 50 mg/d	–
Labetalol	First-line for treatment of hypertension in pregnancy	Oral: F: 25% Onset: 0.3–2 h T_{max}: 1-2h PPB: 50% V_d: 3.2–15 L/kg Metabolism: hepatic glucuronidation (UGT1A1, which is upregulated in pregnancy) $T_{1/2}$: 6–8 h Renal	First-line	Initial dose: 20 mg slow intravenous injection (over >2 min) Dose titration: see **Fig. 2** Maximum: 300 mg intravenously May give labetalol 200 mg orally if intravenous access not yet established; repeat in 30 min if needed	First-line	Initial dose: 100–200 mg orally twice daily Dose titration: Increase every 2–3 d to 200–2400 mg divided in 2–3 doses/d Maximum: 2400 mg/d orally	–

excretion: <5%
Blood pressure response: 8–12h
Intravenous:
F: n/a
Onset: 2–5 min
Tmax: 5–15 min
T1/2: 4–5.5 h
Blood pressure response: 16–18h

Drug	Recommendation	Pharmacokinetics				Dose	Comments
β-blockers – noncardioselective							
Propranolol	Use with caution (available evidence is limited, but without major concerns)	IR: F: 30%–70% Onset: 1.2 h Tmax: 1.5-2h PPB: 93% Vd: 6 L/kg Metabolism: CYP1A2 T1/2: 3-6h Renal excretion: <1%	No	—	Use if potential benefit outweighs risk	Initial dose: 40 mg orally twice daily; Dose titration: up to 120–240 mg/d in 2-3 divided doses; Maximum: 640 mg/d orally	Not considered first-line treatment for hypertension; May be considered for migraine prophylaxis, as needed use for anxiety, and for thyrotoxicosis in pregnancy (0.5–1 mg intravenously to maximum of 2–3 mg over 15 min, repeated every few hours)
Cardio-selective β-blockers							
Metoprolol	Use with caution (available evidence is limited, but without major concerns)	F: 40% Onset: 1.2 h Tmax: 1.5-2h PPB: 10% Vd: 3.2–5.5 L/kg Metabolism:	No	—	Use if potential benefit outweighs risk; Typically reserved for	*Metoprolol tartrate:* Initial dose: 100 mg orally/d in single or divided doses; Dose titration: titrate at weekly interval to	May be considered for migraine prophylaxis and thyrotoxicosis

(continued on next page)

Table 4
(continued)

Antihypertensive Class and Available Medications	Use in Pregnancy	Pharmacokinetic (PK) Characteristics[53,54]	Acute Severe Hypertension in Pregnancy		Nonsevere Hypertension in Pregnancy		Alternative Indications
			Indicated	Dose and Route of Administration	Indicated	Dose and Route of Administration	
		CYP2D6 $T_{1/2}$: 3–7.5 h Renal excretion: 3%–10%			presence of cardiovascular comorbidities (eg, collagen vascular disease, valvular heart disease)	100–400 mg/d; usual dose 100–200 mg/d in 2 divided doses Maximum dose: 400 mg/d *Metoprolol succinate:* Initial dose: 25 mg once daily Dose titration: titrate at weekly interval (or longer) to 25–400 mg/d; usual dose 50–200 mg once daily Maximum dose: 400 mg/d	
Atenolol	Avoid, if possible Atenolol is not recommended in pregnancy because of having strongest association with SGA[12] and association with hypospadias with first trimester use	F: 46%–60% Onset: 3h T_{max}: 2–24h PPB: <5% V_d: 50–75L Metabolism: minimal hepatic $T_{1/2}$: 6–7 h Renal excretion: 40%–50% (unchanged)	No	—	Avoid, if possible	Initial dose: 50 mg orally once daily Dose titration: titrate to 100 mg/d in 1–2 divided doses after 1–2 weeks; further increases are unlikely to be beneficial Maximum dose: 200 mg/d	May be considered for migraine prophylaxis and thyrotoxicosis

Drug	Recommendation	Pharmacokinetics		Dosing		Comments
Esmolol (intravenous only)	Use with caution (available evidence is limited, but without major concerns)	F: n/a (intravenous) Onset: immediate T_{max}: 5 min PPB: 55% V_d: 3.4 L/kg Metabolism: extensively red blood cell esterase $T_{1/2}$: 9 min Renal excretion: <1-2%	Yes, for refractory severe hypertension	Initial dose: 500-1000 µg/kg/min over 1 min Dose titration: 50 µg/kg/min intravenous infusion; for additional dosing, repeat bolus dose and increase infusion in 50-µg/kg/min increments Maximum dose: 200 µg/kg/min	No	May be considered for refractory severe hypertension in pregnancy via intravenous infusion for
Alpha2-adrenergic agonists						
Clonidine (oral, ER)	Use with caution (available evidence is limited, but without major concerns)	F: 95% Onset: <1h T_{max}: 7-8h PPB: 20%-40% V_d: 2.1 L/kg Metabolism: CYP2D6 $T_{1/2}$: 12-16h Renal excretion: 60%	No	—	Use if potential benefit outweighs risk	Initial dose: 0.1 mg orally twice daily Dose titration: Adjust in increments of 0.1 mg/d at weekly intervals; usual dose 0.2-0.6 mg in 2 divided doses Maximum dose: 2.4 mg/d Discontinuation: gradually decrease over 2-4 d → May be considered for management of opioid withdrawal and adjunct for postoperative pain control
Methyldopa (oral)	First-line for treatment of hypertension in pregnancy, but	F: 25%-50% Onset: 3-6h T_{max}: 4-6h PPB: negligible	No	First-line	Initial dose: 250 mg orally 2-3 times daily Dose titration: increase at least at 2 d	—

(continued on next page)

Table 4
(continued)

Antihypertensive Class and Available Medications	Use in Pregnancy	Pharmacokinetic (PK) Characteristics[53,54]	Acute Severe Hypertension in Pregnancy		Nonsevere Hypertension in Pregnancy		Alternative Indications
			Indicated	Dose and Route of Administration	Indicated	Dose and Route of Administration	
	may not be as effective as other first-line agents Safety data available for up to 7.5 y after birth	V_d: 0.6 L/kg Metabolism: decarboxylation $T_{1/2}$: 1.5-2h Renal excretion: 70%	Indicated		Indicated	intervals up to 500–3000 mg/d in 2–4 divided doses Maximum dose: 3000 mg/d	
Nondihydropyridine CCBs							
Verapamil	Use with caution (available evidence is limited, but without major concerns and no evidence of teratogenicity in animal studies)	IR: F: 2%–35% Onset: 1-2h T_{max}: 1-2h PPB: 94% V_d: 3.8 L/kg Metabolism: liver, multiple P450 enzymes $T_{1/2}$: 4–12h (age-dependent) Renal excretion: 70%	No (used IV for paroxysmal SVT and atrial fibrillation)	—	Use if potential benefit outweighs risk	*Immediate release:* Initial dose: 80 mg orally 3 times daily Dose titration: increase at weekly intervals to doses of 120–360 mg orally daily in 3 divided doses Maximum dose: 480 mg/d *Sustained release:* Initial dose: 120 mg once daily in the morning Dose titration: increase at weekly intervals to 360 mg in once or twice daily doses; usual doses 100–300 mg daily Maximum dose:	May be considered for migraine prophylaxis and paroxysmal supraventricular tachycardia prophylaxis

Diltiazem	Avoid, if possible (associated with skeletal anomalies at high-doses in animal studies)	IR: F: 35%–40% Onset: 15–60 min T_{max}: 2-4h PPB: 77%–93% V_d: 5.3 L/kg Metabolism: deacetylation in liver $T_{1/2}$: 3-6.6 h Renal excretion: 35%	No (used intravenously for paroxysmal SVT and atrial fibrillation) —	Avoid, if possible	Extended-release: Initial dose: 180 mg orally once daily Dose titration: increase dose at 1–2 week intervals to 120–540 mg once daily; usual doses 120–360 mg/d Maximum dose: 540 mg/d	May be considered for pulmonary hypertension and atrial arrhythmias
Dihydropyridine CCBs						
Nifedipine	First-line for treatment of hypertension in pregnancy	IR: F: 45%–55% Onset: 20 min T_{max}: 0.5-2h PPB: 96% V_d: 1.4–2.2 L/kg Metabolism: CYP3A4 (activity increased in pregnancy, so dosage increase may be necessary) $T_{1/2}$: 2h Renal excretion: 80% ER: F: 65%–89% Onset: 30–45 min T_{max}: 6 h $T_{1/2}$: 6–11h	First-line Short-acting: Initial dose: 10–20 mg orally Dose titration: see Fig. 2 Maximum dose: 180 mg/d	First-line	Extended-release: Initial dose: 30–60 mg orally once daily Dose titration: increase dose at 1- to 2-week intervals to 60–120 mg daily Maximum dose: 120 mg/d for Procardia XL or 90 mg/d for Adalat	May be considered for tocolysis in preterm labor, Raynaud phenomenon, and esophageal spasm
Nicardipine	Use with caution (available evidence is limited, but	Oral (IR): F: 35% Onset: 20 min T_{max}: 30 min-2 h	Yes, for refractory severe hypertension Initial dose: 5 mg/h intravenous infusion Dose titration:	Use if potential benefit outweighs risk	Immediate release: Initial dose: 20 mg orally 3 times daily Dose titration: increase	May be used for Raynaud phenomenon and for treatment of

(continued on next page)

Table 4
(continued)

Antihypertensive Class and Available Medications	Use in Pregnancy	Pharmacokinetic (PK) Characteristics[53,54]	Acute Severe Hypertension in Pregnancy		Nonsevere Hypertension in Pregnancy		Alternative Indications
			Indicated	Dose and Route of Administration	Indicated	Dose and Route of Administration	
	without major concerns)	PPB: >95% V_d: 8.3 L/kg Metabolism: CYP2C8, CYP2D6, and CYP3A4 $T_{1/2}$: 8.6 h Renal excretion: 60% Intravenous: F: n/a Onset: 1 min T_{max}: – PPB: >95% V_d: 8.3 L/kg Metabolism: CYP2C8, CYP2D6, and CYP3A4 $T_{1/2}$: 14.4 h Renal excretion: 49%		increase by 2.5 mg/h every 5–15 min; rate may be decreased by 3 mg/h once desired blood pressure response achieved Maximum dose: 15 mg/h intravenously May be associated with hypotension, reflex tachycardia, postpartum hemorrhage, tocolysis, headache, nausea, dizziness and flushing when intravenous nicardipine is used in pregnancy	Indicated	dose every 3 d to 20–40 mg orally 3 times daily Maximum dose: 120 mg/d *Sustained release:* Initial dose: 30 mg orally twice daily Dose titration: increase dose every 3 d to 30–60 mg orally twice daily Maximum dose: 120 mg/d	vasospasm (eg, related to subarachnoid hemorrhage or arterial catheterization)
Amlodipine	Use with caution (available evidence is limited, but without major concerns)	F: 64%–90% Onset: 4–8 T_{max}: 6–12 h PPB: 93% V_d: 0.3–8.2 L/kg Metabolism: liver	No	—	Use if potential benefit outweighs risk	Initial dose: 5 mg orally once daily Dose titration: increase dose every 1–2 weeks to 10 mg once daily	May be used for left ventricular hypertrophy, pulmonary hypertension, and

(continued)		$T_{1/2}$: 30–52h; Renal excretion: 10%; Blood pressure response: 24 h				Maximum dose: 10 mg/d	Raynaud phenomenon	May be used in conjunction with isosorbide dinitrate in the setting of heart failure with reduced ejection fraction (ie, peripartum cardiomyopathy)
Vasodilators								
Hydralazine	First-line for treatment of acute severe hypertension in pregnancy; For extended use, use with caution (available evidence is limited, but without major concerns)	Oral: F: 20%–50%; Onset: 20–30 min; T_{max}: 0.5–1.5 h; PPB: 85%–90%; V_d: 0.3–8.2 L/kg; Metabolism: acetylation; $T_{1/2}$: 2-8h; Renal excretion: 10%; IV: Onset: 10–80 min; T_{max}: 0.2–1.4 h; $T_{1/2}$: 2-4 h	First-line	Use if potential benefit outweighs risk	Initial dose: 5 mg intravenously or intramuscularly; Dose titration: see **Fig. 2**; Maximum dose: 20 mg intravenously	Initial dose: 10 mg orally 3–4 times daily; Dose titration: increase dose after 3–4 d to 25 mg orally 3–4 times daily; after 1 week, can increase further to 50 mg orally 4 times daily; Max oral dose: 150 mg/d maximum advised because of risk of drug-induced systemic lupus erythematosus with higher doses; Consider coadministration with labetalol or methyldopa because of risk of reflex tachycardia		
Nitroglycerin (intravenous)	Use with caution for brief periods	F: n/a; Onset: 1–3 min	Yes, for refractory	No	Initial dose: 5 μg/min	—		Intravenous nitroglycerin may be

(continued on next page)

Table 4
(continued)

Antihypertensive Class and Available Medications	Use in Pregnancy	Pharmacokinetic (PK) Characteristics[53,54]	Acute Severe Hypertension in Pregnancy		Nonsevere Hypertension in Pregnancy		Alternative Indications
			Indicated	Dose and Route of Administration	Indicated	Dose and Route of Administration	
	(available evidence is limited, but without major concerns)	T_{max}: 1 min PPB: 60% V_d: 3.3 L/kg Metabolism: Glucuronidation $T_{1/2}$: 1-4 min Renal excretion: <1%	severe hypertension	intravenously Dose titration: increase by 5 µg/min increments at intervals of 3-5 min to blood pressure target Maximum dose: 20 µg/min			considered for brief use in hypertensive emergency in pregnancy, particularly if pulmonary edema present
Nitroprusside (intravenous)	Use with caution for brief periods (available evidence is limited, but without major concerns) because of the risk of cyanide toxicity with prolonged use and large doses	F: n/a Onset: 30 s T_{max}: 2 min PPB: –% V_d: –L/kg Metabolism: $T_{1/2}$: 2-3 h Renal excretion: <1%	Yes, for refractory severe hypertension Can worsen maternal cerebral edema Use with caution in the setting of preeclampsia with severe features	Initial dose: 0.3–0.5 µg/kg/min intravenously Dose titration: increase in increments of 0.5 µg/kg/min to blood pressure target for as short as possible Maximum dose: 10 µg/kg/min	No	–	–
Thiazide diuretics							
HCTZ	Use with caution (available evidence is limited, but	F: 60%–80% Onset: 3–4 d T_{max}: 1.5–2.5 h PPB: 40%	No	–	Second-line for the treatment of chronic	Initial dose: 12.5 mg orally daily Dose titration: increase to	–

Drug	Recommendation	Pharmacokinetics	Breastfeeding	IV / alternative	Use in pregnancy	Dosing	Clinical considerations
	without major concerns)	V_d: 3–4 L/kg Metabolism: none $T_{1/2}$: 10–12h Renal excretion: 50%–70%			hypertension in pregnancy	25–50 mg orally daily in single or 2 divided doses Maximum: 50 mg/d	
Loop diuretics							
Furosemide	Use with caution (available evidence is limited, but without major concerns)	F: 43%–64% Onset: 1 h T_{max}: 50–90 min PPB: 91%–99% V_d: 14 L Metabolism: liver $T_{1/2}$: 1.3–2h Renal excretion: 53%–100%	No	—	Use if potential benefit outweighs risk as adjunct for severe hypertension with renal disease or heart failure in pregnancy	Initial dose: 20 mg orally as a single dose Dose titration: 20–40 mg once or twice daily Maximum dose: 600 mg/d	May be considered for treatment of pulmonary edema and heart failure in pregnancy
ACE inhibitors							
Enalapril	Contraindicated in pregnancy May be considered postpartum because of minimal milk transfer, preferred over captopril because of less frequent dosing	F: 60% Onset: 1–4 h T_{max}: 1 h PPB: 50%–60% V_d: 1–2.4 L/kg Metabolism: hydrolysis in liver $T_{1/2}$: 1.3 h Renal excretion: 40%–61% Blood pressure response: 4 h to several weeks	Consider postpartum	Intravenous enalaprilat Initial dose: 1.25 mg intravenously over a 5-min period Dose titration: can be increased to up to 5 mg intravenously every 6 h as needed Maximum dose: none reported	Use if potential benefit outweighs risk in postpartum period	Initial dose: 5 mg orally once daily Dose titration: increase dose over several days to weeks to 5–40 mg; usual doses 10–40 mg/d in single or divided doses Maximum dose: 40 mg/d	May be considered for hypertensive crisis, heart failure in conjunction with diuretics, diabetic nephropathy and diabetic retinopathy, and left ventricular dysfunction
Captopril	Contraindicated in pregnancy May be considered postpartum because of	F: 75% Onset: 15–30 min T_{max}: 0.5–1.5 h PPB: 25%–30% V_d: 0.7 L/kg Metabolism:	No	—	Use if potential benefit outweighs risk in postpartum period	Initial dose: 25 mg orally 2–3 times daily Dose titration: increase dose to 50 mg orally 2–3 times daily over 1–2 weeks then to	May be considered for hypertensive crisis, heart failure in conjunction with diuretics, diabetic nephropathy and

(continued on next page)

Table 4
(continued)

Antihypertensive Class and Available Medications	Use in Pregnancy	Pharmacokinetic (PK) Characteristics[53,54]	Acute Severe Hypertension in Pregnancy		Nonsevere Hypertension in Pregnancy		Alternative Indications
			Indicated	Dose and Route of Administration	Indicated	Dose and Route of Administration	
	minimal milk transfer	liver (captopril and lisinopril are the only 2 ACE inhibitors that do not need to be activated in the body to be effective) $T_{1/2}$: 1.9 h Renal excretion: >95% Blood pressure response: occurs in stages			Indicated	150–200 mg orally 2–3 times daily Maximum dose: 450 mg/d Take 1 h before meals	diabetic retinopathy, and left ventricular dysfunction
ARBs							
Losartan	Contraindicated in pregnancy May be considered postpartum	F: 33% Onset: 1 week T_{max}: 1 h PPB: 98% V_d: 34 L Metabolism: CYP2C9 and CYP3A4 $T_{1/2}$: 2 h Renal excretion: >35% Blood pressure response: occurs in stages	No	—	Use if potential benefit outweighs risk in postpartum period although limited data exist regarding infant risk	Initial dose: 25 mg orally once daily Dose titration: increase to 50–100 mg orally daily 100 mg/d	May be considered for hypertension in the setting of diabetes mellitus, erythrocytosis, and heart failure

Abbreviations: ER, extended release; F, oral bioavailability; PPB, plasma protein binding; T1/2, drug half-life; Tmax, time to peak plasma levels; Vd, volume of

Published data are not decisive regarding the optimal antihypertensive choice in pregnancy. A thoughtfully designed network meta-analysis published by Bellos and colleagues in 2020 compared the safety and efficacy of antihypertensive agents for chronic hypertension in pregnancy. Pooled results of randomized controlled trials did not show a difference in the risk of preeclampsia between the different agents studied. Of the commonly used antihypertensives, nifedipine and methyldopa demonstrated significantly lower incidences of severe hypertension and placental abruption, while labetalol did not.[12] There were no differences in other outcomes, including gestational age at delivery, cesarean delivery, preterm birth, and perinatal death. With the highest probability score for adverse perinatal events, atenolol ranked as the worst treatment in this analysis.[12] A subsequent systematic review and network meta- and trial sequential analysis concluded that all commonly prescribed antihypertensives reduce the risk of severe hypertension by 30% to 70%, with no single antihypertensive performing better than others. In this analysis, labetalol reduced the risk of proteinuria and preeclampsia, as well as perinatal mortality, compared with methyldopa and CCBs.[9] In the CHAP trial, approximately two-thirds of patients on medication used labetalol, while about one-third used nifedipine.[3] Differential outcomes were not reported by medication used. However, the active treatment group was noted to have a reduced risk of preeclampsia with severe features, suggesting that selection of either agent is reasonable.[3] The authors of the previously discussed Cochrane Review concluded that CCB and ß-blockers appear more effective than methyldopa for preventing severe hypertension.[15] Efficacy data regarding other antihypertensives in pregnancy, such as hydrochlorothiazide and carvedilol, is lacking. One recent meta-analysis of several small randomized, controlled trials comparing amlodipine and nifedipine for hypertension in pregnancy concluded that amlodipine may have slightly better efficacy than nifedipine with decreased maternal side effects and no differences in neonatal outcomes, suggesting amlodipine may warrant further investigation for use in pregnancy.[43]

Until more definitive comparative data are available, nifedipine and labetalol remain first-line antihypertensives for the treatment of nonsevere hypertension in pregnancy. To avoid the teratogenic risks of medications like ACE inhibitors, consideration should be given to switching to a first-line agent in the preconception period for persons with chronic hypertension considering pregnancy and currently using a teratogenic antihypertensive. For those using an antihypertensive with a favorable pregnancy profile and with well-controlled hypertension, it is reasonable to continue that medication through the preconception and early pregnancy period. Individual patient characteristics should be considered in the selection of antihypertensive therapy, including dosing frequency, cost, side effects, and response to therapy. For instance, ß-blockers should be discouraged, if possible, in patients with asthma, and nifedipine has a high frequency (approximately 10%) of headache side effects. The authors propose nifedipine as a reasonable initial choice for the treatment of hypertension in pregnancy given fewer associations with risk of SGA and once daily dosing.

CASE, CONTINUED

Jane now presents to clinic at 28 weeks' gestation with BP of 170/110 mm Hg. Her BP remains 168/105 mm Hg when repeated 15 minutes later, meeting criteria for acute severe hypertension in pregnancy.

- Should antihypertensive therapy be initiated? What medication should be considered first?
- If Jane remains hypertensive despite use of maximum doses of the medications recommended in **Fig. 2**, what additional options should be considered?

ANTIHYPERTENSIVE SELECTION FOR ACUTE SEVERE HYPERTENSION IN PREGNANCY

Fig. 2 outlines a recommended clinical pathway for the management of pregnant patients presenting with acute severe hypertension. **Table 4** further details available dosing regimens. Severe hypertension, defined as an SBP greater than or equal to 160 mm Hg or a DBP greater than or equal to 110 mm Hg, has been associated with increased perinatal morbidity and should be approached more seriously in pregnant than in nonpregnant patients.[5] Treatment should be initiated within 30 to

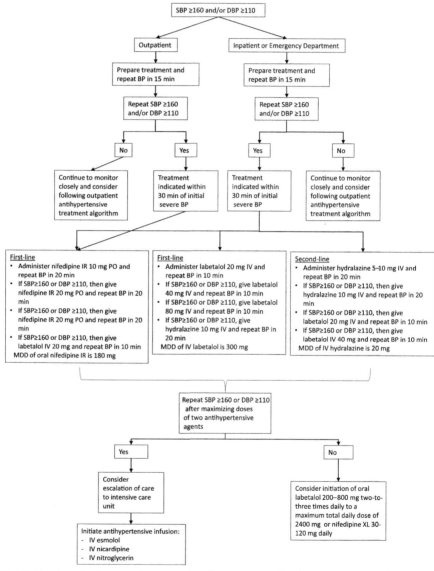

Fig. 2. Treatment of severe hypertension in pregnancy in the outpatient and inpatient setting.[6] BP, blood pressure; DBP, diastolic blood pressure; MDD, maximum daily or cumulative dose; SBP, systolic blood pressure; XL, extended release.

60 minutes of the diagnosis of severe hypertension.[5] Similar to outpatient therapy, no single agent has been definitively identified as superior in terms of efficacy and safety in the acute treatment of severe hypertension in pregnancy. A Cochrane Systematic Review of 35 trials (3573 women) failed to show superiority of 1 agent over another. However, those allocated to CCBs were less likely to have persistent high BP than those allocated to hydralazine, and tended to have fewer side effects than those allocated to labetalol.[31] Other meta-analyses have found that nifedipine immediate release (IR) achieves the target BP more rapidly than hydralazine, while hydralazine is associated with more maternal hypotension, more cesarean sections, more placental abruption, more oliguria, more adverse effects on the fetal heart rate, and more low Apgar scores at 1 minute.[44,45] Similarly, oral nifedipine may also have less risk of persistent hypertension and maternal side effects compared with intravenous labetalol, although existing studies are small.[46,47] Although it is difficult to definitively conclude that labetalol or nifedipine is superior, the data in aggregate support these 2 options as safer and potentially more efficacious than hydralazine.[48] In summary, intravenous labetalol or oral nifedipine IR should be considered first-line for the treatment of acute severe hypertension in the absence of contraindications, and intravenous hydralazine can be reserved for use if either of these treatments is ineffective. Patients who are treated for acute, severe-range hypertension should be considered for initiation of longer-term antihypertensive medications for optimum outcomes.

CASE, CONTINUED

Jane ultimately requires urgent cesarean delivery for refractory hypertension. On postoperative day 3, her blood pressure remains greater than or equal to 140/90. She has initiated breastfeeding and plans to continue to breastfeed on discharge from the hospital.

- Should oral antihypertensive therapy be continued or restarted in the postpartum period?
- Which medications are recommended and how do a patient's breastfeeding goals affect antihypertensive selection?

ANTIHYPERTENSIVE SELECTION IN THE POSTPARTUM PERIOD

Elevated blood pressures in the setting of new-onset hypertensive disorders of pregnancy may persist until 12 weeks postpartum, while unmasked chronic hypertension may continue to manifest at 1 year postpartum.[49,50] Accumulating evidence supports a significantly increased 10-year and lifetime risk of cardiovascular disease in

---

Box 1
Considerations for antihypertensive selection in the postpartum period

Is underlying primary or secondary hypertension suspected and, if so, is long-term antihypertensive therapy anticipated?

Was the patient on an effective antihypertensive regimen prior to pregnancy?

Does the patient have any comorbidities that would benefit from 1 antihypertensive drug over another?

What are the patient's breastfeeding goals, and is there a safe and effective first-line antihypertensive drug that will not interfere with these goals?

individuals who experience hypertensive disorders of pregnancy.[51] These findings highlight the importance of adequate treatment of elevated blood pressure in the postpartum period and continued surveillance well beyond the traditional postpartum visit.

In the absence of evidence supporting selection of one antihypertensive over another in the postpartum period,[52] postpartum antihypertensive therapy should be selected based on the most effective and safe therapies recommended outside of pregnancy. As outlined in **Box 1**, 4 considerations should be addressed when selecting an antihypertensive drug in the postpartum period.

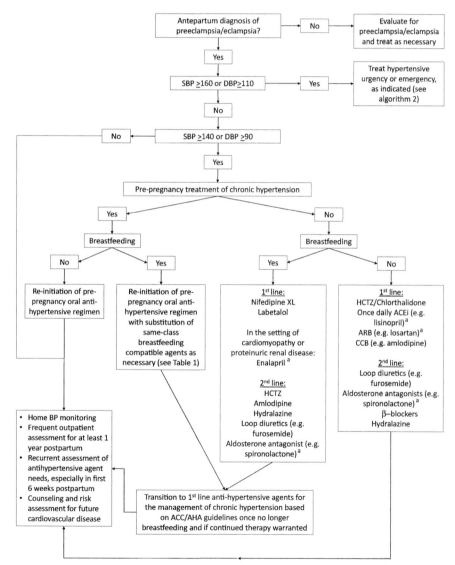

Fig. 3. Postpartum hypertension management algorithm. ACC, American College of Cardiology; ACEi, angiotensin converting enzyme inhibitor; AHA, American Heart Association; DBP, diastolic blood pressure; HCTZ, hydrochlorothiazide; SBP, systolic blood pressure; XL, extended release. [a]Ensure patients has effective contraception.

With regards to the first consideration, it is reasonable to continue labetalol or nifedipine if a patient has no history of hypertension and resolution of her hypertension in the postpartum period is anticipated. Given ease of use with once-daily dosing and inclusion as a first-line agent in the ACC/AHA guidelines, the authors prefer extended-release nifedipine in this scenario.

For those in whom there is concern for possible persistent hypertension beyond the postpartum period (eg, chronic hypertension, persistent severe hypertension postpartum, preterm preeclampsia with severe features, or hypertension at the postpartum visit), it may be worth considering initiation of one of the antihypertensive agents demarcated first-line in the ACC/AHA guidelines (bolded in **Table 3**; **Fig. 3**). If a patient was previously on an effective, first-line antihypertensive regimen prior to pregnancy, reinitiation of this regimen is warranted in the postpartum period. Additionally, comorbid conditions may warrant selection of a specific class of antihypertensives (eg, carvedilol in heart failure) and have a blood pressure treatment goal of less than 130/80 mm Hg. The specific antihypertensive medications recommended for certain comorbid conditions are reviewed in the ACC/AHA guidelines and should be selected in consultation with a specialist.

For those patients with the intention of breastfeeding, a lactation database or lactation specialist, along with the involved pediatrician, may be consulted. A review of lactation compatibility is provided for reference in **Table 3**. Many antihypertensives are considered safe and compatible with breastfeeding and are supported for use during lactation by the American Academy of Pediatrics. It is important to note that individual drug characteristics may impact their compatibility with breastfeeding. Certain medications should be avoided or used with caution. For example, atenolol reaches high concentrations in breastmilk and can result in adverse neonatal effects. Concern has been raised regarding the potential for methyldopa and clonidine to exacerbate postpartum depression.[28] Loop and thiazide diuretics have the potential to decrease milk production.[53] For others, such as ARBs, evidence is inadequate to assess breastfeeding safety.

SUMMARY

A growing body of evidence suggests that chronic hypertension should be treated in pregnancy to prevent maternal morbidity. Several antihypertensives appear to be safe and effective in decreasing the risk of complications from hypertension in pregnancy. Future studies comparing the safety and efficacy of different antihypertensives and pharmacokinetic studies determining the optimal dosing regimens are needed to better guide antihypertensive selection and prescribing in pregnancy.

DISCLOSURE

The authors have no conflicts of interest to disclose.

REFERENCES

1. Bateman BT, Bansil P, Hernandez-Diaz S, et al. Prevalence, trends, and outcomes of chronic hypertension: a nationwide sample of delivery admissions. Am J Obstet Gynecol 2012;206(2):134 e131–138.

2. Freaney PM, Harrington K, Molsberry R, et al. Temporal trends in adverse pregnancy outcomes in birthing individuals aged 15 to 44 years in the United States, 2007 to 2019. J Am Heart Assoc 2022;11(11):e025050.

3. Tita AT, Szychowski JM, Boggess K, et al. Treatment for mild chronic hypertension during pregnancy. N Engl J Med 2022;386(19):1781–92 (1533-4406 (Electronic)).

4. Whelton PK, Carey RM, Aronow WS, et al. 2017 ACC/AHA/AAPA/ABC/ACPM/AGS/APhA/ASH/ASPC/NMA/PCNA guideline for the prevention, detection, evaluation, and management of high blood pressure in adults: a report of the American College of Cardiology/American Heart Association Task Force on Clinical Practice Guidelines. Circulation 2018;138(17):e484–594.

5. American College of Obstetricians and Gynecologists' Committee on Practice Bulletins—Obstetrics. Chronic hypertension in pregnancy: ACOG Practice Bulletin Number 203. Obstet Gynecol 2019;133(1):e26–50.

6. American College of Obstetricians and Gynecologists' Committee on Practice Bulletins—Obstetrics. Gestational hypertension and preeclampsia: ACOG Practice Bulletin, Number 222. Obstet Gynecol 2020;135(6):e237–60.

7. Society for Maternal-Fetal M, Publications Committee. Electronic address pso. Society for Maternal-Fetal Medicine Statement: Antihypertensive therapy for mild chronic hypertension in pregnancy-The Chronic Hypertension and Pregnancy trial. Am J Obstet Gynecol 2022;227(2):B24–7.

8. ACoOa Gynecologists. Clinical Guidance for the Integration of the Findings of the Chronic Hypertension and Pregnancy (CHAP) Study. ACOG. Practice advisory Web site. Available at: https://www.acog.org/clinical/clinical-guidance/practice-advisory/articles/2022/04/clinical-guidance-for-the-integration-of-the-findings-of-the-chronic-hypertension-and-pregnancy-chap-study. . Published 2022. Updated April 2022. Accessed July 11, 2022.

9. Bone JN, Sandhu A, Abalos ED, et al. Oral antihypertensives for nonsevere pregnancy hypertension: systematic review, network meta- and trial sequential analyses. Hypertension 2022;79(3):614–28.

10. Nakhai-Pour HR, Rey E, Berard A. Antihypertensive medication use during pregnancy and the risk of major congenital malformations or small-for-gestational-age newborns. Birth Defects Res B Dev Reprod Toxicol 2010;89(2):147–54.

11. Yakoob MY, Bateman BT, Ho E, et al. The risk of congenital malformations associated with exposure to beta-blockers early in pregnancy: a meta-analysis. Hypertension 2013;62(2):375–81.

12. Bellos I, Pergialiotis V, Papapanagiotou A, et al. Comparative efficacy and safety of oral antihypertensive agents in pregnant women with chronic hypertension: a network metaanalysis. Am J Obstet Gynecol 2020;223(4):525–37.

13. Duan L, Ng A, Chen W, et al. Beta-blocker subtypes and risk of low birth weight in newborns. J Clin Hypertens (Greenwich) 2018;20(11):1603–9.

14. Baggio MR, Martins WP, Calderon AC, et al. Changes in fetal and maternal Doppler parameters observed during acute severe hypertension treatment with hydralazine or labetalol: a randomized controlled trial. Ultrasound Med Biol 2011;37(1):53–8.

15. Abalos E, Duley L, Steyn DW, et al. Antihypertensive drug therapy for mild to moderate hypertension during pregnancy. Cochrane Database Syst Rev 2018; 10:CD002252.

16. Fitton CA, Fleming M, Steiner MFC, et al. In utero antihypertensive medication exposure and neonatal outcomes: a data linkage cohort study. Hypertension 2020;75(3):628–33.

17. von Dadelszen P, Magee LA. Fall in mean arterial pressure and fetal growth restriction in pregnancy hypertension: an updated metaregression analysis. J Obstet Gynaecol Can 2002;24(12):941–5.

18. Orbach H, Matok I, Gorodischer R, et al. Hypertension and antihypertensive drugs in pregnancy and perinatal outcomes. Am J Obstet Gynecol 2013; 208(4):301 e301–306.
19. Davis RL, Eastman D, McPhillips H, et al. Risks of congenital malformations and perinatal events among infants exposed to calcium channel and beta-blockers during pregnancy. Pharmacoepidemiol Drug Saf 2011;20(2):138–45.
20. Weber-Schoendorfer C, Hannemann D, Meister R, et al. The safety of calcium channel blockers during pregnancy: a prospective, multicenter, observational study. Reprod Toxicol 2008;26(1):24–30.
21. Sorensen HT, Czeizel AE, Rockenbauer M, et al. The risk of limb deficiencies and other congenital abnormalities in children exposed in utero to calcium channel blockers. Acta Obstet Gynecol Scand 2001;80(5):397–401.
22. Ariyuki F. Effects of diltiazem hydrochloride on embryonic development: species differences in the susceptibility and stage specificity in mice, rats, and rabbits. Okajimas Folia Anat Jpn 1975;52(2–3):103–17.
23. Bateman BT, Huybrechts KF, Maeda A, et al. Calcium channel blocker exposure in late pregnancy and the risk of neonatal seizures. Obstet Gynecol 2015;126(2): 271–8.
24. Moretti MM, Fairlie FM, Akl S, et al. The effect of nifedipine therapy on fetal and placental Doppler waveforms in preeclampsia remote from term. Am J Obstet Gynecol 1990;163(6 Pt 1):1844–8.
25. Cockburn J, Moar VA, Ounsted M, et al. Final report of study on hypertension during pregnancy: the effects of specific treatment on the growth and development of the children. Lancet 1982;1(8273):647–9.
26. Hoeltzenbein M, Beck E, Fietz AK, et al. Pregnancy outcome after first trimester use of methyldopa: a prospective cohort study. Hypertension 2017;70(1):201–8.
27. Al Khalaf S, Khashan AS, Chappell LC, et al. Role of antihypertensive treatment and blood pressure control in the occurrence of adverse pregnancy outcomes: a population-based study of linked electronic health records. Hypertension 2022; 79(7):1548–58, 10116 1HYPERTENSIONAHA12218920.
28. Wicinski M, Malinowski B, Puk O, et al. Methyldopa as an inductor of postpartum depression and maternal blues: a review. Biomed Pharmacother 2020;127: 110196.
29. Lamont RF, Elder MG. Transfer of hydralazine across the placenta and into breast milk. J Obstet Gynaecol 1986;7(1):47–8.
30. Derham RJ, Robinson J. Severe preeclampsia: is vasodilation therapy with hydralazine dangerous for the preterm fetus? Am J Perinatol 1990;7(3):239–44.
31. Duley L, Meher S, Jones L. Drugs for treatment of very high blood pressure during pregnancy. Cochrane Database Syst Rev 2013;7:CD001449.
32. Collins R, Fau-Yusuf S, Yusuf S, et al. Overview of randomised trials of diuretics in pregnancy. Br Med J 1985;290:0267–623. Print.
33. George JD, Price CJ, Tyl RW, et al. The evaluation of the developmental toxicity of hydrochlorothiazide in mice and rats. Fundam Appl Toxicol 1995;26(2):174–80.
34. Sibai BM, Grossman RA, Grossman HG. Effects of diuretics on plasma volume in pregnancies with long-term hypertension. Am J Obstet Gynecol 1984;150(7): 831–5.
35. Churchill D, Beevers GD, Meher S, et al. Diuretics for preventing pre-eclampsia. Cochrane Database Syst Rev 2007;1:CD004451.
36. Beermann B, Fahraeus L, Groschinsky-Grind M, et al. Placental transfer of hydrochlorothiazide. Gynecol Obstet Invest 1980;11(1):45–8.

37. Robertson RT, Minsker DH, Bokelman DL, et al. Potassium loss as a causative factor for skeletal malformations in rats produced by indacrinone: a new investigational loop diuretic. Toxicol Appl Pharmacol 1981;60(1):142–50.
38. Wang LA, Smith PB, Laughon M, et al. Prolonged furosemide exposure and risk of abnormal newborn hearing screen in premature infants. Early Hum Dev 2018; 125:26–30.
39. Cooper WO, Hernandez-Diaz S, Arbogast PG, et al. Major congenital malformations after first-trimester exposure to ACE inhibitors. N Engl J Med 2006;354(23): 2443–51.
40. Ruys TP, Maggioni A, Johnson MR, et al. Cardiac medication during pregnancy, data from the ROPAC. Int J Cardiol 2014;177(1):124–8.
41. Bateman BT, Patorno E, Desai RJ, et al. Angiotensin-converting enzyme inhibitors and the risk of congenital malformations. Obstet Gynecol 2017;129(1):174–84.
42. Bullo M, Tschumi S, Bucher BS, et al. Pregnancy outcome following exposure to angiotensin-converting enzyme inhibitors or angiotensin receptor antagonists: a systematic review. Hypertension 2012;60(2):444–50.
43. Yin J, Mei Z, Shi S, et al. Nifedipine or amlodipine? The choice for hypertension during pregnancy: a systematic review and meta-analysis. Arch Gynecol Obstet 2022;306(6):1891–900.
44. Sridharan K, Sequeira RP. Drugs for treating severe hypertension in pregnancy: a network meta-analysis and trial sequential analysis of randomized clinical trials. Br J Clin Pharmacol 2018;84(9):1906–16.
45. Magee LA, Cham C, Waterman EJ, et al. Hydralazine for treatment of severe hypertension in pregnancy: meta-analysis. BMJ 2003;327(7421):955–60.
46. Shekhar S, Gupta N, Kirubakaran R, et al. Oral nifedipine versus intravenous labetalol for severe hypertension during pregnancy: a systematic review and meta-analysis. BJOG 2016;123(1):40–7.
47. Shekhar S, Sharma C, Thakur S, et al. Oral nifedipine or intravenous labetalol for hypertensive emergency in pregnancy: a randomized controlled trial. Obstet Gynecol 2013;122(5):1057–63.
48. Alavifard S, Chase R, Janoudi G, et al. First-line antihypertensive treatment for severe hypertension in pregnancy: a systematic review and network meta-analysis. Pregnancy Hypertens 2019;18:179–87.
49. Ditisheim A, Wuerzner G, Ponte B, et al. Prevalence of hypertensive phenotypes after preeclampsia: a prospective cohort study. Hypertension 2018;71(1):103–9.
50. Benschop L, Duvekot JJ, Versmissen J, et al. Blood pressure profile 1 year after severe preeclampsia. Hypertension 2018;71(3):491–8.
51. Ramlakhan KP, Johnson MR, Roos-Hesselink JW. Pregnancy and cardiovascular disease. Nat Rev Cardiol 2020;17(11):718–31.
52. Cairns AE, Pealing L, Duffy JMN, et al. Postpartum management of hypertensive disorders of pregnancy: a systematic review. BMJ Open 2017;7(11):e018696.
53. Tamargo J, Caballero R, Delpon E. Pharmacotherapy for hypertension in pregnant patients: special considerations. Expert Opin Pharmacother 2019;20(8): 963–82.
54. Koren G, Pariente G. Pregnancy-associated changes in pharmacokinetics and their clinical implications. Pharm Res 2018;35(3):61.

Aspirin and Pravastatin for Preeclampsia Prevention in High-Risk Pregnancy

Joe Eid, MD*, Kara M. Rood, MD, Maged M. Costantine, MD

KEYWORDS

- Preeclampsia • Aspirin • Pravastatin

KEY POINTS

- Preeclampsia affects up to 8% of pregnancies and is a major cause of maternal and neonatal morbidities and mortality worldwide.
- Low-dose aspirin use is recommended by professional societies for individuals at high-risk of developing preeclampsia.
- Pravastatin has emerged as a potential agent for the prevention of preeclampsia.

INTRODUCTION AND PATHOGENESIS OF PREECLAMPSIA

Preeclampsia (PE) is a morbid hypertensive disorder that affects up to 8% of all pregnancies.[1,2] PE presents as new onset hypertension in pregnancy, usually after 20 weeks' gestation, and its severe form can be associated with end-organ damage including maternal seizure, stroke, liver injury, coagulopathy, renal failure, pulmonary edema, and death.[2] PE is a leading cause of maternal mortality worldwide.[3,4] It is also one of the most common indications for iatrogenic preterm birth in the United States,[5] accounting for more than one-third of preterm births.[6] Other fetal adverse outcomes include complications related to prematurity, growth restriction, and stillbirth.[7] With this, PE adds a substantial financial burden on the health-care system in the United States, estimated at more than US$1.03 billion in maternal costs and US$1.15 billion in infant costs, in the first year after delivery.[8]

In the United States, marked racial and ethnic disparities exist in the prevalence and burden of PE. Non-Hispanic Black individuals not only develop PE at a much higher rate compared with Non-Hispanic White but also have a 3 times higher case fatality rates and are twice as likely to be readmitted postpartum, with PE a major contributor to all these morbidities.[9,10]

Division of Maternal Fetal Medicine, Department of Obstetrics and Gynecology, The Ohio State University Wexner Medical Center, Columbus, OH, USA
* Corresponding author. 395 West 12th Avenue, Columbus, OH 43210.
E-mail address: Eid07@osumc.edu

Obstet Gynecol Clin N Am 50 (2023) 79–88
https://doi.org/10.1016/j.ogc.2022.10.005
0889-8545/23/© 2022 Elsevier Inc. All rights reserved.

PE is a multifactorial disorder, and its pathogenesis is thought to be the result of interaction between genetic, immunologic, and environmental factors, as well as abnormal placentation.[2,11] During early placental development, abnormal cytotrophoblast invasion and remodeling of the spiral arterioles contribute to the pathogenesis of the disease (**Fig. 1**).[12] This abnormal placentation leads to an imbalance of angiogenic and antiangiogenic factors, endothelial cell dysfunction, increased vascular resistance, enhanced platelet aggregation, and activation of the coagulation system.[2,13] The inflammatory response created by abnormal placentation activates cyclooxygenase (COX) resulting in an increase in thromboxane A2 (TxA2) levels and a reduction in endothelial cell prostacyclin levels (PGI2).[14,15] PGI2 is known for counteracting the effects of TxA2 on vasoconstriction and increased platelet aggregation.[16] Reduced levels of PGI2 occur months before the clinical onset of PE.[17]

Moreover, an imbalance in angiogenic placental mediators is thought to be an important feature in the development of PE.[18] An increase in antiangiogenic factors soluble Fms-like tyrosine kinase-1 (sFlt-1) and soluble endoglin (sEng) is secondary to placental ischemia due to poor placentation.[19–21] Both of these antiangiogenic factors are known to significantly increase several weeks before the onset of the clinical manifestations of the disease.[21] sFlt-1 and sEng have been shown to neutralize and inhibit proangiogenic mediators such as vascular endothelial growth factor (VEGF) and placental growth factor (PlGF), decreasing their circulating levels.[19,20] As a result of this angiogenic imbalance, endothelial dysfunction and maternal vasoconstriction occur leading to an increase in blood pressure and other clinical manifestations of PE.[20,22]

In this review article, we will discuss the use of aspirin and statins for the prevention of PE.

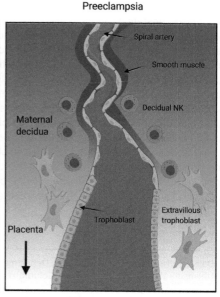

Fig. 1. Abnormal cytotrophoblast invasion and remodeling of the spiral arterioles contribute to the pathogenesis of the disease. (*From* Rana S, Burke SD, Karumanchi SA. Imbalances in circulating angiogenic factors in the pathophysiology of preeclampsia and related disorders. Am J Obstet Gynecol. 2022;226(2S):S1019-S1034; with permission.)

ASPIRIN
Mechanism of Action

Aspirin is a nonselective inhibitor of COX enzymes.[15] COX is a key enzyme in the pathway of prostaglandins (proinflammatory) and thromboxane (proclotting) synthesis.[23] At doses less than 300 mg, aspirin selectively and irreversibly inactivates COX-1 enzyme,[24] which leads to a decrease in thromboxane and prostaglandins production including TxA2 and PGI2.[15,23,24]

PGI2 is a potent vasodilator, an inhibitor of platelet aggregation, and is synthesized and rapidly repleted by endothelial cells lining the cardiovascular system.[15,25] TxA2 is produced by activated platelets during hemostasis. Its prothrombotic effects are manifested by the activation of new platelets, vasoconstriction, and increase in platelet aggregation.[16,26] Aspirin preferentially inhibits TxA2 synthesis as TxA2 is not readily repleted by anuclear platelets.[15] Because the pathogenesis of PE involves vasoconstriction and increased platelet aggregation, aspirin emerged as a drug of interest in the prevention of PE due to its role in decreasing TxA2 levels.[16,27] Furthermore, by inhibiting COX-1, aspirin inhibits the overexpression of sFlt-1 resulting from hypoxic changes in the placenta.[28,29] In addition, by acetylating the active site of COX, aspirin triggers the biosynthesis of anti-inflammatory lipids such as 15-epi-lipoxin A_4 (15-epi-LXA_4).[30] Decreased levels of 15-epi-LXA_4 have been identified in pregnancies affected by PE.[31]

CLINICAL DATA AND IMPLICATIONS

In 1979, the use of aspirin as a medication for the prevention of PE was first reported.[32] Subsequently, different studies showed mixed results in the reduction of PE using daily aspirin with a dose range of 50 to 150 mg.[33-36] A dose–response effect of aspirin in the prevention of PE has been suggested in some meta-analyses and systematic reviews.[37,38] The reduction in risk of PE was shown when aspirin was initiated before 16 weeks of gestation, which corresponds to the completion of placentation, and at a daily dose of at least 100 mg.[36] The current model used to screen and identify pregnant individuals who are candidates for low-dose aspirin (LDA) therapy for PE prevention relies on identification of high-risk factors. More recently, screening tests (done during the 11th to 13th weeks of gestation) to predict and stratify the risk for developing PE have been reported.[39,40] A combination of low maternal serum concentrations of PlGF, high uterine artery pulsatility index, and other maternal parameters, identified 93.1% of patients who would develop preterm PE requiring delivery before 34 weeks of gestation.[41] However, this screening modality is not supported by professional societies in the United States due to lack of data from US population and its low positive predictive value. These tests require a large number of patients identified as high risk by screening, in order to detect one case of early-onset PE.[42] In 2017, the ASPRE trial was published comparing the use of 150 mg aspirin versus placebo in pregnant people at high risk of developing preterm PE.[43] Preterm PE less than 34 weeks occurred in 1.65% of participants in the aspirin group, compared with 4.3% in the placebo group, with an odds ratio 0.38 (95% confidence interval, 0.20–0.74).[43]

In the United States, LDA is available as an 81 mg formulation and is the most used dose in clinical practice. In 2014, US Preventive Services Task Force (USPSTF) concluded that there was adequate evidence supporting the use of LDA (60 to 150 mg/d) for the prevention of PE in individuals at high risk for the disease.[44] In 2019, the American College of Obstetricians and Gynecologists recommended that patients with high-risk factors for PE (previous pregnancy with PE, multifetal gestation, renal disease, autoimmune disease, type 1 or type 2 diabetes mellitus, and chronic hypertension) and those with more than one of the moderate-risk factors (first pregnancy, maternal age of 35 years or older, a body mass index of more than 30, family history of PE, sociodemographic characteristics, and personal history factors) should receive LDA (81 mg/d) for PE prophylaxis, initiated between 12 weeks and 28 weeks of gestation (optimally before 16 weeks of gestation) and continued until delivery.[45] In 2021, USPSTF conducted an updated systematic review on effectiveness of LDA for PE prevention and concluded that LDA (81 mg/d) should be used as preventative medicine for PE after 12 weeks of gestation in persons who are at high risk.[46]

Due to the benefit of LDA in reducing the incidence of PE, its safety profile, and low cost, multiple studies were published suggesting its universal use in pregnancy.[47,48] This practice has not been endorsed by professional societies and the benefits of universal LDA use have not been studied in randomized trials. Previous trials in which LDA was prescribed for low-risk pregnant patients did not show a reduction in the incidence of PE. However, an increased frequency of bleeding episodes and low compliance with LDA were reported.[49,50]

Safety Data

LDA is safe to use in pregnancy. A systematic review from the US Preventative Services Task Force in 2021 concluded that LDA usage was not associated with maternal or neonatal adverse effects, within an 18-year follow-up period.[46] There was no association between LDA use and congenital anomalies, premature closure of the ductus arteriosus, persistent pulmonary hypertension of the newborn, neonatal intracranial hemorrhage, or neonatal bleeding complications.[51,52] Similarly, no association was observed between LDA and placental abruption, postpartum hemorrhage, or estimated blood loss.[51] However, a recent meta-analysis reported higher risk of placental abruption when aspirin was started after 16 weeks of gestation.[53] Clinically, it is preferred to temporarily halt aspirin in pregnant people who have vaginal bleeding until its resolution. There is no contraindication for regional anesthesia in patients on LDA at time of delivery because an increased risk of spinal hematomas in this population was not demonstrated.[54]

PRAVASTATIN
Background and Mechanism of Action

Statins are competitive inhibitors of the enzyme 5-hydroxy-3-methylglutaryl-coenzyme A (HMG-CoA) reductase. HMG-CoA reductase converts HMG-CoA to mevalonate.[55] This reaction is a rate-limiting step in the synthesis of cholesterol. Hence, by inhibiting HMG-CoA reductase, statins play a role in decreasing cholesterol levels.[56] Pravastatin is a first-generation statin. It is one of the most hydrophilic, hepatoselective, and weakest inhibitors of HMG-CoA reductase.[57,58]

Statins decrease the production of TxA2 and inhibit platelet adhesion.[57] In animal models, pravastatin has been shown to play a role in reversing the angiogenic imbalance, which contributes to PE, by increasing the production of PlGF and VEGF while inhibiting the production of sFlt-1 and sEng.[59,60] In addition, pravastatin restores trophoblast invasiveness, improves placental blood flow, and has anti-inflammatory and anticoagulant properties[61,62]; making pravastatin a very promising medication for the prevention of PE.

Clinical Data and Implications

Initial human studies, which were limited to small series, pilot studies, and case reports, were promising.[63–66] Costantine and colleagues, for the *Eunice Kennedy Shriver*

National Institute of Child Health and Human Development Obstetric-Fetal Pharmacology Research Units Network, showed in a multicenter, double-blind, placebo-controlled, randomized pilot trial that the use of 10 mg of pravastatin reduced the rate of PE and preterm delivery in patients with history of PE that required delivery before 34 weeks, compared with placebo. The use of pravastatin was not associated with an increased maternal or fetal/neonatal safety risks.[66] Lefkou and colleagues reported, in a prospective cohort of 21 women with antiphospholipid syndrome and poor obstetric history, that adding 20 mg of pravastatin to LDA and low-molecular weight heparin (LMWH) prolonged pregnancy by almost 10 weeks and improved birthweight and neonatal outcomes.[64] Similarly, Kupferminc and colleagues, showed that the addition of 20 mg of pravastatin to LDA and LMWH was associated with improved outcomes in patients with severe recurrent placenta-mediated complications.[67]

More recently, the INOVASIA trial, a multicenter randomized, open label, controlled trial of pregnant people at high risk of developing PE, randomized participants to pravastatin (2 × 20 mg oral daily) in addition to a standard regimen of aspirin (80 mg) and calcium (1 g) from 14 to 20 weeks until delivery versus aspirin and calcium alone. People who received pravastatin had lower rates of preterm PE (13.8% vs 26.7%) and preterm delivery less than 37 weeks (16.1% vs 36%) as well as improved neonatal outcomes compared with those who received standard of care.[68] Another randomized trial studied the effect of 20 mg of pravastatin on the incidence of PE when started between 35 and 37 weeks of gestation in patients at high risk of term PE.[69] In this trial, pravastatin did not reduce the incidence of delivery with PE, and there was no significant adverse effects with the use of pravastatin when compared with the control group.[69]

Safety Data

In nonpregnant people, statin-associated muscle symptoms have been reported in 0.1% to 0.2% of users. They include myalgias and muscle weakness, and typically affect the thighs, calves, buttocks, and back muscles.[70] In another study, myalgia incidence ranged from 0.6% to 10.9% with pravastatin use.[71] In very rare cases, statins can be associated with drug-induced liver injury, with an incidence of approximately 1 per 100,000 and rhabdomyolysis with an incidence of less than 1%.[70] Data regarding maternal safety of pravastatin use in pregnancy are limited to the more recent trials and cohorts, which showed similar rates of adverse and serious adverse events between pravastatin and placebo groups with the most common side effect among patients who received pravastatin in the US pilot study being headache, heartburn, and musculoskeletal pain.[66]

Statins were initially classified as pregnancy category X by the Food and Drug Administration (FDA) due to theoretic concern for teratogenic effects and lack of indications to use in pregnancy.[57] More recent data, including systematic reviews and meta-analyses, did not show any significant increase in rates of congenital anomalies, stillbirth, or spontaneous abortions with the use of statins in pregnancy.[57,72] Finally, using data from more than 800,000 pregnant women enrolled in the Medicaid program, Bateman and colleagues compared the outcomes of 1152 women exposed to statins during the first trimester with those not exposed. Using propensity score analysis and after controlling for confounders, particularly preexisting diabetes, there was no increased risk of congenital malformation (adjusted odds ratio [aOR] 1.07; 95% CI 0.85–1.37) or organ-specific malformations.[73] Moreover, data from the recent human studies, in which pravastatin was used for a much longer duration, support its safety in pregnancy. These studies did not show any increased rate of fetal or neonatal adverse events. Moreover, neonates exposed to pravastatin in-utero had similar concentrations of cord blood markers for neurologic injury, steroidogenic hormones, and liver enzymes compared with neonates born to women who in the control/placebo groups. Additionally, all newborns exposed to pravastatin passed either an auditory brain stem response or otoacoustic emissions test before discharge from the hospital after birth.[66] Moreover, although statins decrease maternal cholesterol levels, no effect has been shown on fetal cholesterol levels or fetal weight with the use of pravastatin in pregnancy.[66] In July 2021, the FDA removed the strongest warning against using statins during pregnancy.[74]

SUMMARY

PE remains a major cause of maternal and neonatal morbidity and mortality. Advances in research have led to the investigation of multiple agents that can play a role in its prevention and treatment. Although LDA has been used for several years for this purpose, identifying the optimal LDA protocol regarding dosage and timing is still an important target for future studies. Meanwhile, pravastatin has emerged as a potential agent for the prevention of PE, with more randomized trials published in recent years supporting its effectiveness and safety. Research into this topic is still needed, to better elucidate the pathology of the disease and develop targeted therapies with a limited side-effect profile.

CLINICS CARE POINTS

- LDA use is recommended for the prevention of PE in high-risk pregnancies. However, the optimal LDA protocol regarding dosage and timing is yet to be determined.
- Pravastatin is a promising agent for prevention/treatment of PE. Its use has not been recommended yet by professional societies, with more research and evidence being conducted.

DISCLOSURE

M.M. Costantine is supported by a grant from The Eunice Kennedy Shriver National Institute of Child Health and Human Development (grant number: UG1HD027915) and the National Heart, Lung, and Blood Institute, United States (grant number: UG3HL140131). This article does not necessarily represent the official views of the NICHD, NHLBI, or the National Institute of Health. The authors report no conflicts of interest.

REFERENCES

1. Steegers EA, Von Dadelszen P, Duvekot JJ, et al. Pre-eclampsia. Lancet 2010; 376:631–44.
2. Espinoza J, Vidaeff A, Pettker CM, et al. ACOG Practice Bulletin No. 202: Gestational Hypertension and Preeclampsia. Obstet Gynecol 2019;133(1):e1–25.
3. Ronsmans C, Graham WJ. Maternal mortality: who, when, where, and why. Lancet 2006;368:1189–200.
4. Khan KS, Wojdyla D, Say L, et al. WHO analysis of causes of maternal death: a systematic review. Lancet 2006;367:1066–74.
5. Duley L. The Global Impact of Pre-eclampsia and Eclampsia. Semin Perinatol 2009;33:130–7.

6. MacKay AP, Berg CJ, Duran C, et al. An assessment of pregnancy-related mortality in the United States. Paediatr Perinat Epidemiol 2005;19:206–14.
7. Wang A, Rana S, Karumanchi SA. Preeclampsia: the role of angiogenic factors in its pathogenesis. Physiology (Bethesda) 2009;24:147–58.
8. Stevens W, Shih T, Incerti D, et al. Short-term costs of preeclampsia to the United States health care system. Am J Obstet Gynecol 2017;217(3):237–248 e216.
9. Centers for Disease Control and Prevention. Meeting the challenges of measuring and preventing maternal mortality in the United States. Public Health Grand Rounds. Available at: https://www.cdc.gov/grand-rounds/pp/2017/20171114-maternal-mortality.html. Accessed June 6, 2022.
10. Howell EA. Reducing disparities in severe maternal morbidity and mortality. Clin Obstet Gynecol 2018;61(2):387–99.
11. Cunningham F, Leveno K, Bloom F, et al. Williams obstetrics. 24th edition. New York: McGraw-Hill Education; 2014.
12. Roberts JM, Hubel CA. The two stage model of preeclampsia: variations on the theme. Placenta 2009;30(Suppl A):S32–7.
13. Sargent IL, Germain SJ, Sacks GP, et al. Trophoblast deportation and the maternal inflammatory response in pre-eclampsia. J Reprod Immunol 2003;59:153–60.
14. Walsh SW. Eicosanoids in preeclampsia. Prostaglandins Leukot Essent Fatty Acids 2004;70:223–32.
15. Walsh SW. Preeclampsia: an imbalance in placental prostacyclin and thromboxane production. Am J Obstet Gynecol 1985;152(3):335–40.
16. Moncada S, Vane JR. Arachidonic Acid Metabolites and the Interactions between Platelets and Blood-Vessel Walls. N Engl J Med 1979;300:1142–7.
17. Mills JL, DerSimonian R, Raymond E, et al. Prostacyclin and thromboxane changes predating clinical onset of preeclampsia: A multicenter prospective study. J Am Med Assoc 1999;282(4):356–62.
18. Bdolah Y, Sukhatme VP, Karumanchi SA. Angiogenic imbalance in the pathophysiology of preeclampsia: Newer insights. In: Seminars in Nephrology. ; 2004.
19. Zeisler H, Llurba E, Chantraine F, et al. Predictive Value of the sFlt-1:PIGF Ratio in Women with Suspected Preeclampsia. N Engl J Med 2016;374(1):13–22.
20. Herraiz I, Llurba E, Verlohren S, et al. Update on the Diagnosis and Prognosis of Preeclampsia with the Aid of the sFlt-1/PIGF Ratio in Singleton Pregnancies. Fetal Diagn Ther 2018;43(2):81–9.
21. Levine RJ, Lam C, Qian C, et al. Soluble endoglin and other circulating antiangiogenic factors in preeclampsia. N Engl J Med 2006;355:992–1005.
22. Roberts JM. Pathophysiology of ischemic placental disease. Semin Perinatol 2014;38(3):139–45.
23. Atallah A, Lecarpentier E, Goffinet F, et al. Aspirin for prevention of preeclampsia. Drugs 2017;77:1819–31.
24. Vane JR. Inhibition of prostaglandin synthesis as a mechanism of action for aspirin-like drugs. Nat New Biol 1971;231:232–5.
25. Majed BH, Khalil RA. Molecular Mechanisms Regulating the Vascular Prostacyclin Pathways and Their Adaptation during Pregnancy and in the Newborn. Pharmacol Rev 2012;64(3):540–82.
26. Paul BZS, Jin J, Kunapuli SP. Molecular mechanism of thromboxane A2-induced platelet aggregation. J Biol Chem 1999;274(41):29108–14.
27. Patrick J, Dillaha L, Armas D, et al. A randomized trial to assess the pharmacodynamics and pharmacokinetics of a single dose of an extended-release aspirin formulation. Postgrad Med 2015;127:573–80.

28. Lin L, Li G, Zhang W, et al. Low-dose aspirin reduces hypoxia-induced sFlt1 release via the JNK/AP-1 pathway in human trophoblast and endothelial cells. J Cell Physiol 2019;234(10):18928–41.
29. Li C, Raikwar NS, Santillan MK, et al. Aspirin inhibits expression of sFLT1 from human cytotrophoblasts induced by hypoxia, via cyclo-oxygenase 1. Placenta 2015;36(4):446–53.
30. Patrono C, Ciabattoni G, Pinca E, et al. Low dose aspirin and inhibition of thromboxane B2 production in healthy subjects. Thromb Res 1980;17(3–4):317–27.
31. Gonzalez-Brown VM, Ma'ayeh M, Kniss DA, et al. Low-dose aspirin increases 15-epi-lipoxins A4 in pregnancies at high-risk for developing preeclampsia. Pregnancy Hypertens 2021;26:75–8.
32. Crandon AJ, Isherwood DM. Effect of aspirin on incidence of preeclampsia. Lancet 1979;1:1356.
33. Caritis S, Sibai B, Hauth J, et al. Low-dose aspirin to prevent preeclampsia in women at high risk. N Engl J Med 1998;338(11):701–5.
34. CLASP (Collaborative Low-dose Aspirin Study in Pregnancy) Collaborative Group. CLASP: a randomised trial of low-dose aspirin for the prevention and treatment of pre-eclampsia among 9364 pregnant women. Lancet 1994; 343(8898):619–29.
35. Sibai BM, Caritis SN, Thom E, et al. Prevention of preeclampsia with low-dose aspirin in healthy, nulliparous pregnant women. N Engl J Med 1993;329(17): 1213–8.
36. Roberge S, Bujold E, Nicolaides KH. Aspirin for the prevention of preterm and term preeclampsia: systematic review and metaanalysis. Am J Obstet Gynecol 2018;218(3):287–93.e1.
37. Meher S, Duley L, Hunter K, et al. Antiplatelet therapy before or after 16 weeks' gestation for preventing preeclampsia: an individual participant data meta-analysis. Am J Obstet Gynecol 2017;216(2):121–8.e2.
38. Roberge S, Nicolaides K, Demers S, et al. The role of aspirin dose on the prevention of preeclampsia and fetal growth restriction: systematic review and meta-analysis. Am J Obstet Gynecol 2017;216(2):110–20.e6.
39. Rolnik DL, Wright D, Poon LCY, et al. ASPRE trial: performance of screening for preterm pre-eclampsia. Ultrasound Obstet Gynecol 2017;50:492–5.
40. Rolnik DL, O'Gorman N, Roberge S, et al. Early screening and prevention of preterm pre-eclampsia with aspirin: time for clinical implementation. Ultrasound Obstet Gynecol 2017;50:551–6.
41. Poon LCY, Kametas NA, Maiz N, et al. First-trimester prediction of hypertensive disorders in pregnancy. Hypertension 2009;53(5):812–8.
42. Committee Opinion No. 638. American college of obstetricians and gynecologists. first-trimester risk assessment for early-onset preeclampsia. Obstet Gynecol 2015;126:e25–7.
43. Rolnik DL, Wright D, Poon L, et al. Aspirin versus placebo in pregnancies at high risk for preterm pre-eclampsia. N Engl J Med 2017;377(7):613–22.
44. LeFevre ML. Low-dose aspirin use for the prevention of morbidity and mortality from preeclampsia: U.S. Preventive Services Task Force recommendation statement. Ann Intern Med 2014;161(11):819–26.
45. ACOG Practice Bulletin No. 202. Gestational hypertension and preeclampsia. Obstet Gynecol 2019;133(1):1.
46. Henderson JT, Vesco KK, Senger CA, et al. Aspirin use to prevent preeclampsia and related morbidity and mortality: updated evidence report and systematic review for the us preventive services task force. JAMA 2021;326(12):1192–206.

47. Ayala NK, Rouse DJ. A nudge toward universal aspirin for preeclampsia prevention. Obstet Gynecol 2019;133(4):725–8.
48. Werner EF, Hauspurg AK, Rouse DJ. A cost-benefit analysis of low-dose aspirin prophylaxis for the prevention of preeclampsia in the United States. Obstet Gynecol 2015;126(6):1242–50.
49. Subtil D, Goeusse P, Puech F, et al. Aspirin (100 mg) used for prevention of pre-eclampsia in nulliparous women: the Essai Regional Aspirine Mere-Enfant study (Part 1). BJOG 2003;110:475–84.
50. Rotchell YE, Cruickshank JK, Gay MP, et al. Barbados Low Dose Aspirin Study in Pregnancy (BLASP): a randomised trial for the prevention of pre-eclampsia and its complications. Br J Obstet Gynaecol 1998;105:286–92.
51. Henderson JT, Whitlock EP, O'Connor E, et al. Low-dose aspirin for prevention of morbidity and mortality from preeclampsia: a systematic evidence review for the U.S. preventive services task force. Ann Intern Med 2014;160:695–703.
52. Duley L, Henderson-Smart DJ, Meher S, et al. Antiplatelet agents for preventing pre-eclampsia and its complications. Cochrane Database Syst Rev 2007;2: CD004659.
53. Roberge S, Bujold E, Nicolaides KH. Meta-analysis on the effect of aspirin use for prevention of preeclampsia on placental abruption and antepartum hemorrhage. Am J Obstet Gynecol 2018;218:483–9.
54. Horlocker TT, Vandermeulen E, Kopp SL, et al. Regional anesthesia in the patient receiving antithrombotic or thrombolytic therapy: american society of regional anesthesia and pain medicine evidence-based guidelines (4th edition). Reg Anesth Pain Med 2018;43:263–309.
55. Caniggia I, Post M, Ermini L. Statins, Mevalonate Pathway and its Intermediate Products in Placental Development and Preeclampsia. Curr Mol Pharmacol 2016;10:152–60.
56. Istvan ES, Deisenhofer J. Structural mechanism for statin inhibition of HMG-CoA reductase. Science 2001;292(5519):1160–4.
57. Esteve-Valverde E, Ferrer-Oliveras R, Gil-Aliberas N, et al. Pravastatin for preventing and treating preeclampsia: a systematic review. Obstet Gynecol Surv 2018; 73(1):40–55.
58. Nanovskaya TN, Patrikeeva SL, Paul J, et al. Transplacental transfer and distribution of pravastatin. Am J Obstet Gynecol 2013;209(373):e1–5.
59. Kumasawa K, Ikawa M, Kidoya H, et al. Pravastatin induces placental growth factor (PGF) and ameliorates preeclampsia in a mouse model. Proc Natl Acad Sci 2010;108(4):1451–5.
60. Costantine MM, Tamayo E, Lu F, et al. Using pravastatin to improve the vascular reactivity in a mouse model of soluble Fms-like tyrosine kinase-1-induced preeclampsia. Obstet Gynecol 2010;116(116):114–20.
61. Girardi G. Pravastatin to treat and prevent preeclampsia. Preclinical and clinical studies. J Reprod Immunol 2017;124:15–20.
62. Bauer AJ, Banek CT, Needham K, et al. Pravastatin attenuates hypertension, oxidative stress, and angiogenic imbalance in rat model of placental ischemia-induced hypertension. Hypertension 2013;61:1103–10.
63. Lefkou E, Mamopoulos A, Fragakis N, et al. Clinical Improvement and Successful Pregnancy in a Preeclamptic Patient With Antiphospholipid Syndrome Treated With Pravastatin. Hypertension 2014;63:e118–9.
64. Lefkou E, Mamopoulos A, Dagklis T, et al. Pravastatin improves pregnancy outcomes in obstetric antiphospholipid syndrome refractory to antithrombotic therapy. J Clin Invest 2016;126(8):2933–40.

65. Brownfoot FC, Tong S, Hannan NJ, et al. Effects of Pravastatin on Human Placenta, Endothelium, and Women with Severe Preeclampsia. Hypertension 2015;66:687–97.
66. Costantine MM, Cleary K, Hebert MF, et al. Safety and pharmacokinetics of pravastatin used for the prevention of preeclampsia in high-risk pregnant women: A pilot randomized controlled trial. Am J Obstet Gynecol 2016;214(720):e1–17.
67. Kupferminc MJ, Kliger C, Rimon E, et al. Pravastatin is useful for prevention of recurrent severe placenta-mediated complications - a pilot study. J Matern Fetal Neonatal Med 2021;1–7. https://doi.org/10.1080/14767058.2021.1940940.
68. Akbar MIA, Azis MA, Riu DS, et al. INOVASIA study: a multicenter randomized clinical trial of pravastatin to prevent preeclampsia in high-risk patients. Am J Perinatol 2022. https://doi.org/10.1055/a-1798-1925 [published online ahead of print, 2022 Jun 6].
69. Döbert M, Varouxaki AN, Mu AC, et al. Pravastatin Versus Placebo in Pregnancies at High Risk of Term Preeclampsia. Circulation 2021;144(9):670–9.
70. Mach F, Ray KK, Wiklund O, et al. Adverse effects of statin therapy: perception vs. the evidence - focus on glucose homeostasis, cognitive, renal and hepatic function, haemorrhagic stroke and cataract. Eur Heart J 2018;39(27):2526–39.
71. Bruckert E, Hayem G, Dejager S, et al. Mild to moderate muscular symptoms with high-dosage statin therapy in hyperlipidemic patients–the PRIMO study. Cardiovasc Drugs Ther 2005;19(6):403–14.
72. Karalis DG, Hill AN, Clifton S, et al. The risks of statin use in pregnancy: A systematic review. J Clin Lipidol 2016;10(5):1081–90.
73. Bateman BT, Hernandez-Diaz S, Fischer MA, et al. Statins and congenital malformations: cohort study. BMJ 2015;350:h1035.
74. US Food and Drug Administration. FDA requests removal of strongest warning against using cholesterol-lowering statins during pregnancy; still advises most pregnant patients should stop taking statins. Available at: https://www.fda.gov/drugs/drug-safety-and-availability/fda-requests-removal-strongest-warning-against-using-cholesterol-lowering-statins-during-pregnancy. Accessed June 29, 2022.

Magnesium Sulfate Use in Pregnancy for Preeclampsia Prophylaxis and Fetal Neuroprotection

Regimens in High-Income and Low/Middle-Income Countries

Kathleen F. Brookfield, MD, PhD, MPH[a,b,*],
Osinakachukwu Mbata, MD[a]

KEYWORDS

- Pharmacokinetics • Pharmacodynamics • Magnesium sulfate
- Fetal neuroprotection • Preeclampsia

KEY POINTS

- In the setting of preeclampsia and eclampsia, lower dose magnesium regimens that do not reach historically held therapeutic range serum magnesium levels may reduce the likelihood for toxicity without reducing clinical efficacy.
- In the setting of preeclampsia and eclampsia, intramuscular dosing has been shown to be effective therapy in resource-limited countries.
- Multiple IV magnesium sulfate regimens have demonstrated benefit for fetal neuroprotection in the very preterm neonate; however, data are lacking on optimal dosing for this indication.

INTRODUCTION

Magnesium sulfate heptahydrate ($MgSO_4 \cdot 7H_2O$), one of the most commonly used medications in obstetrics, is an inorganic salt. It is manufactured by dissolution of kieserite in water and subsequent crystallization of the heptahydrate. Magnesium sulfate occurs naturally in seawater, mineral springs, and minerals.

[a] Department of Obstetrics and Gynecology, Oregon Health & Science University, 3181 Southwest Sam Jackson Park Road, Portland, OR 97239, USA; [b] Legacy Medical Group, Maternal Fetal Medicine, Legacy Health System, Portland, OR, USA
* Corresponding author. Department of Obstetrics and Gynecology, Oregon Health & Science University, 3181 Southwest Sam Jackson Park Road, Portland, OR 97239.
E-mail address: brookfie@ohsu.edu

Obstet Gynecol Clin N Am 50 (2023) 89–99
https://doi.org/10.1016/j.ogc.2022.10.003
0889-8545/23/© 2022 Elsevier Inc. All rights reserved.

obgyn.theclinics.com

Although standardized magnesium sulfate treatment protocols were initially proposed for eclamptic seizure prophylaxis, magnesium has also been noted to have neuroprotective and tocolytic properties.[1–5] The mechanism by which magnesium works for eclampsia prophylaxis and cerebral palsy prevention is not fully understood but thought to be a consequence of magnesium's effects on smooth muscle relaxation, peripheral vasodilation, and inhibition of calcium channel activity within the N-methyl-D-aspartate (NMDA) receptor resulting in a reflexive increase in cardiac output.[6,7]

Until somewhat recently, knowledge of magnesium pharmacokinetics (PK) and pharmacodynamics (PD) in pregnant women was limited, with standardized protocols administered to all patients, without adjustments for maternal or fetal factors that may affect serum magnesium levels or produce undesirable effects. Through prospective PK/PD modeling, the impact of factors such as mode of magnesium administration, maternal age, renal function, maternal body weight, and indication for magnesium administration has been further elucidated and allowed obstetricians to tailor the administration of the drug in the setting of changes to these covariates.[8–13] Additionally, PK/PD modeling has allowed for the exploration of how regimens might be adjusted in resource-poor areas to maximize desired outcomes of seizure prophylaxis and fetal neuroprotection while minimizing undesired effects or toxicities of the drug.[14,15]

Existing Pharmacokinetic and Pharmacodynamic Modeling

The comparative efficacy of different magnesium sulfate protocols for both preeclampsia and fetal neuroprotection is unclear, with many variations of regimens used in high-income and low and middle-income countries (LMICs).[5,16] Historically, magnesium sulfate dosing was empiric. In the setting of preeclampsia, patients with serum magnesium levels between 4.8 and 8.4 mg/dL demonstrated a low likelihood of eclampsia.[5,17,18] Common regimens that achieved these serum levels for most patients have also been administered for the purposes of fetal neuroprotection; however, there is sparse data to support an optimal therapeutic serum magnesium level for this indication.[14] When magnesium sulfate is administered intravenously, the onset of action is immediate and lasts for approximately 30 minutes. Following intramuscular (IM) administration, the onset of action occurs within 1 hour and the duration of action is 3 to 4 hours.[11,16] The onset of action, half-life, and steady-state concentrations are similar for nonpregnant and pregnant women; however, these parameters are altered by renal impairment in preeclampsia.[9]

The warning signs of toxicity in the mother include the loss of patellar reflexes occurring at plasma concentrations between 3.8 and 5 mmol/L (9.2–12 mg/dL).[19] More serious toxicities include alterations in cardiac conduction and cardiac arrest, which can be expected at serum concentrations greater than 7.5 mmol/L (18 mg/dL) and 12.5 mmol/L (30 mg/dL), respectively.[20]

PK/PD models have used concentration-time profile data of individuals to describe magnesium disposition in pregnant women who received common magnesium sulfate dosing regimens for either preeclampsia or fetal neuroprotection. A summary of PK modeling of magnesium sulfate is demonstrated in **Fig. 1**.

All modeling with reported covariates has concluded that maternal weight and serum creatinine affect magnesium disposition in the setting of preeclampsia. Only one PK model included patients who received magnesium for fetal neuroprotection, and in this setting, weight and creatinine again influenced maternal serum magnesium levels.[9]

Parameter	Model 1	Model 2	Model 3	Model 4	Model 5	Model 6
	(N = 116)	(N = 51)	(N = 258)	(N = 111)	(N = 10,280)	(N = 109)
Clearance (L/hr)	4.28	5.0	4.81	3.98	3.72	1.38
Volume of distribution (L)	32.3	$V_{central}$ = 24 $V_{peripheral}$ = 25	15.6	22.5	$V_{central}$ = 15.4 $V_{peripheral}$ = 17.0	13.3
Intercompartmental clearance (L/hr)	----	5.6	----	----	3.66	--
Covariates	Not reported	Not reported	Weight, serum Cr	Gestational age, pre-eclampsia vs. no pre-eclampsia, weight, serum Cr, antepartum vs. postpartum	Weight, serum Cr	Weight, serum Cr
Reference	Chuan 2001	Lu 2002	Salinger 2013	Brookfield 2016	Du 2019	Da Costa 2020

Fig. 1. Summary of magnesium sulfate PK models. (*Data from* Refs.[8–13])

The application of the existing PK models to explore magnesium PD has been limited but there has been an effort to determine how the dose and duration of magnesium sulfate can be adjusted to maximize eclampsia prevention and prevent cerebral palsy in large cohorts of patients where these outcomes were studied. Two of these studies based on PK modeling are noted in **Fig. 2**.[14,15]

Magnesium for Eclampsia Prevention and Preeclampsia Management

Magnesium sulfate is widely accepted as a life-saving drug for preventing progression of preeclampsia to eclampsia and avoiding associated complications.[21] The recommendation to administer magnesium sulfate for the prevention of eclamptic seizures is based on 2 key publications: the landmark Magpie randomized trial (10,141 women) showing a 58% reduction in eclamptic seizures with standard magnesium sulfate regimens versus placebo (relative risk [RR] 0.42; 95% CI 0.29, 0.60); and a Cochrane review (6 trials, 11,444 women) demonstrating a similar reduction in eclamptic seizures (RR 0.41; 95% CI 0.29, 0.58) with the standard magnesium sulfate regimens versus placebo.[21,22] In both the Magpie trial and the Cochrane review, standard regimens included the Zuspan and the Pritchard regimens. Both regimens have complex dose calculations, and in both, the initial loading dose is administered intravenously. Subsequent maintenance doses are provided either as continuous intravenous (IV) infusion (Zuspan regimen) or as IM injections every 4 hours (Pritchard regimen) for 24 hours. The standard regimens have a 5-fold higher adverse side-effect rate compared with placebo.[22]

High-income countries

Despite the increased costs associated with the IV regimen's requirement for a continuous infusion pump and need for continuous monitoring, the associated injection site pain and rare, but significant, side effect of abscess formation associated with the cheaper IM regimen, make the IV regimen preferred in resource-rich settings.[23]

	Model 1	Model 2
Outcome of interest	Eclampsia	Cerebral palsy
Cohort description to which PK modeling applied	5290 women with preeclampsia (Magpie and Thailand study participants) who received magnesium sulfate, either Zuspan regimen, Pritchard regimen, or 4g IV loading dose followed by 2g/hr x 24 hours. Efficacy criteria of modeling included those regimens with resultant predicted eclampsia rates $\leq 0.7\%$, which was the overall observed eclampsia rate in magnesium sulfate treated women.	1905 women (BEAM Trial) who received magnesium sulfate within 12 hours of delivery, 6g IV loading dose, followed by 2g/hr maintenance dose up to 12 hours.
Risk reduction findings	IV regimens with predicted eclampsia rates $\leq 0.7\%$: 1. 4g in 20 mins, 1g/hr x 24 hrs (Zuspan regimen) 2. 4g in 20 mins, 2g/hr x 24 hrs 3. 6g in 20 mins, 2g/hr x 24 hrs 4. 12g in 120 mins, 3g/hr x 12 hrs 5. 12g in 120 mins, 2g/hr x 8 hrs 6. 8g in 60 mins, 2g/hr x 10 hrs. IM regimens with predicted eclampsia rates $\leq 0.7\%$: 1. 4g IV/10g IM, 5g IM q 4 hrs x 5 doses (Pritchard regimen) 2. 4g IV/10g IM, 8g IM q 6 hrs x 3 doses 3. 4g IV/10g IM, 10g IM Q 8 hrs x 2 doses 4. 4g IV/10g IM, 5g IM Q 4 hrs x 2 doses 5. 10g IM Q 8 hrs x 3 doses	Simulated serum magnesium concentration with lowest probability (95% CI) of cerebral palsy = 4.1 mg/dL (3.7, 4.4). Simulated total dose associated with lowest probability (95% CI) of cerebral palsy = 64g (30, 98).
Covariates	Gestational age, pre-eclampsia vs. no pre-eclampsia, weight, serum Cr, antepartum vs. postpartum	Weight, serum Cr
Reference	Du 2019	Brookfield 2017

Fig. 2. Summary of magnesium sulfate PD models. (*Data from* Refs.[14,15])

Common IV regimens reported in the literature include the following: Zuspan (4 g IV loading dose, followed by maintenance dose of 1 g/h); a 4 g IV loading dose, followed by a maintenance dose of 2 g/h; and a 6 g IV loading dose, followed by a maintenance dose of 2 g/h.[10,11,24–26] A review of these IV regimens and other modified regimens based on these, demonstrated wide variation in the ability to achieve the suggested therapeutic serum magnesium levels and variation in the duration of dosing required to obtain suggested therapeutic serum magnesium levels when the drug was administered for eclamptic seizure prophylaxis.[16] Although the common Zuspan regimen (4 g IV loading dose, followed by maintenance dose of 1 g/h) often did not result in serum magnesium levels of 4.8 mg/dL (or 2 mmol/L), the regimen was still protective against eclampsia.

In an examination of estimated serum magnesium levels when the Zuspan regimen is administered, Du and colleagues[15] applied PK modeling to preeclamptic women participating in the Magpie trial and found serum levels in patients who did not experience eclampsia were significantly lower than those historically reported to be therapeutic for eclampsia prevention.

Hence, although the standard Zuspan regimen does not consistently result in serum levels between 4.8 and 8.4 mg/dL, PK/PD data suggest a likely wider therapeutic window than previously accepted. Dosing regimens using a higher loading or maintenance dose in average-weight patients with normal renal function may increase the likelihood for magnesium toxicity without significantly improving clinical efficacy.[15,16]

Low-income and middle-income countries
The global incidence of preeclampsia ranges between 2% and 10%; however, the rate is up to 7 times higher in LMICs compared with high-income countries.[27,28] Therefore, the use of PK/PD data to address the challenges of selecting appropriate magnesium sulfate dosing regimens in LMICs is of particular interest.

Practical challenges to the administration of magnesium sulfate in LMICs include the relative cost of the drug, the skill required to administer IV regimens, and fears surrounding the drug's toxicity.[28] One specific strategy for expanding the use of magnesium sulfate for preeclampsia and eclampsia in LMICs is to expedite the delivery of the medication in settings without skilled health-care workers or necessary equipment for IV administration. Shifting the use of magnesium sulfate by expansion to facilities attended by health workers with minimal training could optimize pregnancy outcomes for affected women. This makes the examination of IM magnesium regimens particularly important for resource-poor settings.

The Pritchard regimen is the generally accepted regimen in countries with limited resources. It consists of a 4 g IV loading dose given concurrently with a 10 g IM loading dose, followed by a 5 g IM dose administered every 4 hours.[16,22,29] The Magpie trial demonstrated the efficacy of this regimen for eclampsia prevention and determined the regimen was equally efficacious for eclampsia prevention when compared with the IV-only Zuspan regimen.[22] Just as modifications to the IV Zuspan regimen are commonly reported, many practitioners in LMICs omit the IV portion of the Pritchard regimen and administer only the 10 g IM loading dose, followed by the 5 g IM maintenance dose every 4 hours.[16] PK modeling of other IM-predominant or IM-only regimens suggests serum magnesium levels fluctuate greatly over the course of magnesium administration. This often results in serum magnesium levels less than those previously held as therapeutic.[12,16]

Yet, also like IV magnesium administration, the serum magnesium levels achieved by IM dosing seem to be sufficient for the prevention of eclampsia. The exposure–response model published by Du and colleagues,[15] 2019, found that women who received the Pritchard regimen as part of the Magpie trial and had minimal seizure risk had modeled serum magnesium levels between 1.65 and 2.73 mmol/L. Additional adjustments to Du's PK model, which was based on data collection from women receiving IV regimens, were made based on newer concentration–time profile data from women in Nigeria who received the Pritchard regimen. The new model demonstrated little variation when compared with the original model and further supported the findings of the Du and colleagues.[30] The PK/PD data from these reported studies can also be used to predict eclampsia response with other modifications to IM regimens. Although PK/PD modeling point toward alterations in dosing that provide clinical efficacy despite resulting in lower than anticipated serum values necessary for seizure prevention, future studies must also consider the influence of mode of administration and magnesium dosing on other side effects, including injection site pain, infection, and abscess formation. Existing data are also insufficient to highlight differences in efficacy between a standard 24-hour regimen and multiple proposed shorter ones.

Magnesium for Fetal Neuroprotection

Preterm birth is the leading cause of childhood mortality with roughly 1 million deaths occurring annually. This number is likely an underestimation given the difficulty of data acquisition in low-income countries.[31] Several studies have suggested a fetal neuroprotective benefit from the administration of magnesium sulfate when very preterm delivery (before 32 weeks' gestation) is anticipated.[2–4,32,33] These benefits are thought to come from magnesium sulfate's action as a calcium channel antagonist. This property at the neuronal synapse is thought to prevent excessive activation of NMDA receptors, resulting in a cascade of events that inhibit the proinflammatory pathway generally associated with ischemic injury.[34,35] Similar to the data for the use of magnesium sulfate for preeclampsia, magnesium dosing for fetal neuroprotection is variable and has not been traditionally based on PK or PD data. In fact, only one PK study included patients exclusively receiving magnesium sulfate for fetal neuroprotection; therefore, PK-based data for this indication are limited.[9] With nearly 1:1 ratio of maternal to fetal serum concentrations, detectable levels are appreciated in the fetal circulation regardless of the dosing protocol chosen.[9,23]

High-income countries

In resource-rich settings, the current standard of care is to administer IV magnesium sulfate based on findings from 3 large prospective randomized trials concluding there are fetal neuroprotective benefits when delivery is anticipated before 32 weeks' gestation.[2–4] Dosing regimen selection varies by region.

The most commonly accepted regimen for fetal neuroprotection in the United States is based on the BEAM trial, which used a 6 g IV loading dose administered over 20 to 30 minutes followed by an IV maintenance infusion of 2 g/h.[4] BEAM concluded that the rate of moderate or severe cerebral palsy was reduced in the magnesium group compared with the placebo group (1.9% vs 3.5%; $P = .03$). Other reported dosing regimens have included a 4 g IV loading dose administered during 20 minutes followed by a 1 g/h IV maintenance dose (ACTOMgSO4), as well as a 4 g IV bolus dose administered during 30 minutes without a maintenance dose (PREMAG trial).[2,3] The ACTOMgSO$_4$ trial found an association between reduced rates of motor dysfunction and magnesium administration in preterm deliveries before 30 weeks' gestation but did not find a significant difference in cerebral palsy incidence, specifically, between patients who received magnesium sulfate or placebo.[2] The PREMAG trial found reduced rates of white matter injury and mortality in the magnesium group but did not find a significant difference in the incidence of cerebral palsy between patients who received magnesium therapy versus those who received placebo.[3] None of the studies established an effective goal for serum magnesium concentration.

The PK model constructed by Brookfield and colleagues[9] included 23 women who received magnesium sulfate (4 g IV loading dose, followed by 2 g/h IV maintenance dose) for fetal neuroprotection. Nine of these patients had coexisting preeclampsia. The PK model suggested magnesium disposition was altered in patients without preeclampsia compared with those with preeclampsia. The PK model for patients without preeclampsia was then applied to the public use dataset released for participants in the BEAM trial. The incidence of cerebral palsy was minimized in patients who had received a total dose of magnesium sulfate of 64 g and those with a serum magnesium level of 4.1 mg/dL.[14] Although the application of the PK model to this dataset has limitations, the findings highlight that the total dose, duration of administration, and area under the curve are all important factors in exposure–response.

Low-income and middle-income countries

Of the roughly 15 million annual preterm births, 90% of them occur in low-income or middle-income countries.[31] Although the burden of preterm delivery is disproportionately felt by LMICs, most data examining this condition comes from high-income countries.[36,37] One small study looking at the prevalence in LMICs found high rates of severe forms of cerebral palsy, with 86% of cases being acquired in the antenatal or perinatal time.[37] Unlike with preeclampsia, alternate dosing studies have not been conducted in LMICs to specifically evaluate how dose alterations and mode of administration may influence the outcome of cerebral palsy.

No studies of IM magnesium administration have been conducted with fetal neuroprotective benefit as an outcome; however, it stands to reason that PK models based on IV magnesium dosing can be used to predict exposure–response from IM dosing regimens in the same way they have been used in predicting eclampsia. Application of PK modeling to the existing PREMAG and ACTOMgSO$_4$ trials would be useful to lend more robust data on whether alternate magnesium dosing regimens should target total magnesium dose, duration, or serum magnesium levels to maximize cerebral palsy risk reduction. Once this has been determined, alternate IM dosing protocols could be suggested to increase magnesium utilization and coverage for this indication in LMICs.

Important Covariates for Dosing Considerations

Dosing among obese women

Although the therapeutic range of maternal serum magnesium levels is likely wider than previously thought, prior studies have established a therapeutic target for the prevention of eclampsia. As previously stated, a paucity of such data exists for magnesium sulfate protocols in the setting of fetal neuroprotection. Among women with a body mass index (BMI) greater than 35, it has been demonstrated to take roughly twice as long to reach these therapeutic levels based on PK modeling.[9] A prospective randomized trial found that using a 6 g IV loading dose followed by a 2 g/h IV maintenance dose was more likely to achieve the historically held therapeutic serum magnesium levels without significant adverse maternal effects. Of note, no significant differences were observed with respect to neonatal outcomes or maternal side effects when this dosing was used compared with the lower dosing of the Zuspan regimen.[38] No prospective trials have been conducted with IM regimens among different BMI groups; however, PK modeling has accounted for maternal body weight in the assessment of alternate IM dosing.[11,12,15,30] Additional prospective study is needed to

		Preeclampsia	Fetal Neuroprotection
High-income country	BMI > 35 BMI <= 35	6g IV → 2g/hr 4g IV → 1–2g/hr	6g IV → 2g/hr 6g IV → 2g/hr
Low Middle-Income country	Unlimited IV Limited IV	4g IV → 1g/hr 10gIM + 4g IV → 5g IM q 4 h	4-6g IV → 1–2g/hr

- Renal impairment (Cr >1.2 mg/dL), eclampsia, diminished deep tendon reflexes, other concern for magnesium toxicity, check serum magnesium and consider decreasing magnesium maintenance dose or discontinue magnesium maintenance dose. Serum magnesium levels should be checked in these settings every 4 h with magnesium rebolused if serum magnesium is <4.8 mg/dL.

Fig. 3. Common magnesium dosing regimens.

validate an equivalent IM regimen to achieve therapeutic goals among obese women in LMICs. Proposed dosing regimens are outlined in **Fig. 3**.

Magnesium Administration in the Setting of Renal Dysfunction

Magnesium is primarily renally eliminated and when measures of renal function have been included as covariates in PK modeling, they have been found to significantly influence magnesium disposition.[9,11,12] A large PK model evaluating alternate magnesium sulfate regimens in women with preeclampsia by Du and colleagues[12] 2019 found that creatinine was significantly associated with maternal serum magnesium levels after the administration of both IV and IM regimens. The maintenance dose of magnesium sulfate seems to uniquely need adjustment when patients have elevated creatinine, and PK model construction has specifically excluded patients with creatinine elevated above 1.2 mg/dL. It is therefore prudent to exercise caution in any application of standard magnesium sulfate dosing protocols to patients with severely elevated creatinine because a continuous maintenance dose of magnesium sulfate may be associated with an increased risk for magnesium toxicity.

In the setting of normal renal function, the authors do not routinely check serum magnesium levels. Instead, deep tendon reflexes are assessed every hour. If the patient has eclampsia, displays diminished reflexes, complains of excessive symptoms, or has a serum creatinine greater than 1.2 mg/dL, serum magnesium levels are assessed, and magnesium dosing is adjusted. The decision to reduce the rate of the maintenance dosing or discontinue it entirely depends on the running maintenance dose and the level of elevation in serum creatinine. Although there is not sufficient PK data on patients with serum creatinine greater than 1.2 mg/dL to offer definitive recommendations, the authors typically administer a bolus dose only (either 4 g or 6 g depending on BMI), followed by serum magnesium assessment every 4 hours. If the serum magnesium level is less than 4.8 mg/dL 4 hours after the initial bolus is given, an additional magnesium bolus dose is administered at that time. Calcium gluconate should be readily available in all settings that treat obstetric patients to treat cardiac arrest or severe toxicity related to hypermagnesemia. The recommended dose of calcium gluconate is 15 mL 10% solution administered intravenously over 2 to 5 minutes.

SUMMARY

In conclusion, magnesium sulfate PK/PD studies have demonstrated that a variety of IV and IM regimens used consistently provide serum magnesium concentrations below those historically reported as therapeutic for eclampsia prophylaxis, yet are still effective. Additionally, there is a paucity of data on whether total magnesium dose, duration, or serum magnesium levels should be targeted to maximize the fetal neuroprotective benefit of magnesium sulfate administration. Existing models and data can be used to tailor treatment regimens to maximize efficacy and minimize toxicity in patients of different weights and renal function.

CLINICS CARE POINTS

- Multiple IV and IM regimens can be used to achieve therapeutic serum magnesium levels to prevent eclamptic seizures. The target serum level for efficacy is lower than historically reported.
- Therapeutic serum magnesium levels for the prevention of cerebral palsy are unknown but PK/PD data suggest some neuroprotective benefit with total doses of 64 g or serum magnesium levels between 3.7 and 4.4 mg/dL.
- PK modeling demonstrates that magnesium disposition is influenced by maternal weight and serum creatinine and these factors should be considered when choosing appropriate dosing regimens. Patients with higher BMI may need increased magnesium doses to achieve therapeutic serum magnesium levels. Consider limited/lower maintenance dosing to avoid magnesium toxicities in patients with elevated serum creatinine.

DISCLOSURES

Dr K.F. Brookfield has received funds from the NIH Loan Repayment Award, a departmental Mission Support Award, and the World Health Organization for past magnesium sulfate research and travel. Dr O. Mbata has no financial disclosures to make.

REFERENCES

1. American College of Obstetricians and Gynecologists Committee on Obstetric Practice Society for Maternal-Fetal Medicine. Committee Opinion No. 573: magnesium sulfate use in obstetrics. Obstet Gynecol 2013;122(3):727–8.
2. Crowther CA, Hiller JE, Doyle LW, et al. Australasian Collaborative Trial of Magnesium Sulphate Collaborative G. Effect of magnesium sulfate given for neuroprotection before preterm birth: a randomized controlled trial. JAMA 2003;290(20): 2669–76.
3. Marret S, Marpeau L, Zupan-Simunek V, et al. Magnesium sulphate given before very-preterm birth to protect infant brain: the randomised controlled PREMAG trial. BJOG 2007;114(3):310–8.
4. Rouse DJ, Hirtz DG, Thom E, et al. A randomized, controlled trial of magnesium sulfate for the prevention of cerebral palsy. N Engl J Med 2008;359(9):895–905.
5. Pritchard JA. The use of the magnesium ion in the management of eclamptogenic toxemias. Surg Gynecol Obstet 1955;100(2):131–40.
6. Tang J, He A, Li N, et al. Magnesium Sulfate-Mediated Vascular Relaxation and Calcium Channel Activity in Placental Vessels Different From Nonplacental Vessels. J Am Heart Assoc 2018;7(14). https://doi.org/10.1161/JAHA.118.009896.
7. Sibai BM, Spinnato JA, Watson DL, et al. Effect of magnesium sulfate on electroencephalographic findings in preeclampsia-eclampsia. Obstet Gynecol 1984; 64(2):261–6.
8. Lu J, Pfister M, Ferrari P, et al. Pharmacokinetic-pharmacodynamic modelling of magnesium plasma concentration and blood pressure in preeclamptic women. Clin Pharmacokinet 2002;41(13):1105–13.

9. Brookfield KF, Su F, Elkomy MH, et al. Pharmacokinetics and placental transfer of magnesium sulfate in pregnant women. Am J Obstet Gynecol 2016;214(6):737 e1-e9.

10. Chuan FS, Charles BG, Boyle RK, et al. Population pharmacokinetics of magnesium in preeclampsia. Am J Obstet Gynecol 2001;185(3):593-9.

11. Salinger DH, Mundle S, Regi A, et al. Magnesium sulphate for prevention of eclampsia: are intramuscular and intravenous regimens equivalent? A population pharmacokinetic study. BJOG 2013;120(7):894-900.

12. Du L, Wenning L, Migoya E, et al. Population Pharmacokinetic Modeling to Evaluate Standard Magnesium Sulfate Treatments and Alternative Dosing Regimens for Women With Preeclampsia. J Clin Pharmacol 2019;59(3):374-85.

13. da Costa TX, Azeredo FJ, Ururahy MAG, et al. Population pharmacokinetics of magnesium sulfate in preeclampsia and associated factors. Drugs R D 2020; 20(3):257-66.

14. Brookfield KF, Elkomy M, Su F, et al. Optimization of maternal magnesium sulfate administration for fetal neuroprotection: application of a prospectively constructed pharmacokinetic model to the BEAM cohort. J Clin Pharmacol 2017; 57(11):1419-24.

15. Du L, Wenning LA, Carvalho B, et al. Alternative magnesium sulfate dosing regimens for women with preeclampsia: a population pharmacokinetic exposure-response modeling and simulation study. J Clin Pharmacol 2019;59(11):1519-26.

16. Okusanya BO, Oladapo OT, Long Q, et al. Clinical pharmacokinetic properties of magnesium sulphate in women with pre-eclampsia and eclampsia. BJOG 2016; 123(3):356-66.

17. Chesley LC, Tepper I. Plasma levels of magnesium attained in magnesium sulfate therapy for preeclampsia and eclampsia. Surg Clin North Am 1957;37(2):353-67.

18. Sibai BM, Lipshitz J, Anderson GD, et al. Reassessment of intravenous MgSO4 therapy in preeclampsia-eclampsia. Obstet Gynecol 1981;57(2):199-202.

19. Smith JM, Lowe RF, Fullerton J, et al. An integrative review of the side effects related to the use of magnesium sulfate for pre-eclampsia and eclampsia management. BMC Pregnancy Childbirth 2013;13:34.

20. Nick JM. Deep tendon reflexes, magnesium, and calcium: assessments and implications. J Obstet Gynecol Neonatal Nurs 2004;33(2):221-30.

21. Duley L, Gulmezoglu AM, Henderson-Smart DJ, et al. Magnesium sulphate and other anticonvulsants for women with pre-eclampsia. Cochrane Database Syst Rev 2010;10(11):CD000025.

22. Do women with pre-eclampsia, and their babies, benefit from magnesium sulphate? The Magpie Trial: a randomised placebo-controlled trial. Lancet 2002; 359(9321):1877-90.

23. Lu JF, Nightingale CH. Magnesium sulfate in eclampsia and pre-eclampsia: pharmacokinetic principles. Clin Pharmacokinet 2000;38(4):305-14.

24. Sibai BM, Graham JM, McCubbin JH. A comparison of intravenous and intramuscular magnesium sulfate regimens in preeclampsia. Am J Obstet Gynecol 1984; 150(6):728-33.

25. Abbade JF, Costa RA, Martins AM, et al. Zuspan's scheme versus an alternative magnesium sulfate scheme: Randomized clinical trial of magnesium serum concentrations. Hypertens Pregnancy 2010;29(1):82-92.

26. Guzin K, Goynumer G, Gokdagli F, et al. The effect of magnesium sulfate treatment on blood biochemistry and bleeding time in patients with severe pre-eclampsia. J Matern Fetal Neonatal Med 2010;23(5):399-402.

27. Wang W, Xie X, Yuan T, et al. Epidemiological trends of maternal hypertensive disorders of pregnancy at the global, regional, and national levels: a population-based study. BMC Pregnancy Childbirth 2021;21(1):364.
28. Osungbade KO, Ige OK. Public health perspectives of preeclampsia in developing countries: implication for health system strengthening. J Pregnancy 2011;2011:481095.
29. Pratt JJ, Niedle PS, Vogel JP, et al. Alternative regimens of magnesium sulfate for treatment of preeclampsia and eclampsia: a systematic review of non-randomized studies. Acta Obstet Gynecol Scand 2016;95(2):144–56.
30. Brookfield K, Hadiza G, Lihong D, et al. Magnesium sulfate pharmacokinetics after intramuscular dosing in women with preeclampsia. AJOG Glob Rep 2021; 1(4):100018.
31. Walani SR. Global burden of preterm birth. Int J Gynaecol Obstet 2020; 150(1):31–3.
32. Bain E, Middleton P, Crowther CA. Different magnesium sulphate regimens for neuroprotection of the fetus for women at risk of preterm birth. Cochrane Database Syst Rev 2012;15(2):CD009302.
33. Brookfield KF, Vinson A. Magnesium sulfate use for fetal neuroprotection. Curr Opin Obstet Gynecol 2019;31(2):110–5.
34. Lingam I, Robertson NJ. Magnesium as a neuroprotective agent: a review of its use in the fetus, term infant with neonatal encephalopathy, and the adult stroke patient. Dev Neurosci 2018;40(1):1–12.
35. Jahnen-Dechent W, Ketteler M. Magnesium basics. Clin Kidney J 2012;5(Suppl 1):i3–14.
36. Dan B, Paneth N. Making sense of cerebral palsy prevalence in low-income countries. Lancet Glob Health 2017;5(12):e1174–5.
37. Jahan I, Muhit M, Hardianto D, et al. Epidemiology of cerebral palsy in low- and middle-income countries: preliminary findings from an international multi-centre cerebral palsy register. Dev Med Child Neurol 2021;63(11):1327–36.
38. Brookfield KF, Tuel K, Rincon M, et al. Alternate dosing protocol for magnesium sulfate in obese women with preeclampsia: a randomized controlled trial. Obstet Gynecol Dec 2020;136(6):1190–4.

Obstetric Indications for Progestin Therapy

Rupsa C. Boelig, MD, MS[a,b,*]

KEYWORDS

- Progestin • Progesterone • 17-OHPC • 17-hydroxyprogesterone caproate
- Preterm birth

KEY POINTS

- Progestin therapy is beneficial for prevention of preterm birth in selected high-risk pregnancies. Evidence of benefit varies by progestin type.
- The strength of evidence for preterm birth prevention is greatest for vaginal progesterone in prevention of early preterm birth in singletons or twins with asymptomatic mid-trimester short cervix ≤25 mm on transvaginal ultrasound.
- Vaginal progesterone has been studied in prevention of recurrent pregnancy loss and may be beneficial in selected pregnancies.

INTRODUCTION

Progesterone has long been studied as a therapy in obstetrics for prevention of pregnancy loss and prematurity. Csapo initially identified the hormone's functions in pregnancy with studies on rabbits demonstrating progesterone's impact on uterine myometrial activity.[1] The name of the hormone itself conveys its function, *progestation*, supporting pregnancy. The purpose of this article is to review the obstetric indications for progestin therapy in pregnancy. Both natural and synthetic progestins will be addressed, but the use of progestin therapy in the setting of assisted reproductive techniques will not be included. **Table 1** presents a summary of indications for progestin therapy in the prevention of adverse perinatal outcomes.

PROGESTIN PHARMACOLOGY

There are two commonly used formulations of progesterone, natural progesterone, often micronized for improved absorption, and a synthetic progestin, 17-hydroxyprogesterone caproate (17-OHPC). The 17-OHPC is a synthetic progestin that is lipophilic

[a] Division of Maternal Fetal Medicine, Department of Obstetrics and Gynecology, Sidney Kimmel Medical College, Thomas Jefferson University, 833 Chestnut Street, Level 1, Philadelphia, PA 19107, USA; [b] Department of Clinical Pharmacology and Therapeutics, Sidney Kimmel Medical College, Thomas Jefferson University, Philadelphia, PA, USA
* Corresponding author.
E-mail address: rupsa.boelig@jefferson.edu

Obstet Gynecol Clin N Am 50 (2023) 101–107
https://doi.org/10.1016/j.ogc.2022.10.004
0889-8545/23/© 2022 Elsevier Inc. All rights reserved.

obgyn.theclinics.com

Table 1
Summary of evidence for progestins in improving perinatal outcomes

Indication	Formulation/Dose	Selected Benefits	GRADE Quality of Evidence
• Singleton • ≥1 spontaneous miscarriage • Early pregnancy bleeding	400 mg vaginal micronized progesterone twice daily	*Increased live birth rate* RR vs placebo 1.08 (1.02–1.15)[15]	Moderate[e]
• Singleton • Prior spontaneous preterm birth and/or short cervix	Vaginal progesterone daily from 16 to 36 wk[a] 17-OHPC 250 mg IM weekly from 16 to 36 wk	*Reduced preterm birth rate <34 wk* RR vs placebo 0.78 (0.68–0.90)[6] *Reduced preterm birth rate<34 wk* RR vs placebo 0.83 (0.68–1.01)[6]	High Moderate[c]
• Singleton • Prior spontaneous preterm birth	200 mg vaginal progesterone daily from 16 to 36 wk[b] 17-OHPC 250 mg weekly (IM) from 16 to 36 wk	*Reduced preterm birth rate <37 wk* RR (vs placebo) 0.43 (0.23–0.74)[17] RR (vs 17-OHPC) 0.76 (0.69–0.85) *Increased latency* MD (vs 17-OHPC) 1.02 (0.01–2.01)wk *Reduced preterm birth rate <37 wk* RR (vs placebo) 0.53 (0.27–0.95)[17]	Moderate[d] Low[d,e] Low[e] Moderate [d]
• Singleton • Short cervix on transvaginal ultrasound (≤25 mm) diagnosed <24 weeks	200 mg vaginal progesterone or 8% vaginal progesterone gel daily from diagnosis to 36 wk[b]	*Reduced preterm birth <33 weeks* RR 0.62 (0.47–0.81)[24]	High
• Twin • Short cervix on transvaginal ultrasound (≤25 mm) diagnosed <24 weeks	200 mg vaginal progesterone from diagnosis to 36 wk[b]	*Reduced preterm birth <33 weeks* RR (vs placebo) 0.60 (0.38–0.95)[25]	High

Data presented as relative risk (RR) or mean difference (MD) with (95% confidence interval).
Abbreviation: GRADE, Grading of recomendations, assessment, development, and evaluations; IM, intramuscular.[28]
[a] Multiple doses and formulations.
[b] Most commonly used dose/formulation(s), although multiple studied.
[c] Reduced for wide confidence interval.
[d] Reduced for inconsistency in randomized trial results.
[e] Reduced for risk of bias in randomized trial results.

and highly protein bound. The 17-OHPC has a long half-life ($\sim$16 days), likely related to the slow release from the depot preparation and maternal adipose tissue.[2]

Micronized progesterone can be administered vaginally or orally. Oral progesterone undergoes a hepatic first-pass effect, which reduces systemic exposure and results in many of the side effects. Vaginal progesterone, in contrast, undergoes a "uterine" first-pass effect, resulting in increased concentration in the uterus relative to its systemic exposure.[3–5] Vaginal formulations of progesterone include gels and suppositories. Both of these formulations use micronized progesterone and have been found to be effective in the prevention of preterm birth.[6] There may be a difference in vaginal absorption of gel formulation compared with suppository, although this may vary by specific formulations.[7] Finally, although oral micronized progesterone has been studied, the benefit of oral progesterone in the prevention of preterm birth or other adverse perinatal outcomes is limited,[6,8] and as such when discussing micronized progesterone this review specifically focuses on the vaginal route.

Although both micronized progesterone and 17-OHPC are often grouped together under the umbrella of progestin therapy, there are some important distinctions. Both act on progesterone receptors, but 17-OHPC has reduced affinity compared with vaginal progesterone.[5] The mechanism of action of 17-OHPC is theorized to be via its activity at the progesterone receptors, although the precise mechanism of action is not clear.[5] In contrast, there are more data available regarding the mechanism of action of vaginal progesterone in prematurity prevention. A series of experiments in murine and in vitro models found that vaginal progesterone, but not 17-OHPC, reinforces cervical stromal integrity,[9,10] amniotic membrane integrity,[11] and attenuates inflammatory pathways in the uterus/cervix.[12]

PREVENTION OF RECURRENT FIRST TRIMESTER PREGNANCY LOSS

Progesterone formulations have been studied in several randomized trials for the prevention of first trimester pregnancy loss, including two recent high-quality large randomized trials[13,14] as well as a recent network meta-analysis.[15] The summation of evidence finds little benefit in the administration of any progestin formulation for the prevention of pregnancy loss for those with either threatened miscarriage or recurrent pregnancy loss. However, there may be limited benefit of vaginal progesterone in increasing the live birth rate compared with placebo in those with one or more prior miscarriage and early vaginal bleeding in the first trimester (relative risk [RR] 1.08, 95% confidence interval [CI] 1.02 to 1.15).[15,16] This finding is largely driven by the results of one trial using 400 mg vaginal progesterone twice daily.[14]

Summary: Vaginal micronized progesterone 400 mg twice daily may improve the live birth rate in people with singleton pregnancy, prior spontaneous miscarriage, and current early pregnancy bleeding.

PREVENTION OF PRETERM BIRTH IN SINGLETON PREGNANCIES

Both vaginal progesterone and 17-OHPC have been found to be effective in the prevention of preterm birth in high-risk singleton pregnancies (prior spontaneous preterm birth and/or current short cervix). A recent large meta-analysis found both vaginal progesterone (RR 0.78 [0.68–0.90]) and 17-OHPC (RR 0.83 [0.68–1.01]) reduced the rate of preterm birth less than 34 weeks compared with placebo in these high-risk individuals.[6] The totality of evidence is greater for vaginal progesterone in the prevention of preterm birth[6,17,18] and improving neonatal outcomes, including reduced low and very low birth weight, intensive care admission, respiratory distress, and need for respiratory support.[6]

Prior Spontaneous Preterm Birth

Singletons with a prior spontaneous preterm birth of a singleton pregnancy are recommended progesterone therapy from 16 to 36 weeks' to prevent recurrent preterm birth.[19] The specific dose/formulation is not specified. There is evidence to support the benefit of both vaginal progesterone and 17-OHPC.

In 2003, a large randomized trial found 17-OHPC reduced the risk of preterm birth compared with placebo in singletons with prior preterm birth,[20] although these findings were not reproduced in a subsequent confirmatory trial.[21] Given the mixed data, limitations identified in both trials, and meta-analysis demonstrating benefit, both American College of Obstetrics and Gynecology (ACOG) and Society for Maternal Fetal Medicine (SMFM) continue to support offering 17-OHPC for the prevention of recurrent preterm birth.[19,22]

Regarding vaginal progesterone, the most common vaginal progesterone dose/formulation studied is 200 mg micronized progesterone daily.[6,18] Similar to 17-OHPC, randomized trial data are mixed in their findings of benefit compared with placebo. A meta-analysis found vaginal progesterone reduced the risk of recurrent preterm birth less than 34 weeks (RR 0.29 [0.12–0.68]) and less than 37 weeks (RR 0.43 [0.23–0.74]) compared with placebo in singletons with prior spontaneous preterm birth.[17]

A head-to-head comparison of vaginal progesterone and 17-OHPC favor vaginal progesterone in the prevention of recurrent preterm birth, although results are low quality due to the risk of bias in included trials. Specifically, one recent randomized trial in the United States did not find that vaginal progesterone significantly reduced the rate of preterm birth but found later gestational age of delivery compared with 17-OHPC (mean difference 1.02 [0.01–2.01] weeks).[23] A subsequent meta-analysis directly comparing vaginal progesterone and 17-OHPC in prevention of recurrent preterm birth found vaginal progesterone reduced the rates of preterm birth less than 37 weeks (RR 0.76 [0.69–0.85]) and early preterm birth less than 34 weeks (RR 0.74 [0.57–0.96]) compared with 17-OHPC, but these results were no longer statistically significant when restricted to high-quality studies.[18]

Summary: Vaginal progesterone daily (most commonly 200 mg daily) or 17-OHPC 250 mg intramuscular weekly from 16 to 36 weeks should be offered to reduce the risk of recurrent preterm birth; the strength of evidence seems to be greater for vaginal progesterone.

Short Mid-Trimester Cervical Length

Regardless of preterm birth history, multiple randomized trials, and meta-analyses have found that vaginal progesterone reduces the risk of preterm birth in the setting of asymptomatic short cervix identified on transvaginal ultrasound. Although individual trials have used a range of cervical length cutoffs to define short cervix, as well as a variety of micronized progesterone doses and formulations, a meta-analysis identified that vaginal progesterone reduced the risk of early preterm birth less than 33 weeks (RR 0.62 [0.47–0.81]) as well as reduced adverse neonatal outcomes including composite neonatal morbidity, respiratory distress syndrome, intensive care admission.[24] Given the strength of evidence, ACOG recommends vaginal progesterone for prevention of preterm birth and associated neonatal morbidity/mortality in singleton pregnancies with an asymptomatic short cervix identified on transvaginal ultrasound.[19]

Summary: Vaginal micronized progesterone (most commonly 8% gel or 200 mg daily) is recommended in the setting of an asymptomatic mid-trimester (<24 weeks) short cervix ≤25 mm in singletons to prevent preterm birth and associated neonatal morbidity/mortality.

PREVENTION OF PRETERM BIRTH IN TWIN PREGNANCIES

No progesterone formulation has been found to be effective in preterm birth prevention in unselected twin, or other multiple, gestations.[6] However, vaginal progesterone seems to be effective in prevention of early preterm birth in twin gestation with a short cervix. A recent analysis found vaginal progesterone reduced the rate of early preterm birth less than 33 weeks (RR 0.60 [0.38–0.95]) and composite neonatal morbidity (RR 0.59 [0.33–0.98]) in twins with asymptomatic mid-trimester transvaginal cervical length ≤25 mm compared with placebo.[25] Vaginal progesterone dosing in these studies ranged from 100 to 600 mg daily with 200 mg daily being the most commonly used dose.

Summary: Vaginal micronized progesterone (most commonly 200 mg daily) is recommended in the setting of asymptomatic mid-trimester (<24 weeks) short cervix ≤25 mm in twin gestation to prevent preterm birth and associated neonatal morbidity/mortality.

OTHER INDICATIONS

Progestin therapy has been studied in a number of settings for prevention of preterm birth but has not been found to be effective in those settings. These commonly studied indications include unselected multiple gestations,[6] twin pregnancy with prior preterm birth,[26] and preterm labor.[27]

CLINICS CARE POINTS

- Vaginal progesterone 400 mg twice daily may improve live birth rate in singletons with prior recurrent early pregnancy loss history and current early pregnancy bleeding.
- Vaginal progesterone (most commonly 200 mg daily) or 17-hydroxyprogesterone caproate (17-OHPC) (weekly 250 mg) administered intramuscularly may reduce the risk of recurrent preterm birth in singletons with prior spontaneous preterm birth. The strength of evidence seems greater for vaginal progesterone.
- Vaginal progesterone (most commonly 200 mg suppository daily or 8% gel) reduces the risk of preterm birth and improves neonatal outcomes in singletons with an asymptomatic short cervix ≤25 mm diagnosed on transvaginal ultrasound less than 24 weeks' gestation.
- Vaginal progesterone (most commonly 200 mg suppository daily) reduces the risk of preterm birth and improves neonatal outcomes in twins with asymptomatic short cervix ≤25 mm diagnosed on transvaginal ultrasound less than 24 weeks' gestation.

FUNDING

There was no funding for this article

CONFLICTS OF INTEREST

No conflicts of interest, financial or otherwise, to disclose.

REFERENCES

1. Csapo AI, Pinto-Dantas CA. The effect of progesterone on the human uterus. Proc Natl Acad Sci U S A 1965;54(4):1069–76.
2. Caritis SN, Feghali MN, Grobman WA, et al. What we have learned about the role of 17-alpha-hydroxyprogesterone caproate in the prevention of preterm birth. Semin Perinatol 2016;40(5):273–80.
3. Cicinelli E, de Ziegler D, Bulletti C, et al. Direct transport of progesterone from vagina to uterus. Obstet Gynecol 2000;95(3):403–6. Available at: http://www.ncbi.nlm.nih.gov/pubmed/10711552. Accessed October 3, 2017.

4. Boelig RC, Zuppa AF, Kraft WK, et al. Pharmacokinetics of Vaginal Progesterone in Pregnancy. Am J Obstet Gynecol 2019;221(3). https://doi.org/10.1016/j.ajog.2019.06.019.

5. O'Brien JM, Lewis DF. Prevention of preterm birth with vaginal progesterone or 17-alpha-hydroxyprogesterone caproate: A critical examination of efficacy and safety. Am J Obstet Gynecol 2016;214(1):45–56.

6. Stewart LA, Simmonds M, Duley L, et al. Evaluating Progestogens for Preventing Preterm birth International Collaborative (EPPPIC): meta-analysis of individual participant data from randomised controlled trials. Lancet 2021;397(10280): 1183–94.

7. Blake EJ, Norris PM, Dorfman SF, et al. Single and multidose pharmacokinetic study of a vaginal micronized progesterone insert (Endometrin) compared with vaginal gel in healthy reproductive-aged female subjects. Fertil Steril 2010; 94(4):1296–301.

8. Boelig RC, Della Corte L, Ashoush S, et al. Oral progesterone for the prevention of recurrent preterm birth: systematic review and metaanalysis. Am J Obstet Gynecol MFM 2019;1(1):50–62.

9. Nold C, Maubert M, Anton L, et al. Prevention of preterm birth by progestational agents: what are the molecular mechanisms? Am J Obstet Gynecol 2013;208(3): 223.e1–7.

10. Nold C, Jensen T, O'Hara K, et al. Replens prevents preterm birth by decreasing type I interferon strengthening the cervical epithelial barrier. Am J Reprod Immunol 2020;83(1). https://doi.org/10.1111/aji.13192.

11. Kumar D, Springel E, Moore RM, et al. Progesterone inhibits in vitro fetal membrane weakening. Am J Obstet Gynecol 2015;213:520.e1–9. Mosby Inc.

12. Furcron A, Romero R, Plazyo O, et al. Vaginal progesterone, but not 17-ahydroxyprogesterone caproate, has antiinflammatory effects at the murine maternal-fetal interface. Am J Obstet Gynecol 2015;213(6):e1–35. Vaginal.

13. Coomarasamy A, Williams H, Truchanowicz E, et al. PROMISE: First-trimester progesterone therapy in women with a history of unexplained recurrent miscarriages – A randomised, double-blind, placebo-controlled, international multicentre trial and economic evaluation. Health Technol Assess (Rockv) 2016; 20(41):7–91.

14. Coomarasamy A, Harb HM, Devall AJ, et al. Progesterone to prevent miscarriage in women with early pregnancy bleeding: The PRISM RCT. Health Technol Assess (Rockv) 2020;24(33):1–70.

15. Devall AJ, Papadopoulou A, Podesek M, et al. Progestogens for preventing miscarriage: a network meta-analysis. Cochrane Database Syst Rev 2021; 2021(4). https://doi.org/10.1002/14651858.CD013792.pub2.

16. Coomarasamy A, Devall AJ, Brosens JJ, et al. Micronized vaginal progesterone to prevent miscarriage: a critical evaluation of randomized evidence. Am J Obstet Gynecol 2020;223(2):167–76.

17. Jarde A, Lutsiv O, Beyene J, et al. Vaginal progesterone, oral progesterone, 17-OHPC, cerclage, and pessary for preventing preterm birth in at-risk singleton pregnancies: an updated systematic review and network meta-analysis. BJOG An Int J Obstet Gynaecol 2019;126(5):556–67.

18. Boelig RC, Locci M, Saccone G, et al. Vaginal progesterone compared with intramuscular 17-alpha-hydroxyprogesterone caproate for prevention of recurrent preterm birth in singleton gestations: a systematic review and meta-analysis. Am J Obstet Gynecol MFM 2022;4(5). https://doi.org/10.1016/j.ajogmf.2022.100658.

19. ACOG. Prediction and Prevention of Spontaneous Preterm Birth: ACOG Practice Bulletin, Number 234. Obstet Gynecol 2021;138(2):e65–90.
20. Meis PJ, Klebanoff M, Thom E, et al. Prevention of recurrent preterm delivery by 17 alpha-hydroxyprogesterone caproate. N Engl J Med 2003;348(24):2379–85.
21. Blackwell SC, Gyamfi-Bannerman C, Biggio JR, et al. 17-OHPC to Prevent Recurrent Preterm Birth in Singleton Gestations (PROLONG Study): A Multicenter, International, Randomized Double-Blind Trial. Am J Perinatol 2019;1(212). https://doi.org/10.1055/s-0039-3400227.
22. Society of Maternal Fetal Medicine. SMFM Statement: Use of 17-Alpha Hydroxyprogesterone Caproate for Prevention of Recurrent Preterm Birth. https://els-jbs-prod-cdn.literatumonline.com/pb/assets/raw/Health Advance/journals/ymob/SMFM_Statement_PROLONG-1572023839767.pdf. Accessed November 15, 2022.
23. Boelig RC, Schoen CN, Frey HA, et al. Vaginal versus Intramuscular Progesterone for Prevention of Recurrent Preterm Birth (VIP): a randomized controlled trial. Am J Obstet Gynecol 2022;226(1):S26.
24. Romero R, Conde-Agudelo A, Da Fonseca E, et al. Vaginal Progesterone for Preventing Preterm Birth and Adverse Perinatal Outcomes in Singleton Gestations with a Short Cervix: A Meta-Analysis of Individual Patient Data. Am J Obstet Gynecol 2018;218(2):161–80.
25. Romero R, Conde-Agudelo A, Rehal A, et al. Vaginal progesterone for the prevention of preterm birth and adverse perinatal outcomes in twin gestations with a short cervix: an updated individual patient data meta-analysis. Ultrasound Obstet Gynecol 2022;59(2):263–6.
26. Ward A, Greenberg V, Valcarcel B, et al. Intramuscular progesterone in women with twins and a prior singleton spontaneous preterm birth. Am J Obstet Gynecol MFM 2020;2. https://doi.org/10.1016/j.ajogmf.2020.100124. Elsevier Inc.
27. Su L-L, Samuel M, Chong Y-S. Progestational agents for treating threatened or established preterm labour. Cochrane Database Syst Rev 2014. https://doi.org/10.1002/14651858.CD006770.pub3.
28. Guyatt GH, Oxman AD, Akl EA, et al. GRADE guidelines: 1. Introduction-GRADE evidence profiles and summary of findings tables. J Clin Epidemiol 2011;64(4):383–94.

Antenatal Steroids and Tocolytics in Pregnancy

Kelsey Pinson, MD*, Cynthia Gyamfi-Bannerman, MD, MS

KEYWORDS

- Tocolysis • Antenatal corticosteroids • Preterm birth • Preterm labor

KEY POINTS

- Antenatal corticosteroids reduce morbidity and mortality associated with preterm birth in neonates.
- Antenatal corticosteroids should be offered to all pregnant people at risk of preterm birth within 7 days who are between 24 weeks 0 days and 33 weeks 6 days gestational age.
- Antenatal corticosteroids can be offered to all pregnant people at risk of preterm birth within 7 days who are between 34 weeks 0 days and 36 weeks 6 days if they have not received a prior corticosteroid course.
- Additional data are needed to understand the long-term risks and benefits of antenatal corticosteroid administration in the periviable and late-preterm periods.
- Tocolysis can be considered to temporarily slow uterine activity and allow the administration of antenatal corticosteroids or transfer to a higher level of care for individuals at risk of preterm birth.

ANTENATAL CORTICOSTEROIDS
Introduction

Antenatal corticosteroid administration is one of the most important obstetric interventions to reduce the morbidity and mortality of the neonate associated with preterm birth and has become the standard of care for pregnant individuals with anticipated preterm delivery, particularly before 34 weeks gestational age.[1–4] Owing to the rising rates of preterm birth in the United States, with an estimated 12% to 15% of births occurring before 37 weeks' gestation, the administration of antenatal steroids has the potential to remarkably reduce morbidity in the neonatal period.[5,6]

As demonstrated in a large meta-analysis of 30 randomized controlled trials with over 8000 participants, infants whose mothers received antenatal corticosteroids have significantly reduced risks of developing respiratory distress syndrome (RDS) (relative risk [RR] = 0.66; 95% confidence interval [CI] 0.56–0.77), necrotizing

University of California, San Diego, 9300 Campus Point Drive, Mail Code 7433, La Jolla, CA 92037, USA
* Corresponding author.
E-mail address: kapinson@health.ucsd.edu

Obstet Gynecol Clin N Am 50 (2023) 109–119
https://doi.org/10.1016/j.ogc.2022.10.006
0889-8545/23/© 2022 Elsevier Inc. All rights reserved.

obgyn.theclinics.com

enterocolitis (RR = 0.50; 95% CI, 0.32–0.78), intraventricular hemorrhage (RR = 0.55; 95% CI, 0.40–0.76), and neonatal death (RR = 0.69; 95% CI, 0.59–0.81) when compared with infants born at the same gestational ages to mothers who did not receive corticosteroids.[1–4,7,8]

Although the ultimate minimization of these morbidities likely lies in the reduction of preterm birth, both spontaneous and indicated, antenatal corticosteroid treatment remains a mainstay for the reduction of these morbidities.

Discussion

Physiology

After first demonstration in a sheep model in the 1960s, the benefits of antenatal corticosteroids have been established in dozens of human studies and have become the standard of care in the treatment of gravid people at risk of preterm delivery.[9] In the fetal lung, antenatal steroids primarily function by means of the induction of structural and biochemical changes to improve lung compliance, surfactant production, and gas exchange.[5,10] In the early preterm period, the effect is primarily through the induction of type II pneumocytes, which produce surfactant, a substance that reduces surface tension in the lung and prevents the collapse of alveoli during expiration.[5,6,10] In late preterm and early term infants, antenatal corticosteroids are also thought to have a significant effect on ENaC, sodium channels within the lung that facilitate clearance of fetal alveolar fluid.[5,6]

Choice of medication

The 2 steroids with demonstrated fetal benefit for prenatal use are dexamethasone and betamethasone. The 2 drugs are structurally similar epimers and differ in their biochemical structure only in the orientation of a single methyl group. In the United States, betamethasone is typically administered as a 1:1 mixture of 2 prodrugs: betamethasone acetate and betamethasone phosphate. Betamethasone phosphate is rapidly metabolized by dephosphorylation, while betamethasone acetate undergoes a slower deacetylation process. This allows for rapid effect of the betamethasone phosphate with a delayed metabolism and effect from betamethasone acetate. Because of this combination of rapid and delayed-onset actions, betamethasone is typically dosed at 24-hour intervals. Dexamethasone is usually administered as dexamethasone sodium phosphate, which in similar fashion to betamethasone phosphate is rapidly dephosphorylated and has a rapid onset of action. Because of this rapid metabolism, dexamethasone is usually dosed every 6 hours.[11]

Although there are some limited pharmacokinetic data, the optimal dosing of either medication is unknown, as the well-studied doses were chosen arbitrarily. Nonetheless, the standard dosing for betamethasone is 2 intramuscularly administered 12 mg doses, 24 hours apart. Dexamethasone is administered as 4 intramuscular doses of 6 mg, 12 hours apart. Neither has clearly been established as preferred over the other, with some studies favoring betamethasone and others favoring dexamethasone.[5,6]

Maternal effects

Both agents have demonstrated benefit in the reduction of complications of prematurity as previously discussed. From a maternal perspective, the most common side effect of either medication is hyperglycemia, which may require additional monitoring and blood glucose control. For people with pregestational diabetes, a continuous insulin infusion may be required for acceptable serum glucose control while receiving treatment with antenatal corticosteroids. Because of this transient hyperglycemia effect, screening for gestational diabetes should be delayed at least 1 week after administration of corticosteroids, if not completed before administration. A transient maternal leukocytosis has been associated with corticosteroid administration, but typically does not exceed $20,000 \times 10^3$ cells/mL.[6] A 2020 meta-analysis suggested that the rates of maternal death, chorioamnionitis, and endometritis are not affected by the administration of antenatal corticosteroids.[8]

Current recommendations

The American College of Obstetricians and Gynecologists (ACOG), the Society for Maternal-Fetal-Medicine (SMFM), and Royal College of Obstetricians and Gynecologists (RCOG) all support a course of antenatal corticosteroids under the following circumstances[1,12,13]:

- For pregnant people between 24 weeks 0 days and 33 weeks 6 days gestational age at risk of preterm delivery in the next 7 days
- For pregnant people between 24 weeks 0 days and 33 weeks 6 days gestational age at risk of preterm birth within 7 days who have received 1 prior course of antenatal corticosteroids and for whom at least 7 days have passed since the first course
- Consideration of a single course of antenatal corticosteroids for patients between 34 weeks 0 days gestational age and 36 weeks 6 days gestational age who have not received a prior course of corticosteroids, after discussion of the risks and benefits of late-preterm administration

Special Populations and Controversies

Repeat courses

As previously noted, a single rescue course of steroids is recommended for pregnant people who are less than 34 weeks gestational age, at risk for preterm birth within 7 days, and who have received 1 prior course at least 7 days prior. This is based on meta-analysis data demonstrating that there was no longer a statistically significant reduction in rates of RDS more than 7 days after exposure to antenatal steroids and that a repeat course reduces the risk of neonatal respiratory morbidity without significantly increasing the risk of other maternal and neonatal complications including neonatal death, neonatal major disability, maternal chorioamnionitis or sepsis, and cesarean delivery.[4,6,8,14,15]

Several studies have since examined serial courses of corticosteroids, at either 7- or 14-day intervals, and their effects on the neonate. Although scheduled serial courses likely reduce the risk of short-term respiratory morbidity, both 7- and 14-day serial courses have been associated with lower birth weight and smaller head size in infants exposed to multiple courses across several randomized-controlled trials.[5,16] In 2007, a Cochrane review, including more than 2000 participants, assessed repeat courses of betamethasone and found a reduction in occurrence of neonatal lung disease (RR 0.82, 95% CI 0.72–0.93) but did not demonstrate a difference in mean birthweight.[17] Long-term data are mixed; however, because of concerns regarding fetal growth and lack of demonstrated long-term benefit of scheduled repeat courses of corticosteroids, administering more than 2 courses during a single pregnancy is not currently recommended by any major organization in the United States.

Multiple gestation

Further study is needed to clearly demonstrate the benefits of antenatal corticosteroid administration in twin gestations; however, in the setting of likely benefit and unlikely harm, it is reasonable to administer antenatal corticosteroids to twin and higher order multiple gestations for the same indications as singletons.[1,4]

Administration in the periviable period

Corticosteroids in the periviable period, typically defined as 22 to 24 weeks gestational age, should be considered if treatment would be aligned with a family's goals of care for the neonate. Data from an NICHD Neonatal Research Network observational cohort demonstrated a reduction in neonatal death and neurodevelopmental impairment in infants exposed to corticosteroids who were born at 23 weeks through 25 weeks 6 days gestational age. No clear benefit was demonstrated in infants born 22 weeks 0 days to 22 weeks 6 days, and the outcomes in this group were poor regardless of exposure to antenatal steroids.[2] If resuscitation of an infant born in the periviable period is pursued, steroids should be offered, as they are likely to reduce complications in this population, while acknowledging that periviable birth is still associated with high rates of respiratory distress and long-term neurodevelopmental disability.

Administration in the late preterm period

As noted previously, a single course of corticosteroids in the late preterm period (34 0/7–36 6/7 weeks gestational age) should be considered for patients who have not received a prior course and who are at risk for delivery within 7 days. This recommendation was derived from the Antenatal Betamethasone for Women at Risk for Late Preterm Delivery (ALPS) trial, the largest trial at the time of publication assessing steroids in late preterm infants. This study randomized 2831 people at high risk for delivery between 34 0/7 to 36 6/7 weeks gestational age to receive a single course of antenatal corticosteroids or placebo. This group found a reduction in the primary composite outcome, which included any of: continuous positive airway pressure (CPAP) or high-flow nasal cannula for at least 2 hours, supplemental oxygen for at least 4 hours, mechanical ventilation, extracorporeal membrane oxygenation (ECMO), and neonatal death.[18] Exposed neonates also demonstrated lower rates of need for resuscitation at birth, transient tachypnea of the newborn (TTN), and bronchopulmonary dysplasia. No differences were seen in RDS, and exposed neonates were more likely to require treatment for hypoglycemia, although this was usually not severe. Meta-analyses including the various late preterm trials have reinforced these findings, and demonstrated reductions in RDS, mechanical ventilation, and TTN but an increase in neonatal hypoglycemia.[8,19]

Although exposure to antenatal corticosteroids in the early preterm period (before 34 weeks) has been associated with decreased risk of long-term neurodevelopmental impairment, fewer data are available regarding exposure in the late-preterm period. Animal studies have suggested that exposure to steroids in the late preterm period may alter fetal brain development, with structural effects seen primarily in the hippocampus in addition to altered postnatal behaviors.[20] In people, a retrospective cohort study of Finnish children analyzed term born sibling pairs and found that children exposed to antenatal steroids were more likely to exhibit any childhood mental or behavioral disorder compared with their unexposed siblings, although gestational age at administration of steroids was not known.[21] Long-term follow-up data from randomized trials of a single course of late preterm steroids are scarce, but the available data are reassuring.

In 2013, a long-term follow-up study of the Antenatal Steroids for Term Elective Caesarean Section (ASTEC) trial demonstrated no differences in behavioral, cognitive, or developmental outcomes among school-aged children whose mothers received a single course of antenatal corticosteroids before delivery at 37 to 38 weeks' gestation.[22] The 30-year follow-up of the first landmark trial demonstrating effectiveness of betamethasone for reduction of neonatal morbidity examined 192 adults (87 exposed to antenatal betamethasone, 105 exposed to placebo). No differences were found on neurocognitive assessment between groups exposed or unexposed to betamethasone, including cognitive function, working memory and attention, psychiatric morbidity, handedness, and health-related quality of life. Notably, most of these participants were exposed in the late-preterm period during fetal life.[23,24] The ALPS neurocognitive follow-up study is currently being conducted, and results are expected by 2023.

Summary

Antenatal corticosteroids are highly effective to reduce neonatal morbidity and mortality associated with preterm birth.

Clinics Care Points

- Antenatal corticosteroids can reduce morbidity and mortality of preterm birth in neonates, including RDS, necrotizing enterocolitis, intraventricular hemorrhage, and neonatal death.
- Antenatal corticosteroids cause transient maternal leukocytosis and hyperglycemia but do not appear to increase maternal morbidity, including chorioamnionitis, sepsis, endometritis, and maternal death.
- Antenatal corticosteroids should be offered to all pregnant people at risk of preterm birth within 7 days who are between 24 weeks 0 days and 33 weeks 6 days gestational age.
- Antenatal corticosteroids can be offered to select pregnant individuals at risk of preterm birth within 7 days who are between 34 weeks 0 days and 36 weeks 6 days if they have not received a prior corticosteroid course.
- Additional data are needed to understand the long-term risks and benefits of antenatal corticosteroid administration in the periviable and late-preterm periods, particularly regarding long-term neurodevelopment in the late-preterm exposed fetuses.

TOCOLYTICS
Introduction

Preterm labor, diagnosed in the setting of regular uterine contractions with cervical change before 37 weeks gestation, accounts for approximately 50% of preterm births in the United States. As such, much research has gone into identifying predictors, methods of prevention, and possible treatments for preterm labor in order to prevent the known neonatal mortality and morbidity associated with it.[25] Tocolytics, medications administered to inhibit uterine contractions, have been studied for short- and long-term use for the prolongation of pregnancies affected by preterm labor.

Overall, less than half of women who are hospitalized for preterm labor ultimately deliver preterm, so identifying which women will benefit from short-term tocolysis to allow for the administration of antenatal corticosteroids is challenging. As a general rule, tocolysis should be used when the fetal risks of prematurity outweigh the fetal and maternal risks of prolonging a pregnancy in the setting of preterm labor. Typically, tocolysis is only used prior to 34 weeks 0 days gestational age.[25]

Discussion

Clinical use

A number of different agents have been studied to inhibit uterine contractions and those with the most data include calcium channel blockers, nonsteroidal anti-inflammatory drugs (NSAIDs), beta-adrenergic receptor agonists, and magnesium sulfate.[25]

Overall, the evidence supports the short-term use of tocolytic agents to allow the administration of antenatal corticosteroids, magnesium sulfate for fetal neuroprotection, and possible transfer to a higher acuity care setting for maternal and neonatal benefit.[25,26] Long-term use of tocolytics (ie, over more than 48 hours or for consecutive weeks) has not been proven to be effective and is generally avoided because of risks of maternal and fetal adverse effects.[27]

Tocolysis is not recommended beyond 34 weeks 0 days gestational age and is typically not recommended prior to 24 weeks 0 days gestational age unless neonatal resuscitation is being considered before that time.[26] Additional contraindications to tocolysis include intrauterine fetal demise or lethal fetal anomaly, heavy vaginal bleeding or suspected placental abruption, nonreassuring fetal status, severe preeclampsia or eclampsia, maternal instability, and chorioamnionitis.[25]

Calcium channel blockers

Calcium Channel blockers, most commonly nifedipine, inhibit voltage-gated calcium channels in smooth muscle cells, resulting in decreased release of stored calcium, which leads to myometrial relaxation via inhibition of calcium-dependent myosin light-chain kinase phosphorylation.[6]

A 2003 Cochrane review supported the use of calcium channel blockers as short-term tocolytics over other available agents (primarily beta-mimetics), with significantly reduced rates of preterm birth occurring within 7 days of treatment (RR = 0.76; 95% CI, 0.60–0.97) and before 34 weeks (RR = 0.83; 95% CI, 0.69–0.99).[28] More recently, a small randomized, placebo-controlled trial of 90 participants found no significant difference in the rate of preterm birth before 37 weeks (52% vs 48%, RR 1.1, 95% CI 0.7–1.7), or in delivery at least 48 hours from randomization (78% vs 71%, RR 1.1, 95% CI 0.9–1.4) for people who presented in preterm labor and were randomized to receive either nifedipine or placebo for 48 hours, although this study was likely underpowered to detect small differences in rates of preterm birth.[29]

Overall, although there are some conflicting data, the sum of the evidence supports the short-term use of calcium channel blockers for tocolysis before 34 weeks' gestation.[25]

Nonsteroidal anti-inflammatory medications

Nonsteroidal anti-inflammatory drugs (NSAIDs) are used to reduce prostaglandin synthesis via inhibition of cyclooxygenase (COX). Prostaglandins are known to mediate uterine muscle contraction and are used for ripening the cervix and induction of labor.[6]

A 2005 Cochrane Review concluded the COX inhibitors (primarily indomethacin) were associated with a reduction in preterm birth before 37 weeks gestation, but that data were insufficient to recommend use because of overall small numbers and the potential for adverse fetal effects.[30] Reported adverse effects associated with NSAID use in pregnancy include maternal nausea, gastritis, and renal impairment, as well as fetal risks including oligohydramnios, premature closure of the ductus arteriosus, and increased risk of necrotizing enterocolitis in preterm neonates. These risks can be mitigated by restricting indomethacin use to pregnancies before 32 weeks gestation and limiting use to 48 hours of therapy.[6,25]

Magnesium sulfate

Magnesium sulfate acts at the motor end plate and the cell membrane by competition with calcium and resulting inhibition of myometrial contractility.[6]

Magnesium sulfate, despite having limited evidence of benefit, is often used as a tocolytic owing its benefits for fetal neuroprotection.[6,31,32] A 2002 Cochrane meta-analysis including over 2000 women found no difference in rates of preterm birth within 48 hours (RR 0.85, 95% CI 0.58–1.25) or before 34 or 37 weeks in women given magnesium sulfate over controls, and the rates of neonatal death were significantly increased in those who received magnesium therapy (RR 2.82, 95% CI 1.20–6.62).[33] This association with neonatal death is poorly understood. Two additional randomized trials comparing magnesium sulfate to nifedipine and celecoxib (COX inhibitor) found no difference in the number of women who delivered within 48 hours.[6]

Because of potentially serious maternal adverse effects including the development of pulmonary edema or hypotension, the use of concurrent nifedipine or terbutaline tocolysis in combination with magnesium sulfate should be cautioned.[25]

Beta-adrenergic receptor agonists

Terbutaline, a beta agonist occasionally used for tocolysis in the United States, acts via beta receptors in the myometrium to relax smooth muscle and inhibit myometrial contractions.[6] Owing to the widespread presence of beta receptors throughout the body, terbutaline has many reported side effects (**Table 1**) and thus is not recommended for long-term and repeated use.[6,25]

In 2011, the US Food and Drug Administration (FDA) issued a warning regarding the use of terbutaline for the treatment of preterm labor because of serious maternal adverse effects including maternal cardiac events and death.[34] Neither ACOG nor the most recent Cochrane review support the use of terbutaline for longer than 48 hours, and this medication should generally be reserved for the treatment of acute uterine tachysystole.[6,35]

Maintenance therapy

The only tocolytic medication that has demonstrated efficacy in the prolongation of pregnancy as a maintenance therapy is atosiban, an oxytocin and vasopressin receptor inhibitor. This medication is not available in the United States.[36] As mentioned previously, because of the risk of maternal side effects and lack of evidence supporting efficacy, tocolysis is typically reserved for short-term use in the United States, although atosiban is still frequently used in other parts of the world.

SUMMARY

Several agents are used for short-term tocolysis, primarily with the goal of obtaining sufficient time for administration of antenatal corticosteroids or transfer of care to a higher acuity care center. The data in support of maintenance tocolysis are poor, and data supporting short-term use are mixed with regard to efficacy.

CLINICS CARE POINTS

- Short-term tocolysis with calcium channel blockers and NSAIDs (before 32 weeks' gestation) can be used for the short-term prolongation of pregnancies in the setting of preterm labor.
- Magnesium sulfate, although beneficial for fetal neuroprotection, should be avoided for tocolytic therapy alone, and combined use with calcium channel blockers and beta mimetic agents is cautioned because of the risk of maternal side effects.
- Maintenance tocolysis for greater than 48 hours is not recommended.

Table 1
Tocolytic medications and dosages in pregnancy

Agent or Medication Class	Typical Dosing	Fetal Adverse Effects	Maternal Adverse Effects	Contraindications
Calcium Channel Blockers	Nifedipine: 10–20 mg every 3–6 h	None known	Hypotension, headache, nausea, dizziness	• Hypotension • Severe maternal cardiac disease
NSAID	Indomethacin: 50 mg load (rectally or orally) followed by 25 mg every 6 h for up to 48 h	• Oligohydramnios • Increased risk of necrotizing enterocolitis in preterm neonates • Premature closure of the ductus arteriosus	Nausea, kidney injury, gastritis	• Gestational age ≥ 32 weeks • Maternal bleeding disorder or thrombocytopenia • Gastrointestinal ulcer • Caution with maternal renal disease and maternal history of bariatric surgery
Oxytocin receptor antagonist	Atosiban: 6.75 mg bolus injection followed by 300 µg/min infusion for 3 h, followed by 100 µg/min infusion for up to 45 additional hours	None known	Injection site reactions	• No absolute contraindications • Not available in the United States
Beta-adrenergic receptor agonists	Terbutaline: 0.25 mg subcutaneous injection every 4 h	Neonatal hypoglycemia, fetal tachycardia	Tachycardia, palpitations, tremor, headache, hypokalemia, hyperglycemia	Maternal cardiac disease with sensitivity to tachycardia
Magnesium sulfate	Intravenous MgSO4: 4 or 6 g bolus followed by 1–2 g/h for up to 12 h	None known, possible temporary neonatal depression although data are inconsistent	Flushing, headache, respiratory depression, cardiac arrhythmia or arrest, pulmonary edema	Myasthenia gravis *Caution with renal insufficiency because of impaired clearance

DISCLOSURE

Dr C. Gyamfi-Bannerman received payment for lectures given for Medela and Hologic. Dr K. Pinson receives research support from Dexcom, Inc, United States.

REFERENCES

1. Committee on Obstetric Practice. Committee Opinion No. 713: Antenatal corticosteroid therapy for fetal maturation. Obstet Gynecol 2017;130(2):e102–9.
2. Carlo WA, McDonald SA, Fanaroff AA, et al. Association of antenatal corticosteroids with mortality and neurodevelopmental outcomes among infants born at 22 to 25 weeks' gestation. Eunice Kennedy Shriver National Institute of Child Health and Human Development Neonatal Research Network. JAMA 2011;306:2348–58.
3. Management of preterm labor. Practice Bulletin No. 171. American College of Obstetricians and Gynecologists. Obstet Gynecol 2016;128:e155–64.
4. Roberts D, Dalziel SR. Antenatal corticosteroids for accelerating fetal lung maturation for women at risk of preterm birth. Cochrane Database Syst Rev 2006;3: CD004454.
5. Bonanno C, Wapner RJ. Antenatal corticosteroid treatment: what's happened since Drs Liggins and Howie? Am J Obstet Gynecol 2009;200(4):448–57.
6. Copel J, Silver R. Creasy and Resnik's maternal-fetal medicine: principles and practice E-book. 8th edition. Elsevier - OHCE; 2018. Available from: Elsevier eBooks+.
7. Roberts D, Brown J, Medley N, et al. Antenatal corticosteroids for accelerating fetal lung maturation for women at risk of preterm birth. Cochrane Database Syst Rev 2017;3:CD004454.
8. McGoldrick E, Stewart F, Parker R, et al. Antenatal corticosteroids for accelerating fetal lung maturation for women at risk of preterm birth. Cochrane Database Syst Rev 2020;12(12):CD004454.
9. Liggins GC. Premature delivery of foetal lambs infused with glucocorticoids. J Endocrinol 1969;45:515–23.
10. Bolt RJ, van Weissenbruch MM, Lafeber HN, et al. Glucocorticoids and lung development in the fetus and preterm infant. Pediatr Pulmonol 2001;32:76–91.
11. Kemp MW, Newnham JP, Challis JG, et al. The clinical use of corticosteroids in pregnancy. Hum Reprod Update 2015;22(2):240–59.
12. Stock SJ, Thomson AJ, Papworth S. Antenatal corticosteroids to reduce neonatal morbidity and mortality. BJOG 2022;129(8):e35–60.
13. Reddy UM, Deshmukh U, Dude A, et al. Society for Maternal-Fetal Medicine Consult Series #58: Use of antenatal corticosteroids for individuals at risk for late preterm delivery: Replaces SMFM Statement #4, Implementation of the use of antenatal corticosteroids in the late preterm birth period in women at risk for preterm delivery, 2016. Am J Obstet Gynecol 2021;225(5):B36–42.
14. Crowther CA, McKinlay CJ, Middleton P, et al. Repeat doses of prenatal corticosteroids for women at risk of preterm birth for improving neonatal health outcomes. Cochrane Database Syst Rev 2015;2015(7):CD003935.
15. Gyamfi-Bannerman C, Son M. Preterm premature rupture of membranes and the rate of neonatal sepsis after two courses of antenatal corticosteroids. Obstet Gynecol 2014;124(5):999–1003.
16. Murphy K, for the MACS Collaborative Group. Multiple courses of antenatal corticosteroids for preterm birth study. Am J Obstet Gynecol 2007;197:S2.

17. Crowther CA, Harding JE. Repeat doses of prenatal corticosteroids for women at risk of preterm birth for preventing neonatal respiratory disease. Cochrane Database Syst Rev 2007;3:CD003935.

18. Gyamfi-Bannerman C, Thom EA, Blackwell SC, et al. NICHD Maternal–Fetal Medicine Units Network. Antenatal betamethasone for women at risk for late preterm delivery. N Engl J Med 2016;374(14):1311–20.

19. Saccone G, Berghella V. Antenatal corticosteroids for maturity of term or near term fetuses: systematic review and meta-analysis of randomized controlled trials. BMJ 2016;355(i5044):e1.

20. van der Merwe J, van der Veeken L, Inversetti A, et al. Neurocognitive sequelae of antenatal corticosteroids in a late preterm rabbit model. Am J Obstet Gynecol 2022;226(6):850.e1–21. Epub 2021 Dec 4. PMID: 34875248.

21. Räikkönen K, Gissler M, Kajantie E. Associations between maternal antenatal corticosteroid treatment and mental and behavioral disorders in children. JAMA 2020;323:1924–33.

22. Stutchfield PR, Whitaker R, Gliddon AE, et al. Behavioural, educational and respiratory outcomes of antenatal betamethasone for term caesarean section (AS-TECS trial). Arch Dis Child Fetal Neonatal Ed 2013;98:F195–200.

23. Dalziel SR, Lim VK, Lambert A, et al. Antenatal exposure to betamethasone: psychological functioning and health related quality of life 31 years after inclusion in randomised controlled trial. BMJ 2005;331(7518):665.

24. Liggins GC, Howie RN. (1972). A controlled trial of antepartum glucocorticoid treatment for prevention of the respiratory distress syndrome in premature infants. Pediatrics 1972;50(4):515–25.

25. American College of Obstetricians and Gynecologists' Committee on Practice Bulletins—Obstetrics. Practice bulletin no. 171: management of preterm labor. Obstet Gynecol 2016;128(4):e155–64.

26. Committee Opinion No. 455: Magnesium sulfate before anticipated preterm birth for neuroprotection. Obstet Gynecol 2010;115(3):669–71.

27. Anotayanonth S, Subhedar NV, Garner P, et al. Betamimetics for inhibiting preterm labour. Cochrane Database Syst Rev 2004;4:CD004352.

28. King JF, Flenady VJ, Papatsonis DN, et al. Calcium channel blockers for inhibiting preterm labour. Cochrane Database Syst Rev 2002;2:CD002255.

29. Hawkins J, Seth MD, Wells C, et al. Nifedipine for acute tocolysis of preterm labor. Obstet Gynecol 2021;138(1):73–8.

30. King J, Flenady V, Cole S, et al. Cyclo-oxygenase (COX) inhibitors for treating preterm labour. Cochrane Database Syst Rev 2005;2:CD001992.

31. Lyell DJ, Pullen K, Campbell L, et al. Magnesium sulfate compared with nifedipine for acute tocolysis of preterm labor: a randomized controlled trial. Obstet Gynecol 2007;110(1):61–7.

32. Borna S, Saeidi FM. Celecoxib versus magnesium sulfate to arrest preterm labor: randomized trial. J Obstet Gynecol Res 2007;33:631–4.

33. Crowther CA, Hiller JE, Doyle LW. Magnesium sulphate for preventing preterm birth in threatened preterm labour. Cochrane Database Syst Rev 2002;4:CD001060.

34. FDA Drug Safety Communication. New warnings against use of terbutaline to treat preterm labor. 2-2011. Available at: https://www.fda.gov/drugs/drug-safety-and-availability/fda-drug-safety-communication-new-warnings-against-use-terbutaline-treat-preterm-labor. Accessed June 15, 2022.

35. Nanda K, Cook LA, Gallo MF, et al. Terbutaline pump maintenance therapy after threatened preterm labor for preventing preterm birth. Cochrane Database Syst Rev 2002;4:CD003933.

36. Valenzuela GJ, Sanchez-Ramos L, Romero R, et al. Maintenance treatment of preterm labor with the oxytocin antagonist atosiban. The Atosiban PTL-098 Study Group. Am J Obstet Gynecol 2000;182(5):1184–90.

Medications for Managing Preexisting and Gestational Diabetes in Pregnancy

Michaela Rickert, PA-C, RDN, CDCES*,
Aaron B. Caughey, MD, MPH, PhD, Amy M. Valent, DO, MCR

KEYWORDS

- Diabetes and pregnancy • Medications and pregnancy • Diabetes and breastfeeding
- Metformin • Glyburide • Insulin • Acarbose • Pregnancy

KEY POINTS

- Glycemia is influenced by multiple factors which include nutritional health, physical activity, mental health, stress, social determinants of health, and sleep quality.
- Pregnant and lactating persons should be *educated* on the benefits, potential risks, and limitations of the medications available for managing glucose in pregnancy.
- Medical management should be *individualized* to determine the safest regimen to achieve pregnancy glycemic targets. Gestational age, insulin resistance factors (glucose tolerance test, A1C, prepregnancy and current body mass index, degree of glycemic control before initiating medications, and so forth), health literacy, and perinatal factors (ultrasound fetal measurements, prior pregnancy history, and so forth) should all be considered to develop a patient-centered pharmacologic regimen.
- Professional guidelines for glycemic management during pregnancy vary, in part because of limited studies among pregnant and lactating persons. The American College of Obstetricians and Gynecologists and the American Diabetes Association recommend insulin for first-line management. The Society for Maternal Fetal Medicine advises either metformin or insulin can be used as first-line agents over glyburide.

INTRODUCTION

Diabetes impacts nearly one in 10 pregnancies in the United States.[1] The glycemic management of diabetes in pregnancy is challenging with dynamic metabolic and physiologic changes across gestation. Glycemic targets during pregnancy are much tighter than nonpregnant targets because even small glucose elevations have been associated with significant adverse perinatal and neonatal consequences.[2] Although many patients with gestational diabetes (GDM) can be managed with medical nutrition

Division of Maternal-Fetal Medicine, Department of Obstetrics and Gynecology, School of Medicine
* Corresponding author. 3181 Southwest Sam Jackson Park Road, L-466, Portland, OR 97239.
E-mail address: covelli@ohsu.edu

Obstet Gynecol Clin N Am 50 (2023) 121–136
https://doi.org/10.1016/j.ogc.2022.10.007
0889-8545/23/Published by Elsevier Inc.

therapy (MNT) and lifestyle modifications, up to 30% require pharmacologic therapy to achieve pregnancy glycemic targets.[3] In addition, almost all patients with type 2 diabetes (T2DM) before pregnancy will require medical therapy.

The increasing fetal and placental demands with advancing gestation require maternal adaptations and rising insulin resistance to ensure adequate fuel delivery for normal fetal growth and development. Pharmacologic agents are initiated when pregnancy glycemic targets are not achieved with MNT and lifestyle modifications. In a systematic review and meta-analysis of observational studies of persons with GDM, the need for insulin treatment was associated with a body mass index (BMI) ≥ 30 kg/m^2, family history of T2DM, a prior history of GDM, and a higher hemoglobin A1C level (but still below diabetes cutoff range) at the time of GDM diagnosis.[4] At what point or degree of relative hyperglycemia pharmacotherapy should be considered is variable in practice, and the data are limited to provide quality guidance. In a meta-analysis that included 15 randomized controlled trials (RCT; $n = 4307$), 87% initiated pharmacologic therapy if either 1 or 2 values per 1- or 2-week period were higher than the target values.[5]

Medications available for optimizing glycemic control during pregnancy are limited. Before the 1990s, the medical management of diabetes in pregnancy predominantly used Neutral Protamine Hagedorn (NPH) and regular insulin. However, over the past several decades, rapid-acting insulin has become first-line therapy, often accompanied by an NPH or a longer acting insulin such as detemir. Although insulin has been shown to be safely used in pregnancy and does not cross the placenta, some oral agents have been investigated to expand the pool of available medications to manage hyperglycemia in pregnancy.

An RCT comparing glyburide and insulin, published in the New England Journal of Medicine in 2000,[6] demonstrated that glyburide and insulin similarly achieved pregnancy glucose targets (82% vs 88%) with only 4% in the glyburide group requiring transition to insulin to improve glycemic control. Although the study was not sufficiently powered to investigate neonatal outcomes, there was a higher incidence of macrosomia and hypoglycemia among the glyburide users. Despite the inadequate power of the study and misperception that glyburide did not cross the placenta well, it was rapidly adopted by many clinicians to manage pregnant patients with GDM. More recently, recommendations from the American College of Obstetricians and Gynecologists and the Society for Maternal Fetal Medicine have moved away from the use of glyburide due to its inferiority to both metformin and insulin when comparing maternal and neonatal outcomes in persons with GDM.[7]

Metformin has gained popularity over the years. The metformin in gestational (MiG) diabetes was the largest RCT of persons with GDM randomized to metformin or insulin, showing metformin alone or with supplemental insulin was not associated with adverse perinatal outcomes.[8] In this review, the authors examine the evidence surrounding the use of a wide range of insulin and oral agents most commonly used for the medical management of glucose among pregnancies complicated by diabetes, highlighting key points and considerations for use (**Box 1**).

Insulin

Insulin is a hormone (51-residue anabolic protein) that is secreted by the β-cells of the pancreatic islets of Langerhans. It is an important metabolic regulator that stimulates glucose uptake, suppresses hepatic gluconeogenesis, and regulates protein, fat, DNA, and RNA synthesis. The goal of insulin therapy is to mimic normal patterns of insulin secretion by the endocrine pancreas, which helps achieve glycemic control among patients with diabetes. Various insulin formulations are available on the market

---

Box 1
Key points and considerations for pharmacologic management of glucose during pregnancy

Insulin
- Rapid-acting insulin is used for prandial hyperglycemia and should be given 15 to 30 minutes before meals.
- Insulin absorption may be delayed with advancing gestation, and patients may need to administer rapid-acting insulin 30 to 45 minutes before a meal in the third trimester or consider switching to ultra-rapid insulin.[44]
- If rapid-acting insulin is *not* available, regular human insulin can be considered for prandial hyperglycemia and be given at least 30 to 60 minutes before meals.
- NPH insulin can be dosed at bedtime to improve fasting hyperglycemia. With its peak at 4 to 6 hours, NPH can target early morning insulin resistance and lower fasting glycemia.
- Consider a morning NPH injection for postprandial glucose elevations after a midday meal only if the patient has a structured eating schedule. It is important to time the morning NPH dose so that its peak lines up with a person's midday meal (ideally, 4–5 hours before eating lunch).
- Multidose injectables using detemir or glargine among patients who need long-acting glucose treatment and rapid-acting insulin coverage for meals are preferred for patients with an erratic eating schedule or who prefer to have more autonomy when insulin is required for prandial hyperglycemia.

Oral medications
- Oral agents should *not* be considered for pregnancies at <20 weeks gestation that require pharmacologic therapy for glycemic optimization
- Metformin can be considered for fasting or postprandial hyperglycemia. It crosses the placenta after approximately 12 weeks gestation and the long-term effects of fetal exposure to metformin in utero are unclear.
- Glyburide can be considered for postprandial hyperglycemia. It has been shown to cross the placenta using more sensitive assays. Owing to the increased clearance in pregnancy, it should be ideally taken 60 minutes before breakfast and/or dinner.
- Glyburide should *not* be prescribed at bedtime to help fasting hyperglycemia. It can cause hypoglycemia by stimulating release of insulin from the pancreatic beta cells, particularly if not administered timely.
- Acarbose can be considered for postprandial hyperglycemia, and it is still unknown whether it crosses the placenta.

---

and are primarily administered subcutaneously via syringe, pen, or an insulin pump. The different pharmacokinetic profiles of insulin products result from the properties of the tissue through which it must pass and the properties of the insulin molecule complex (**Table 1**).

Insulin pump systems
An insulin pump is a wearable device that is inserted subcutaneously and delivers continuous and customized doses of rapid-acting or ultra-rapid-acting insulin. The "basal" rate(s) is the programed rate (units per hour) at which small background doses of rapid-acting insulin are continuously delivered. To cover prandial glucose excursions, a larger "bolus" dose of insulin is administered before meals and/or snacks based on the anticipated grams of carbohydrate consumption.

Because the pump technology is complex and accurate carbohydrate counting is fundamental for appropriate insulin dosing, initiating an insulin pump during pregnancy should be considered with caution. The continuous metabolic changes in pregnancy and the steep learning curve required to manage an insulin pump can lead to delayed and prolonged periods of suboptimal glycemic control in pregnancy. The CONCEPTT trial compared continuous subcutaneous insulin infusion (CSII) with

Table 1
Insulin therapies commonly used during pregnancy

Insulin Type	Medication	Dosing	Peak and Duration	Key Considerations
Rapid-Acting	Lispro	• Administer 15–30 min before meals • Consider dosing 30–45 min before meals, 2nd and 3rd trimester	Peak: 30–90 min Duration: 3–4 h	• Used for postprandial hyperglycemia • Mimics physiologic prandial response with a faster onset and shorter duration of action than short-acting insulin, resulting in less hypoglycemia and improved prandial coverage • Approved for insulin pump use • Ultra-rapid acting lispro is an available bolus insulin option that contains excipients that enhance absorption and accelerate onset of action
	Aspart	• Administer 15–30 min before meals • Consider dosing 30–45 min before meals 2nd and 3rd trimester	Peak: 40–45 min Duration 3–5 h	• Used for postprandial hyperglycemia • Mimics physiologic prandial response with a faster onset and shorter duration of action than short-acting insulin, resulting in less hypoglycemia and improved prandial coverage • Approved for insulin pump use • Ultra-rapid acting aspart is an available bolus insulin option that contains excipients that enhance absorption and accelerate onset of action
	Glulisine	• Administer 15–30 min before meals	Peak: 55 min Duration: 3–5 h	• Used for postprandial hyperglycemia

			Peak / Duration	
		• Consider dosing 30–45 min before meals 2nd and 3rd trimester		• Mimics physiologic prandial response with a faster onset and shorter duration of action than short-acting insulin, resulting in less hypoglycemia and improved prandial coverage • Approved for limited insulin pumps
Short-Acting	Regular (U-100)	• Administer 30–60 min before meals • Consider administering at least 60 min before meals in the 2nd and 3rd trimester	Peak: 3 h Duration: 8 h	• Used for postprandial hyperglycemia • Risk for hypoglycemia if administration is timed poorly • Administering at least 30–60 min before meals can be challenging for some patients
	Regular (U-500)	• Administer 30–45 min before breakfast and dinner • Can titrate up to 30–45 min before all meals	Peak: 3–6 h Duration: 8–24 h (dose-dependent)	• Used for patients requiring >200 units total daily dose of insulin • Risk for hypoglycemia if administration is timed poorly
Intermediate-acting	Neutral Protamine Hagedorn	• Morning dose: Administer 4–6 h before the peak of a midday/lunch meal for midday prandial coverage • Bedtime dose: Administer at bedtime to help cover early morning insulin resistance	Peak: 4–8 h Duration: 10–20 h	• Used for fasting hyperglycemia and both midday prandial and basal daytime hyperglycemia • Best used during the day for people who have a structured eating schedule • Caution to use for nocturnal/fasting hyperglycemia among persons with T1DM who may be more sensitive to nocturnal hypoglycemia

(continued on next page)

Table 1
(continued)

Insulin Type	Medication	Dosing	Peak and Duration	Key Considerations
Long-acting	Detemir	• Daily at bedtime • Commonly administered every 12 h in pregnancy	No definitive peak Duration: 20 h	• Twice a day dosing allows for differing insulin dose concentrations during the day and night • Lesser degree over insulin overlap/stacking when used twice a day compared with glargine
	Glargine	• Daily at bedtime • May consider administration every 12 h in pregnancy but higher risk for insulin overlap/stacking and hypoglycemia	No definitive peak Duration: 24 h	• Higher risk for insulin overlap/stacking and hypoglycemia when administered twice a day

multiple daily injections (MDI) among patients with type 1 diabetes (T1DM). A secondary analysis demonstrated that the CSII group resulted in better first trimester glycemic control and lower overall insulin requirements than MDI users. However, the MDI users were more likely to have better glycemic outcomes and less likely to have gestational hypertension, neonatal hypoglycemia, and neonatal intensive care unit (NICU) admissions than pump users.[9]

Hybrid closed-loop systems combine continuous glucose monitoring (CGM) data, an insulin pump, and proprietary algorithms to automatically deliver variable basal insulin concentrations to keep glucose within a specific target range. CGM technology is commonly used among patients with T1DM using MDI or an insulin pump to characterize glycemia in real-time or intermittent scan. The CONCEPTT trial demonstrated lower rates of maternal hyperglycemia and neonatal adverse outcomes among participants using CGM. Both CGM technology and hybrid closed-loop systems are considered off-label use in pregnancy, as the accuracy of CGM across gestation has not been studied and current hybrid closed-loop models cannot lower the glucose target level to achieve a pregnancy-specific range (average glucose = 100). Providers should caution their patients to confirm CGM data with self-capillary blood glucose checks, particularly if the glucose value is discrepant from clinical symptomatology.

Rapid-Acting Insulin

Insulin aspart, lispro, and glulisine
Insulin analogs better mimic endogenous insulin secretion as compared with regular insulin and have become first-line therapy to treat prandial hyperglycemia. High-quality comparisons of insulin analogs and regular insulin to determine differences in glycemic control are limited.[10] However, an RCT comparing insulin aspart and regular insulin in basal–bolus therapy with NPH insulin (n = 322, T1DM) demonstrated aspart to be at least as safe and effective as human insulin with less major hypoglycemic episodes per year (1.4% vs 2.1%; Relative risk [RR] 0.720 [95% Confidence interval [CI] 0.36–1.46]).[11] Participants using aspart had a 28% lower risk for major hypoglycemia, and a 52% lower risk for major nocturnal hypoglycemia when compared with human/regular insulin users.[11] Insulin analogs have not been shown to be associated with any congenital malformations and are approved for use in pregnancy.[11]

Short-Acting Insulin

Regular or U-100 insulin
Although there are no safety restrictions to the use of regular insulin in pregnancy, regular insulin should only be considered if rapid-acting insulin is not available. Educating patients on the importance of *timing* regular insulin to avoid hypoglycemia is imperative and often the biggest challenge for patients. Moreover, the duration of regular insulin is longer than insulin analogs so there is greater potential for insulin stacking, which could further contribute to an increased risk of unintended hypoglycemia.

U-500 insulin
Regular U-500 insulin is five times more concentrated than U-100 human insulin. It is often used outside of pregnancy in patients requiring greater than 200 units of insulin daily. It differs from U-100 insulin in that it has a delayed peak of action and a longer duration of action (see **Table 1**). Among patients requiring large insulin concentrations to achieve glycemic pregnancy targets, U-500 may be the preferable approach to insulin dosing. With a longer duration and potential for insulin stacking, patients using

U-500 have a higher risk of hypoglycemic events. Currently, there is a paucity of data on the utility and effectiveness of U-500 insulin in pregnancy.[12]

Intermediate-Acting Insulin

Neutral Protamine Hagedorn

Insulin isophane (NPH) is considered an intermediate-acting insulin and is commonly used in pregnancy. NPH is valuable at addressing fasting hyperglycemia. When administered at bedtime, the 4 to 8 hour peak can effectively lower blood sugars overnight when the naturally rising levels of cortisol and growth hormone can challenge early morning glycemia. Consider morning or daytime NPH only for patients who have structured meal timing with midday hyperglycemia. NPH is not an optimal choice for shift-workers, sensitive to overnight hypoglycemia, or persons with erratic meal timing.

Long-Acting Insulin

Detemir

Detemir has Food Drug Administration (FDA) approval for use in pregnancy and is a favorable option for basal insulin coverage in pregnancy. In an RCT of insulin detemir versus NPH for the treatment of pregnant women with GDM and T2DM, the time to achieve glycemic control between the two groups was similar with no differences in maternal weight gain or perinatal outcomes.[13] However, the NPH group experienced more hypoglycemic events than the detemir group.[13] Detemir is a particularly important option to consider if patients have unpredictable schedules or meal timing, as it has less of a peak than NPH and does not depend on food consumption to prevent hypoglycemia.

Glargine

Similar to detemir, glargine insulin has a long duration ($\sim$24 hours) of action without a defined peak. With its increased use outside of pregnancy, it is more common to see pregnant or persons planning pregnancy taking glargine for basal coverage. A systematic review and meta-analysis that included 702 women reported no evidence of increased adverse fetal outcomes with the use of glargine in comparison to NPH in persons with GDM or preexisting diabetes.[14] Higher insulin concentrations may benefit from twice daily dosing, but caution a higher potential for insulin stacking due to glargine's longer duration (22–24 hours) versus detemir's shorter duration (18–20 hours) of action. Consider switching from glargine to detemir if the patient is experiencing episodes of hypoglycemia that cannot otherwise be explained.

Degludec

Many patients with diabetes outside of pregnancy are taking long-acting insulin degludec due to its longer half-life and less of a peak than other basal insulins making the flexibility with injection timing very convenient for patients. Although there are a few case studies published showing successful outcomes when taking degludec in pregnancy, there are currently no RCTs to determine safety and optimal strategies for use in pregnancy.[15]

Oral Agents

Metformin

Metformin is increasingly being used as first-line therapy for GDM after failure to achieve pregnancy glycemic targets with MNT and lifestyle modifications. However, recent clinical evidence and basic research suggest caution when using metformin during pregnancy.[16] Metformin has been associated with increased rates of spontaneous

Table 2
Oral antidiabetic medications used during pregnancy

Medication	Benefits	Limitations	Fetal Risk	Key Considerations and Dosing Administration
Metformin	• Oral formulation • Low cost • No need for refrigeration • Lower gestational weight gain	• Crosses the placenta with fetal concentrations similar or higher than maternal levels • GI intolerance • Lactic acidosis (rare) • Vitamin B12 insufficiency (long-term use) • Approximately half started on metformin may require insulin to achieve pregnancy targets	• No evidence of congenital malformations • Potential risk for small for gestational age (SGA) • Potential risk for higher childhood weight and altered body composition	• May be used for fasting or postprandial hyperglycemia • Starting dose 500 or 850 mg with meal and/or bedtime • Titration every 5–7 d, incrementally by 500 mg until maximum dose 2000–2500 mg
Glyburide	• Oral formulation • Low cost • No need for refrigeration	• Crosses the placenta • Hypoglycemia • Weight gain • Approximately one in five will require insulin to achieve pregnancy targets	• No evidence of congenital malformations • Neonatal hypoglycemia • Unknown long-term risks for fetal drug exposure	• May be used for postprandial hyperglycemia • Starting dose 2.5 mg and taken 30–60 min before breakfast and/or 30–60 min before dinner • Titration every 5–7 d, incrementally by 2.5 mg until maximum dose 20 mg
Acarbose	• Oral medication • Low cost • No need for refrigeration	• GI intolerance	• Limited studies of acarbose use in pregnancy	• May be used for postprandial hyperglycemia • Starting dose 25 mg taken with meal(s) • Titration every 5–7 d, incrementally by 25 mg until maximum dose 300 mg

(continued on next page)

Table 2
(continued)

Medication	Benefits	Limitations	Fetal Risk	Key Considerations and Dosing Administration
SGLT2 inhibitors	• Oral medication	• No human pregnancy studies	• Unknown	• Medication should be discontinued during pregnancy and lactation
GLP-1 agonists	• Subcutaneous injection	• No human pregnancy studies	• Unknown	• Medication should be discontinued during pregnancy and lactation
DPP-4 inhibitors	• Oral medication	• No human studies conducted in pregnancy	• Unknown	• Medication should be discontinued during pregnancy and lactation

preterm birth and small for gestational age infants, but also with lower gestational weight gain.[17,18] Moreover, the MiG trial demonstrated almost half (46%) of the participants randomized to metformin required supplemental insulin to achieve pregnancy glucose targets.[18] Follow-up studies of offspring exposed to metformin are limited but suggest offspring born to individuals using metformin during pregnancy have increased subcutaneous fat, BMI, and adverse metabolic profiles compared with offspring pregnancies that were not exposed to metformin.[16,19–21] Metformin crosses the placenta through highly expressed organic cation transporters 3 (OCT3) and have been demonstrated to have similar or even higher fetal concentrations as maternal levels of metformin.[22] Although metformin has not been demonstrated to be associated with congenital anomalies, safety of use in pregnancy should consider the potential long-term implications on offspring health with *in utero* exposure to the medication.

Metformin is an inexpensive, oral medication with maximum dose of 2500 mg daily and does not contribute to hypoglycemia (**Table 2**). It should be titrated every 5 to 7 days in increments of 500 or 850 mg to a therapeutic dose of 2000 to 2500 mg. Although not required to be taken with food, metformin's side effects may be better tolerated when taken with food. Titration can occur more gradually if GI side effects continue but switching agents should also be considered if GI intolerance persists. Metformin is the only oral medication used in pregnancy that can treat both fasting and postprandial hyperglycemia. The published studies on metformin concentrations in breast milk involve small sample sizes but demonstrate metformin concentrations in breast milk is overall low.[23–25] The mean infant exposure to the drug was 0.28% of the weight-normalized maternal dose, which is well below the 10% level of concern for breastfeeding.[24]

Metformin versus insulin

A recent systematic review and meta-analysis of 21 RCTs ($n = 4545$) compared the efficacy and safety of metformin alone or as add-on therapy to insulin versus insulin alone in pregnancy in persons with GDM or T2DM.[26] Metformin users had significantly reduced maternal weight gain, gestational hypertension, maternal hypoglycemia, neonatal hypoglycemia, NICU admissions, birth weight $\geq$4000 g, and large for gestational age (LGA) compared with insulin therapy alone.[26] However, metformin-exposed pregnancies have been associated with higher rates of spontaneous preterm birth and small for gestational age infants compared with insulin therapy.[17,26,27] To achieve pregnancy glycemic targets, pregnant persons who require insulin have a more severe metabolic phenotype, particularly in the setting of preexisting diabetes, early onset hyperglycemia, or persons who failed to achieve targets with oral agents. Therefore, retrospective analyses need to be interpreted with caution.

Glyburide

Glyburide is a controversial sulfonylurea in the nonpregnant population, causing more hypoglycemia and interfering with ischemic preconditioning compared with other types of sulfonylureas.[28] In a meta-analysis of 32 RCTs of persons with GDM, including 6 kinds of treatments (metformin, metformin plus insulin, insulin, glyburide, acarbose, and placebo), glyburide was found to have the highest incidence of macrosomia, preeclampsia, hyperbilirubinemia, neonatal hypoglycemia, preterm birth, and low birth weight compared with other interventions.[29] In a pharmacokinetic study of glyburide, pregnant persons with GDM were shown to have doubled the rate of oral clearance than in nonpregnant persons and glyburide crossed the placenta more than was previously assumed.[30] Plasma concentrations increase 1 hour after drug ingestion, peak at 2 to 3 hours and return to baseline levels by 8 hours.[30] The pharmacokinetics is important to recognize when considering glyburide for glycemic management. The existing studies describe taking glyburide at the start of meals or bedtime, but it may be more effective if dosed 60 minutes before eating and prescribing at bedtime is avoided to prevent unintended hypoglycemia.[31–33] Considering the challenges of dosing glyburide appropriately, risks of hypoglycemia, and unknown long-term implications of drug exposure in the offspring, glyburide should not be considered first line for pharmacologic therapy of GDM.

Glyburide versus metformin

A systematic review and meta-analysis of 15 RCTs demonstrated a lower fasting blood glucose during treatment but a higher incidence of maternal weight gain, birth weight, macrosomia, large-for-gestational-age newborn, and neonatal hypoglycemia among pregnancies treated with glyburide compared with metformin.[7] A more recent meta-analysis did not show differences in glucose levels or birth weight between pregnancies treated with glyburide compared with metformin, but the glyburide treated participants had higher rates of gestational weight gain.[34] Although studies have demonstrated a significantly lower risk for macrosomia and lower birth weights among metformin-treated pregnancies compared with glyburide, these data need to be interpreted with caution as the MiTy trial demonstrated higher rates of SGA among people treated with metformin.[21] Long-term studies of glyburide and metformin are needed to understand the health and safety risks of fetal drug exposure to these medications.

Glyburide versus insulin

Although an RCT meta-analysis comparing glyburide and insulin in persons with GDM demonstrated no significant differences in glycemia (82% glyburide and 88% insulin-treated pregnancies achieved glycemic pregnancy ranges), the glyburide-treated group had higher rates of neonatal hypoglycemia.[6] Moreover, Balsells and colleagues'[7] systematic review and meta-analysis of 15 RCT ($n = 2509$) demonstrated persons who took glyburide for GDM management had higher birth weights, macrosomia, neonatal hypoglycemia studies since that meta-analysis have had conflicting conclusions to the risks of glyburide compared with insulin.[35,36] A retrospective cohort study of 11,321 patients with GDM by Hedderson and colleagues[37] used inverse probability weighting estimation to separately compare perinatal outcomes between pregnancies initiating glyburide and insulin while combining Super Learning for propensity score estimation to evaluate sustained exposure to the same therapy. Their analysis showed similar rates of infant hypoglycemia, hyperbilirubinemia, appropriate size-for-gestational age, and cesarean delivery among glyburide and insulin-treated pregnancies. An open-label, feasibility study in five UK antenatal clinics randomized metformin-treated pregnant persons with GDM who failed to achieve pregnancy targets to glyburide or insulin. Glyburide was 8.3 times more likely to fail to achieve pregnancy targets in pregnancies less than 25 weeks gestation than those diagnosed after 25 weeks gestation.[38]

Similar to studies comparing metformin and insulin, observational and retrospective cohort studies must be interpreted with caution when comparing glyburide and insulin, acknowledging provider bias in prescribing glyburide versus insulin and accounting for the addition of insulin when glyburide therapy fails to achieve pregnancy targets. A retrospective cohort study of persons with GDM who required medication therapy found that women who either did not attend high school or did not speak English as their primary language were more likely to receive glyburide versus insulin.[39] Palatnik and colleagues[40] conducted a retrospective cohort study ($n = 437$) of persons with GDM requiring medications and found that women of Hispanic ethnicity and no

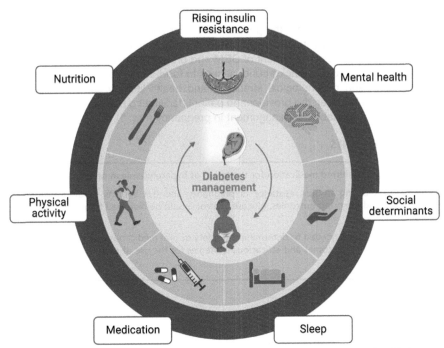

Fig. 1. Factors that influence diabetes management in pregnancy. Metabolic health in pregnancy is complicated by many factors that not only influence glycemia but also the ability to manage diabetes effectively in pregnancy. Understanding these factors and individualizing therapy with each patient is imperative for patients to achieve pregnancy glucose targets and health goals. (Created with BioRender.com.)

insurance were more likely be prescribed an oral antidiabetic medication for GDM management. Recognizing unconscious prescribing patterns and individualizing medication regimens with shared decision-making is encouraged.

Acarbose

Acarbose is a complex oligosaccharide that acts as a competitive, reversible inhibitor of pancreatic alpha-amylase and membrane-bound intestinal alpha-glucoside hydrolase, slowing glucose absorption and lowering *postprandial* glycemia.[41] There is limited data for use of acarbose in pregnancy and few studies in regard to its use in pregnancy. One prospective, open-label study (*n* = 100) demonstrated comparable glycemic control among patients with GDM treated with acarbose and insulin.[42] There were no significantly different adverse neonatal or maternal outcomes or congenital anomalies in the acarbose treated group.[42] When acarbose was added to glyburide in patients with GDM, there were low rates of failure and transition to insulin, while maintaining similar rates of cesarean delivery and neonatal outcomes as the insulin treatment group.[43]

SUMMARY

Management of pregestational and GDM is complicated, and more studies using oral medications in pregnancy need to be conducted. Regardless of one's own practice, it is important to individualize therapy, aiming for a regimen with the lowest immediate and long-term health risks for the gestational carrier and offspring. The goal as providers is to educate patients on benefits, potential risks, and limitations of the different options available. The management of GDM and pregestational diabetes is complex. Understanding a patient's background, access to food, medications, care resources, mental health and psychological stressors, and health literacy can help open the communication between the provider and patient, facilitating patient-centered strategies for optimizing diabetes management in pregnancy (**Fig. 1**).

CLINICS CARE POINTS

- Insulin is the preferred medication for treatment of hyperglycemia in pregnancy.
- Due to increasing insulin resistance in pregnancy and the impacts of dysglycemia on perinatal and offspring outcomes, glucose control should be reviewed frequently during pregnancy.
- Further research is needed to determine the safety of oral medication use in pregnancy on offspring health outcomes and efficacious strategies for the use of different insulin types during pregnancy.

DISCLOSURE

There are no financial disclosures.

REFERENCES

1. Deputy NP, Kim SY, Conrey EJ, et al. Prevalence and Changes in Preexisting Diabetes and Gestational Diabetes Among Women Who Had a Live Birth - United States, 2012-2016. MMWR Morb Mortal Wkly Rep 2018;67(43):1201-7.
2. Coustan DR, Lowe LP, Metzger BE, et al. The Hyperglycemia and Adverse Pregnancy Outcome (HAPO) study: paving the way for new diagnostic criteria for gestational diabetes mellitus. Am J Obstet Gynecol 2010;202(6):654.e1-6.
3. SMFM Statement: Pharmacological treatment of gestational diabetes. Am J Obstet Gynecol 2018;218(5):B2-4.
4. Alvarez-Silvares E, Bermúdez-González M, Vilouta-Romero M, et al. Prediction of insulin therapy in women with gestational diabetes: a systematic review and meta-analysis of observational studies. J Perinat Med 2022;50(5):608-19.
5. Caissutti C, Saccone G, Khalifeh A, et al. Which criteria should be used for starting pharmacologic therapy for management of gestational diabetes in pregnancy? Evidence from randomized controlled trials. J Matern Fetal Neonatal Med 2019;32(17):2905-14.
6. Langer O, Conway DL, Berkus MD, et al. A comparison of glyburide and insulin in women with gestational diabetes mellitus. N Engl J Med 2000;343(16):1134-8.
7. Balsells M, García-Patterson A, Solà I, et al. Glibenclamide, metformin, and insulin for the treatment of gestational diabetes: a systematic review and meta-analysis. BMJ 2015;350:h102.
8. Tripathi R, Tyagi S, Goel V. Metformin in gestational diabetes mellitus. Indian J Med Res 2017;145(5):588-91.
9. Feig DS, Donovan LE, Corcoy R, et al. Continuous glucose monitoring in pregnant women with type 1 diabetes (CONCEPTT): a multicentre international randomised controlled trial. Lancet 2017;390(10110):2347-59.

10. Santos LL, Santos JL, Barbosa LT, et al. Effectiveness of Insulin Analogs Compared with Human Insulins in Pregnant Women with Diabetes Mellitus: Systematic Review and Meta-analysis. Rev Bras Ginecol Obstet 2019;41(2):104–15. Efetividade dos análogos da insulina comparados às insulinas humanas em gestantes com diabetes mellitus: Revisão sistemática com metanálise.
11. Mathiesen ER, Kinsley B, Amiel SA, et al. Maternal glycemic control and hypoglycemia in type 1 diabetic pregnancy: a randomized trial of insulin aspart versus human insulin in 322 pregnant women. Diabetes Care 2007;30(4):771–6.
12. Zuckerwise LC, Werner EF, Pettker CM, et al. Pregestational diabetes with extreme insulin resistance: use of U-500 insulin in pregnancy. Obstet Gynecol 2012;120(2 Pt 2):439–42.
13. Herrera KM, Rosenn BM, Foroutan J, et al. Randomized controlled trial of insulin detemir versus NPH for the treatment of pregnant women with diabetes. Am J Obstet Gynecol 2015;213(3):426.e1–7.
14. Pollex E, Moretti ME, Koren G, et al. Safety of insulin glargine use in pregnancy: a systematic review and meta-analysis. Ann Pharmacother 2011;45(1):9–16.
15. Hiranput S, Ahmed SH, Macaulay D, et al. Successful outcomes with insulin degludec in pregnancy: a case series. Diabetes Ther 2019;10(1):283–9.
16. Barbour LA, Scifres C, Valent AM, et al. A cautionary response to SMFM statement: pharmacological treatment of gestational diabetes. Am J Obstet Gynecol 2018;219(4):367.e1–7.
17. Feig DS, Donovan LE, Zinman B, et al. Metformin in women with type 2 diabetes in pregnancy (MiTy): a multicentre, international, randomised, placebo-controlled trial. Lancet Diabetes Endocrinol 2020;8(10):834–44.
18. Rowan JA, Hague WM, Gao W, et al. Metformin versus insulin for the treatment of gestational diabetes. N Engl J Med 2008;358(19):2003–15.
19. Rø TB, Ludvigsen HV, Carlsen SM, et al. Growth, body composition and metabolic profile of 8-year-old children exposed to metformin in utero. Scand J Clin Lab Invest 2012;72(7):570–5.
20. Rowan JA, Rush EC, Plank LD, et al. Metformin in gestational diabetes: the offspring follow-up (MiG TOFU): body composition and metabolic outcomes at 7-9 years of age. BMJ Open Diabetes Res Care 2018;6(1):e000456.
21. Tarry-Adkins JL, Aiken CE, Ozanne SE. Neonatal, infant, and childhood growth following metformin versus insulin treatment for gestational diabetes: A systematic review and meta-analysis. PLoS Med 2019;16(8):e1002848.
22. Eyal S, Easterling TR, Carr D, et al. Pharmacokinetics of metformin during pregnancy. Drug Metab Dispos 2010;38(5):833–40.
23. Gardiner SJ, Kirkpatrick CM, Begg EJ, et al. Transfer of metformin into human milk. Clin Pharmacol Ther 2003;73(1):71–7.
24. Hale TW, Kristensen JH, Hackett LP, et al. Transfer of metformin into human milk. Diabetologia 2002;45(11):1509–14.
25. Briggs GG, Ambrose PJ, Nageotte MP, et al. Excretion of metformin into breast milk and the effect on nursing infants. Obstet Gynecol 2005;105(6):1437–41.
26. He K, Guo Q, Ge J, et al. The efficacy and safety of metformin alone or as an add-on therapy to insulin in pregnancy with GDM or T2DM: A systematic review and meta-analysis of 21 randomized controlled trials. J Clin Pharm Ther 2022;47(2):168–77.
27. Gui J, Liu Q, Feng L. Metformin vs insulin in the management of gestational diabetes: a meta-analysis. PLoS One 2013;8(5):e64585.

28. Zeller M, Danchin N, Simon D, et al. Impact of type of preadmission sulfonylureas on mortality and cardiovascular outcomes in diabetic patients with acute myocardial infarction. J Clin Endocrinol Metab 2010;95(11):4993–5002.

29. Liang HL, Ma SJ, Xiao YN, et al. Comparative efficacy and safety of oral antidiabetic drugs and insulin in treating gestational diabetes mellitus: An updated PRISMA-compliant network meta-analysis. Medicine (Baltimore) 2017;96(38): e7939.

30. Caritis SN, Hebert MF. A pharmacologic approach to the use of glyburide in pregnancy. Obstet Gynecol 2013;121(6):1309–12.

31. Rochon M, Rand L, Roth L, et al. Glyburide for the management of gestational diabetes: risk factors predictive of failure and associated pregnancy outcomes. Am J Obstet Gynecol 2006;195(4):1090–4.

32. Anjalakshi C, Balaji V, Balaji MS, et al. A prospective study comparing insulin and glibenclamide in gestational diabetes mellitus in Asian Indian women. Diabetes Res Clin Pract 2007;76(3):474–5.

33. Silva JC, Pacheco C, Bizato J, et al. Metformin compared with glyburide for the management of gestational diabetes. Int J Gynaecol Obstet 2010;111(1):37–40.

34. Oliveira MM, Andrade KFO, Lima GHS, et al. Metformin versus glyburide in treatment and control of gestational diabetes mellitus: a systematic review with meta-analysis. Einstein (Sao Paulo). 2022;20:eRW6155.

35. Song R, Chen L, Chen Y, et al. Comparison of glyburide and insulin in the management of gestational diabetes: a meta-analysis. PLoS One 2017;12(8): e0182488.

36. Moretti ME, Rezvani M, Koren G. Safety of glyburide for gestational diabetes: a meta-analysis of pregnancy outcomes. Ann Pharmacother 2008;42(4):483–90.

37. Hedderson MM, Badon SE, Pimentel N, et al. Association of Glyburide and Subcutaneous Insulin With Perinatal Complications Among Women With Gestational Diabetes. JAMA Netw Open 2022;5(3):e225026.

38. Kahn BF, Davies JK, Lynch AM, et al. Predictors of glyburide failure in the treatment of gestational diabetes. Obstet Gynecol 2006;107(6):1303–9.

39. Cheng YW, Chung JH, Block-Kurbisch I, et al. Treatment of gestational diabetes mellitus: glyburide compared to subcutaneous insulin therapy and associated perinatal outcomes. J Matern Fetal Neonatal Med 2012;25(4):379–84.

40. Palatnik A, Harrison RK, Thakkar MY, et al. Correlates of Insulin Selection as a First-Line Pharmacological Treatment for Gestational Diabetes. Am J Perinatol 2022;39(1):8–15.

41. McIver LA, Preuss CV, Tripp J. Acarbose. StatPearls. Treasure Island, FL: StatPearls Publishing Copyright © 2022, StatPearls Publishing LLC.; 2022.

42. Jayasingh S, Sr, Nanda S, et al. Comparison of fetomaternal outcomes in patients with gestational diabetes mellitus treated with insulin versus acarbose: results of a prospective, open label, controlled study. Cureus 2020;12(12):e12283.

43. Wang X, Liu W, Chen H, et al. Comparison of insulin, metformin, and glyburide on perinatal complications of gestational diabetes mellitus: a systematic review and meta-analysis. Gynecol Obstet Invest 2021;86(3):218–30.

44. Murphy HR, Elleri D, Allen JM, et al. Pathophysiology of postprandial hyperglycaemia in women with type 1 diabetes during pregnancy. Diabetologia 2012; 55(2):282–93.

Antibiotics in Labor and Delivery

Joanna M. Izewski, MD, Brandon Z. Bell, DO, David M. Haas, MD, MS*

KEYWORDS

- Antibiotics • Pregnancy • Infection

KEY POINTS

- Antibiotic use in labor and delivery is recommended for Group B streptococcus prophylaxis, PPROM latency, cesarean deliveries, obstetric anal sphincter injuries, infections during labor (chorioamnionitis and endometritis), and for urinary tract infections.
- Antibiotics are not indicated for routine labor and delivery or for operative vaginal delivery.
- Decision and treatment algorithms can guide clinicians in areas of obstetric antibiotic use.

INTRODUCTION

Nearly two-thirds of all pregnant individuals report at least one infection during pregnancy.[1] Severe infections can contribute to maternal morbidity and mortality.[2] Thus, the prevention and treatment of infections during labor and delivery are crucial in reducing adverse perinatal outcomes.

Antibiotics are taken by approximately 1 in every 4 pregnant individuals during their pregnancy or delivery.[3,4] Antibiotics are not only used to treat active infections but also as prophylactic medications to prevent severe peripartum infections.[5] This review will discuss clinical situations where antibiotics are used in labor and delivery care, as well as specific considerations for dosing antibiotics in pregnant individuals.

Prophylactic Antibiotics in Labor

Routine use during labor

Routine use of antibiotics during labor is not recommended.[5] Existing evidence shows that up to 50% of antibiotics prescribed in US hospitals are prescribed inappropriately, contributing to the growing epidemic of antibiotic resistance and its associated morbidity.[6] Thus, antibiotics are only indicated in particular clinical scenarios and administration should follow guidelines for antimicrobial stewardship outlined by individual institutions.[5,6]

The authors report no conflict of interest and no funding for this study.
Indiana University School of Medicine
* Corresponding author. Department of OB/GYN, 550 North University Boulevard, UH2440, Indianapolis, IN 46202.
E-mail address: dahaas@iupui.edu

Obstet Gynecol Clin N Am 50 (2023) 137–150
https://doi.org/10.1016/j.ogc.2022.10.011
0889-8545/23/© 2022 Elsevier Inc. All rights reserved.

Group B Streptococcus prophylaxis

Group B *Streptococcus* (GBS), or *Streptococcus agalactiae*, is a gram-positive bacterium, which colonizes the gastrointestinal and genitourinary tracts and is present in approximately 10% to 30% of pregnant patients at any given time.[7] Vertical transmission to the infant occurs in up to 50% of women colonized with GBS, and GBS remains the leading infectious cause of neonatal morbidity and mortality in the United States.[8,9]

National screening and antibiotic prophylaxis guidelines developed during the past 20 years are aimed mainly at prevention of early-onset disease (EOD), defined as neonatal sepsis, pneumonia, or meningitis within the first 7 days of life.[7] The leading risk factor for vertical transmission is vaginal-rectal colonization of the pregnant patient at the time of labor, and risk further increases with rupture of membranes. Approximately 1% to 2% of neonates born to pregnant persons with a GBS-colonized genital tract will develop clinically apparent GBS EOD without antibiotic prophylaxis. Implementation of national guidelines for screening of pregnant patients during pregnancy, as well as intrapartum antibiotic prophylaxis guidelines, has reduced the incidence of GBS EOD in neonates by more than 80%.[7,8,10]

Universal culture-based antepartum screening for pregnant patients is superior to risk-based screening and is currently recommended by leading national organizations such as the American College of Obstetricians and Gynecologists (ACOG) and The Centers for Disease Control.[8,9] Studies also suggest that GBS cultures have a high degree of accuracy in predicting GBS colonization status at delivery if collected within 5 weeks of birth.[11,12] In a recent update, ACOG recommends universal screening for all pregnant persons between 36 0/7 and 37 6/7 weeks of gestation, unless the patient already qualifies for antibiotic prophylaxis by other criteria. These criteria include (1) a positive urine culture in the current pregnancy, (2) preterm labor before 37 0/7 weeks with unknown GBS status, or (3) a prior child affected by GBS EOD.[8] Full criteria for intrapartum antibiotic prophylaxis are summarized in **Box 1**.

Infection prophylaxis with antibiotics during labor aims to decrease the colonization load in the pregnant patient thereby lowering the risk of vertical transmission to the neonate, as well as to provide adequate antibiotic levels in the fetus through placental perfusion.[8,13] Current therapeutic regimen recommendations have been developed with these goals in mind (**Fig. 1**).

Box 1
Indications for Group B Streptococcus antimicrobial prophylaxis

- GBS-positive culture in current pregnancy (obtained within 5 weeks of presentation)
- GBS-positive urine culture in current pregnancy
- Prior child affected with GBS EOD
- Unknown GBS status if intrapartum and:
  - Gestational age less than 37 0/7
  - Membrane rupture greater than 18 h
  - Intrapartum fever of 100.4 F or more
  - Known GBS-positive culture in prior pregnancy
  - Intrapartum-positive NAAT GBS result

Abbreviation: NAAT, nucleic acid amplification test.

Data from Prevention of Group B Streptococcal Early-Onset Disease in Newborns: ACOG Committee Opinion, Number 797 [published correction appears in Obstet Gynecol. 2020 Apr;135(4):978-979]. Obstet Gynecol. 2020;135(2):e51-e72; with permission.

Intravenous administration of penicillin (PCN) or ampicillin remains the first-line agent for prophylaxis because these agents have a narrow therapeutic window for gram-positive bacteria and resistance is uncommon.[8] Alternatives are suggested for those individuals with a PCN allergy. It is recommended to investigate a patient's specific allergies before presentation to labor and delivery. GBS susceptibilities should also be analyzed in PCN-allergic patients (with specific focus on cefazolin and clindamycin) to better tailor alternative therapy. Up to 80% to 90% of women who report a PCN allergy do not have true allergy, or the allergic reaction is not an IgE-mediated, anaphylactic type, reaction.[14,15] PCN allergy testing can be used in pregnancy to help delineate risk.[16] For those patients who are at high-risk for an IgE-mediated reaction and susceptibilities of the GBS isolate to clindamycin are not known, vancomycin remains the agent of choice.[8,17] Regardless of the chosen agent, current recommendation is for treatment to continue for at least *4 hours* before delivery whenever clinically safe and possible, which is the minimal treatment time needed to significantly decrease the risk of neonatal GBS EOD.[8,18]

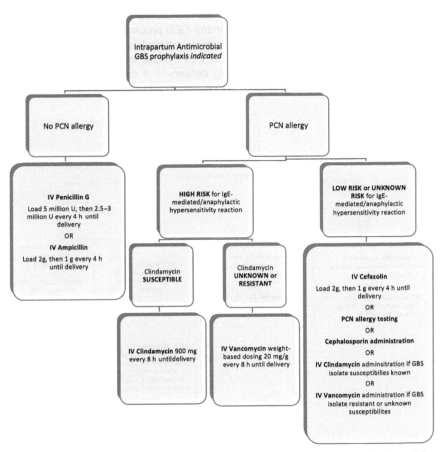

Fig. 1. Antibiotic prophylaxis treatment algorithm for GBS-positive status. (*Adapted from* Prevention of Group B Streptococcal Early-Onset Disease in Newborns: ACOG Committee Opinion, Number 797 [published correction appears in Obstet Gynecol. 2020 Apr;135(4):978-979]. Obstet Gynecol. 2020;135(2):e51-e72; with permission.)

Preterm prelabor rupture of membranes latency

Preterm prelabor rupture of membranes (PPROM) is defined as clinical evidence of rupture of membranes before 37 0/7 weeks.[19] Approximately 50% of patients with PPROM will ultimately proceed to delivery within 7 days.[20] Clinically evident intra-amniotic infection occurs in 15% to 35% of patients with PPROM,[21] with the incidence of infection inversely proportional to gestational age, and notably higher at earlier gestational ages.[22] Current recommendations by ACOG and The Society for Maternal-Fetal Medicine (SMFM) includes initiation of antibiotic prophylaxis (in the absence of clinical contraindications) if rupture of membranes occurs before 34 0/7 weeks of gestation.[19] Additionally, SMFM advises that latency antibiotics can be considered as early as 20 0/7 weeks.[23] Initiation of prophylaxis has been shown to increase latency, or the time from rupture of membranes until delivery, and to decrease the neonatal morbidity and mortality associated with sepsis and prematurity.[19] No one specific antibiotic regimen has been shown to be superior to another.[5,24] Treatment should be tailored to include coverage of GBS, aerobic gram-negative bacilli, anaerobic species, as well as *Ureoplasma* and *Chlamydia trachomatis*.[25]

Regardless of regimen, recommended duration of treatment is for *7 days after first presentation*.[19,24] Following this initial 7 days, treatment should be guided by clinical signs and symptoms of intra-amniotic infection and/or GBS prophylaxis guidelines.[5,8] **Fig. 2** summarizes evidence-based regimens for antibiotic prophylaxis to help increase latency.

Clinical contraindications to latency antibiotics include evidence of intra-amniotic infection, fetal compromise, or impending delivery.[19] If delivery seems imminent, GBS prophylaxis should be administered instead of latency antibiotics. Similarly, if

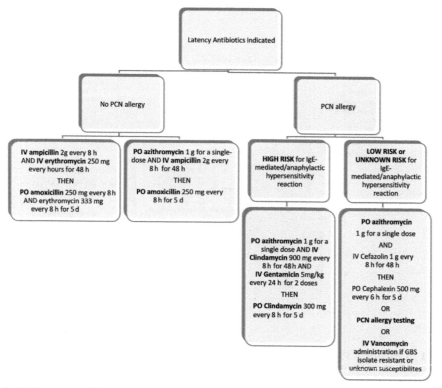

Fig. 2. Latency antibiotic prophylaxis treatment algorithm for PPROM.

intra-amniotic infection is suspected or confirmed, antibiotic therapy for chorioamnio-nitis should be started.[19]

Operative Delivery

Operative vaginal delivery

Operative vaginal delivery (OVD) is performed by using a vacuum extractor or forceps to assist the delivery of the fetal head. OVD accounts for 3.3% of US deliveries and is associated with an increased risk of maternal infection compared with spontaneous delivery.[26] Contributive factors to the increased infection risk associated with OVD include insertion of instruments, bladder catheterization, and increased risk of extensive perineal lacerations.[27] Because up to approximately 16% of patients with an OVD develop an infection,[28] prophylactic postdelivery antibiotics are often prescribed for these individuals.

Current Guidelines

The American College of Obstetrics and Gynecology (ACOG) currently does not recommend routine use of prophylactic antibiotics in the setting of OVD.[26] However, the Royal College of Obstetrics and Gynecology (RCOG) does recommend a single prophylactic dose of intravenous amoxicillin and clavulanic acid be administered following assisted vaginal birth because it significantly reduces confirmed or suspected maternal infection compared with placebo.[29]

Current Evidence

A 2020 study from the United Kingdom in 2019 involving more than 3000 participants assessed infection rates following OVD at 36 weeks gestation or later.[30] This study, titled "Prophylactic Antibiotics in the Prevention of Infection After Operative Vaginal Delivery (ANODE)", randomly assigned patients to receive antibiotics or placebo, with a primary outcome of confirmed or suspected maternal infection within 6 weeks of delivery. The trial showed that fewer women provided amoxicillin and clavulanic acid had a confirmed or suspected infection than women allocated to placebo (11% vs 19%; risk ratio 0.58, 95% CI 0.49–0.69).[30] This trial significantly affected the RCOG recommendation for using prophylactic antibiotics. ACOG states that because 89% of patients in the trial underwent episiotomy, routine in the United Kingdom but not in the United States, it may be reasonable to consider antibiotic prophylaxis if episiotomy is performed in conjunction with OVD.

Cesarean Delivery

Incidence and risk factors

Cesarean delivery is the most important risk factor for puerperal infection, increasing the incidence by 5-fold to 20-fold compared with a vaginal birth. This includes infections of the pelvic organs, the incision, and the urinary tract. The use of antibiotics can reduce the infection rate by 60% to 70% for both planned and unplanned cesarean delivery.[31] The estimated cost of cesarean delivery associated infection in the United States is US$2500 to US$3800 per case.[32] With more than 1.2 million cesarean deliveries performed annually, these infections represent a significant source of hospitalization and health-care utilization.[33]

Medication choice

Antibiotic use for cesarean delivery should be effective against both gram-negative and gram-positive organisms. Although many antibiotics are effective, a single dose of a first-generation cephalosporin remains the first-line choice due to low cost, low toxicity potential, and the convenience of one time administration.[5] The addition of azithromycin (500 mg IV over 1 hour) has been recommended for nonelective cesareans because it further reduces postoperative infectious morbidity.[5] In patients with severe allergy (anaphylaxis, urticaria, angioedema, or respiratory distress) to PCNs or cephalosporins, a combination of an aminoglycoside and clindamycin is recommended.[5] **Fig. 3** displays a diagram of steps to select appropriate prophylactic antibiotics for patients undergoing cesarean delivery.

Timing

Prophylaxis antibiotic administration for cesarean deliveries should be given within 60 minutes before skin incision.[34] This recommendation is supported by multiple studies and is part of the Society for Obstetric Anesthesia and Perinatology's guidelines for enhanced recovery after cesarean. Timing for redosing is also an important consideration. In cases where surgery extends beyond 2 half-lives of the antibiotic (eg, 4 hours for cefazolin) or with excessive blood loss (>1500 mL), additional dosing should be provided.[5]

Obesity

In a study evaluating postoperative antibiotics to reduce postoperative infection in obese individuals (prepregnancy body mass index [BMI] $\geq$30), a 48-hour course of 500 mg metronidazole and 500 mg cephalexin every 8 hours significantly improved outcomes compared with placebo.[35] However, this trial was performed before recommendations to add azithromycin for nonelective deliveries. Thus, it is difficult to separate the role that each individual intervention played. However, additional

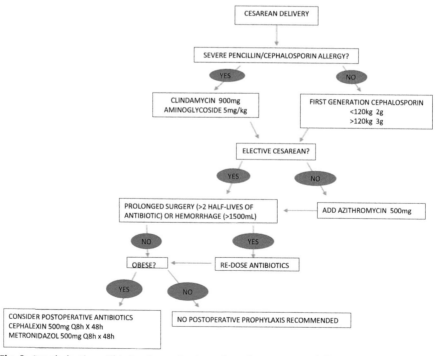

Fig. 3. Prophylactic antibiotics for patients undergoing cesarean delivery.

postoperative medications may be considered as an adjunct in obese postoperative patients.

Obstetric Anal Sphincter Injuries

High-degree perineal trauma at the time of vaginal delivery involves injury to the anal sphincter (third degree) or the anal mucosa (fourth degree).[36] The reported incidence of obstetric anal sphincter injuries (OASIS) is extremely variable among published data with ranges as wide as 0% to 24%[37,38] but it is thought that a reasonable estimate is somewhere between 4% and 7% of all vaginal deliveries.[36]

There are limited data assessing the effectiveness of prophylactic antibiotics with patients who sustained OASIS using a one-time dose of a second-generation cephalosporin. Those patients were followed for 2 weeks postpartum and the treated group saw a significant decrease in perineal wound complications compared with the untreated group, 8.2% versus 24.1%, respectively.[39] ACOG states that a single dose of antibiotic at the time of OASIS repair is reasonable.[36]

TREATMENT OF PERIPARTUM INFECTIONS
Chorioamnionitis

Intra-amniotic infection, commonly referred to as chorioamnionitis, is an infection and inflammation within the uterine cavity.[40] Intra-amniotic infection is typically polymicrobial in origin with involvement of both aerobic and anaerobic bacteria, commonly originating from the vagina flora. Thus, treatment of intra-amniotic infection often involves combinations of antibiotics providing broad-spectrum coverage.[40] Without treatment, intra-amniotic infection is associated with acute neonatal and maternal morbidity, including pneumonia, meningitis, sepsis, and death. There can also be long-term consequences of intra-amniotic infection to the infant and pregnant individual. Intra-amniotic infection is diagnosed clinically by the presence of a fever with a combination of one or more of the following: maternal leukocytosis, purulent cervical drainage, or fetal tachycardia.[41]

The currently recommended antibiotic regimen for intra-amniotic infection from both the World Health Organization (WHO) and ACOG is a combination of ampicillin 2 g IV every 6 hours along with gentamicin, either 2 mg/kg IV load followed by 1.5 mg/kg every 8 hours or 5 mg/kg IV every 24 hours (**Table 1**).[5,40,42] Alternative regimens for individuals with mild PCN allergy substitute cefazolin for the ampicillin. For individuals with severe PCN allergy, clindamycin or vancomycin is substituted for ampicillin (see **Table 1**). There is no convincing evidence that one regimen is superior to another regimen.[43] After a vaginal delivery, no additional doses of antibiotics are required. However, after a cesarean delivery, one additional dose of the chosen antibiotic regimen is advised plus a single dose of clindamycin 900 mg IV or metronidazole 500 mg IV.[40]

The neonatal implications of intra-amniotic infection are beyond the scope of this review. Timely diagnosis and maternal management, together with notification of neonatal health-care providers, will facilitate the appropriate evaluation and empiric antibiotic treatment of the neonate when indicated.

Postpartum Endometritis

Postpartum endometritis, infection of the uterus after delivery, is a clinical diagnosis based on the presence of fever and other clinical signs of infection in the absence of other causes.[42,44] Rates of endometritis vary based on the type of delivery. Similar to intra-amniotic infection, endometritis is typically polymicrobial, with a mixture of

Table 1
Antibiotic regimens recommended to treat intra-amniotic infections

Recommended drugs	Dosage and Administration
Primary regimens	
Ampicillin and gentamicin	2 g IV every 6 h
	2 mg/kg IV load followed by 1.5 mg/kg every 8 h
	Or 5 mg/kg IV every 24 h
If mild PCN allergy:	2 g IV every 8 h
Cefazolin, and gentamicin	2 mg/kg IV load followed by 1.5 mg/kg every 8 h
	Or 5 mg/kg IV every 24 h
If severe PCN allergy:	2 mg/kg IV load followed by 1.5 mg/kg every 8 h
Gentamicin, and either	5 mg/kg IV every 24 h
Clindamycin, or vancomycin	900 mg IV every 8 h
	1 g IV every 12 h
Alternative Regimens	
Ampicillin-sulbactam	3 g IV every 6 h
Piperacillin-tazobactam	3.375 g IV every 6 h or 4.5 g IV every 8 h
Cefotetan	2 g IV every 12 h
Cefoxitin	2 g IV every 8 h
Ertapenem	1 g IV every 24 h

Notes: After a cesarean delivery-one additional dose of antibiotic of choice recommended. If Primary Regimen used, add 900 mg clindamycin IV or metronidazole 500 mg IV with the additional dose. If Alternative Regimen is used, no clindamycin needed. After vaginal delivery, no additional doses after delivery recommended. If a patient is colonized with GBS resistant to either clindamycin or erythromycin, or antibiotic sensitivities are not known, vancomycin is recommended in the patient with severe PCN allergy.
Committee Opinion No. 712: Intrapartum Management of Intraamniotic Infection. Obstetrics & Gynecology: August 2017 - Volume 130 - Issue 2 - p e95-e101 https://doi.org/10.1097/AOG.0000000000002236.

aerobic and anaerobic flora. Bacteremia and sepsis are potential complications of postpartum endometritis and contribute to severe maternal morbidity and mortality.[44]

The recommended antibiotic regimen is a combination of clindamycin 600 mg IV every 6 to 8 hours plus an aminoglycoside, such as gentamicin (1.0–1.5 mg/kg or 60–80 mg IV or IM every 8 hours or 5 mg/kg IV every 24 hours). There is no good evidence that any one regimen is associated with fewer side effects, although the clindamycin and gentamicin combination demonstrated superior effectiveness to regimens consisting of PCNs and cephalosporins.[45] The WHO guideline suggests that antibiotics should be continued for at least 24 to 48 hours after complete resolution of clinical signs and symptoms.[42] Individuals receiving antibiotics for postpartum endometritis are still able to provide breast milk for their newborns.

In resource-limited countries or situations where intravenous access is not available, clindamycin oral therapy plus gentamicin intramuscular therapy may be acceptable.[46] Other options may include cefotetan intramuscularly or amoxicillin-clavulanic acid orally.

OTHER OBSTETRIC INFECTIONS
Urinary Tract Infections and Pyelonephritis

Multiple physiologic changes that occur during pregnancy predispose pregnant patients to urinary tract infections (UTI). First, the increase in progesterone slows the smooth muscle components of the urinary tract, including the ureter, thus inhibiting transit and increasing the chance for vesicoureteral reflux. Second, the growing uterus applies pressure to the bladder, making complete evacuation of the bladder more difficult leading to urinary stasis. Third, pregnancy causes an increase in the amount of sugar and proteins in urine that can further increase propensity toward bacterial growth.[47]

Clinical significance

Acute cystitis occurs in approximately 1% to 2% of pregnancies and pyelonephritis in 0.5% to 2%. In one study, 3.5% of antepartum admissions were accounted for by UTI.[48] Additionally, pyelonephritis is the most common cause of septic shock in pregnancy.[47] Untreated pyelonephritis is associated with significant maternal and fetal morbidities including fever, acute renal failure, acute respiratory distress, preterm birth, low birth weight, chorioamnionitis, primary cesarean section, and intrauterine fetal demise.[49]

Asymptomatic bacteriuria

Asymptomatic bacteriuria (ASB), defined as a urine culture containing greater than 100,000 cfu/mL, is the most significant predisposing factor for the development of a UTI. It is suggested that if untreated in pregnancy, approximately 1 in 4 patients with ASB will progress to subsequent UTI but if treated that number drops to 3 to 4 in 100. Rates of ASB in pregnancy are around 2% to 7% of all pregnancies.[47]

The optimal duration of treatment of ASB is uncertain, and multiple antibiotic regimens are effective. Short-course regimens (3–7 days) are preferred and effective but single-dose options are often not as successful at bacterial eradication.[50,51] For common treatment options, see **Table 2**.

Lower urinary tract/cystitis

Symptomatic infection of the urinary bladder in the pregnant patient typically presents in the same manner as the nonpregnant patient with symptoms including dysuria, frequency, and urgency. Often, empiric therapy should be started at the onset of symptoms and therapy tailored by urinary culture results. Additionally, in those patients with recurrent infection, defined as 3 or more infections during the pregnancy, prophylactic antibiotics is a reasonable recommendation. There is no current consensus on the best antibiotic for prophylaxis but effective choices are nitrofurantoin 50 mg daily and cephalexin 250 mg daily, among others (see **Table 2**).[52]

PYELONEPHRITIS

Given the limited data on efficacy and safety of outpatient treatment and the associated risk for maternal and fetal complication, hospitalization for intravenous antibiotics and patient monitoring is suggested until clinical improvement is seen, typically a 24-hour to 48-hour period of being afebrile with resolving symptoms.[52]

There are insufficient data to suggest a specific treatment regimen as superior. Commonly used and proven regimens typically include PCNs, aminoglycosides, cephalosporins, and broad-spectrum regimens.[53] Following parenteral therapy, an oral regimen should be completed for 10 to 14 days. A urine culture should be obtained after completion for assurance of bacterial eradication. To reduce recurrence risk, pregnant patients are recommended to receive prophylactic daily antibiotics for the remainder of their pregnancy.[47]

Subacute Bacterial Endocarditis Prophylaxis

Subacute bacterial endocarditis (SBE) is an infection of the endocardial surfaces of the heart, most often including one or more heart valves.[54] Clinical presentation may be delayed and nonspecific but can be fatal if not recognized and treated in a timely manner. Antibiotic prophylaxis before surgical procedures has been show to help

Table 2
Effective treatments for asymptomatic bacteriuria and cystitis

Medication	Dose/Regimen	Duration[a]	Precautions
Sulfisoxazole	500–1000 mg by mouth TID-QID	3–7 d	Contraindicated in term pregnancies
Erythromycin	500 mg by mouth QID	7–14 d	
Cephalosporin		3–7 d	
Cephalexin	250 mg by mouth QID		
Cefpodoxime	100 mg by mouth BID		
Nitrofurantoin	50–100 mg by mouth QID	3–7 d	
Trimethoprim-sulfamethoxazole	160/180 mg by mouth BID	3–7 d	Avoid in first trimester and at term
Amoxicillin	500 mg by mouth TID	3–7 d	
Amoxicillin-Clavulanic acid	250 mg by mouth QID	3–7 d	
Fosfomycin	3 g by mouth one dose	One time	

Abbreviations: TID, three times daily; QID, four times daily.

[a] Shorter courses acceptable for asymptomatic cases but longer for symptomatic cases (up to 7–10 d).

Data from Smaill FM, Vazquez JC. Antibiotics for asymptomatic bacteriuria in pregnancy. Cochrane Database of Systematic Reviews. 2019;(11); and Delzell JE, Jr., Lefevre ML. Urinary tract infections during pregnancy. Am Fam Physician. 2000;61(3):713-21.

prevent SBE in at-risk patient populations.[54–56] Prophylaxis is not universally recommended in pregnancy but is recommended in a small subset of high-risk pregnant patients.[5,54–56] These include patients with (1) unrepaired cyanotic heart disease, (2) repaired cyanotic disease with residual valve dysfunction, (3) prosthetic heart valves or any cardiac repair involving prosthetic material, (4) a history of infectious endocarditis, and (5) cardiac transplant patients with any residual valve defects or dysfunction.

Most cases of SBE are caused by PCN-sensitive *Streptococcus viridans*. If antibiotic prophylaxis is indicated, the recommended regimen is ampicillin 2g IV or ceftriaxone or cefazolin 1g IV or amoxicillin 2g oral if the patient is able to tolerate oral treatment. Ideal timing is to administer a single dose of antibiotic therapy 30 to 60 minutes before a procedure (such as a cesarean section) or anticipated vaginal delivery. If the patient is allergic to PCN, an alternate regimen is ceftriaxone or cefazolin 1g IV or clindamycin 600 mg IV. Alternative oral regimens include clindamycin 600 mg oral or azithromycin 500 mg oral or cephalexin 2 g oral.[5,54–56]

SUMMARY

Antibiotics are key components of complete care during labor and delivery. Antibiotic use both prophylactically and therapeutically is important for reducing severe maternal morbidity and mortality and improving perinatal outcomes. The prevention and treatment of infections also improves newborn outcomes. Understanding the indications and usage of antibiotics during pregnancy is important for the care of pregnant individuals.

CLINICS CARE POINTS

- Antibiotics are safe and effective for both prevention and treatment of infections in labor and delivery settings. As infectious morbidity can impact maternal and child outcomes, it is crucial to appropriately treat these according to evidence-based guidelines.

REFERENCES

1. Collier SA, Rasmussen SA, Feldkamp ML, et al. Prevalence of self-reported infection during pregnancy among control mothers in the National Birth Defects Prevention Study. Birth Defects Res A Clin Mol Teratol 2009;85(3):193–201.
2. Obstetric Care Consensus No. 5: Severe Maternal Morbidity: Screening and Review. Obstet Gynecol 2016;128(3):e54–60.
3. Haas DM, Marsh DJ, Dang DT, et al. Prescription and Other Medication Use in Pregnancy. Obstet Gynecol 2018;131(5):789–98.
4. Palmsten K, Hernández-Díaz S, Chambers CD, et al. The Most Commonly Dispensed Prescription Medications Among Pregnant Women Enrolled in the U.S. Medicaid Program. Obstet Gynecol 2015;126(3):465–73.
5. ACOG Practice Bulletin No. 199. Use of Prophylactic Antibiotics in Labor and Delivery. Obstet Gynecol 2018;132(3):e103–19.
6. Centers for Disease Control and Prevention. Core Elements of hospital antibiotic stewardship Programs. US Department of Health and Human Services; 2022. Available at: https://www.cdc.gov/antibiotic-use/healthcare/implementation/core-elements.html. Accessed June 9 2022.
7. Morgan JA, Zafar N, Cooper DB. Group B Streptococcus and pregnancy. StatPearls; 2022.

8. Prevention of Group B. Streptococcal Early-Onset Disease in Newborns: ACOG Committee Opinion, Number 797. Obstet Gynecol 2020;135(2):e51–72.

9. Verani JR, McGee L, Schrag SJ, Division of Bacterial Diseases NCfI, Respiratory Diseases CfDC, Prevention. Prevention of perinatal group B streptococcal disease–revised guidelines from CDC. MMWR Recomm Rep 2010; 59(RR-10):1–36.

10. Phares CR, Lynfield R, Farley MM, et al. Epidemiology of invasive group B streptococcal disease in the United States, 1999-2005. JAMA 2008;299(17): 2056–65.

11. Kwatra G, Cunnington MC, Merrall E, et al. Prevalence of maternal colonisation with group B streptococcus: a systematic review and meta-analysis. Lancet Infect Dis 2016;16(9):1076–84.

12. Towers CV, Rumney PJ, Asrat T, et al. The accuracy of late third-trimester antenatal screening for group B streptococcus in predicting colonization at delivery. Am J Perinatol 2010;27(10):785–90.

13. Muller AE, Oostvogel PM, Steegers EA, et al. Morbidity related to maternal group B streptococcal infections. Acta Obstet Gynecol Scand 2006;85(9):1027–37.

14. Paccione KA, Wiesenfeld HC. Guideline adherence for intrapartum group B streptococci prophylaxis in penicillin-allergic patients. Infect Dis Obstet Gynecol 2013;2013:917304.

15. Shenoy ES, Macy E, Rowe T, et al. Evaluation and Management of Penicillin Allergy: A Review. JAMA 2019;321(2):188–99.

16. Macy E, Vyles D. Who needs penicillin allergy testing? Ann Allergy Asthma Immunol 2018;121(5):523–9.

17. Hamel MS, Has P, Datkhaeva I, et al. The Effect of Intrapartum Vancomycin on Vaginal Group B Streptococcus Colony Counts. Am J Perinatol 2019;36(6): 555–60.

18. Fairlie T, Zell ER, Schrag S. Effectiveness of intrapartum antibiotic prophylaxis for prevention of early-onset group B streptococcal disease. Obstet Gynecol 2013; 121(3):570–7.

19. Prelabor Rupture of Membranes: ACOG Practice Bulletin, Number 217. Obstet Gynecol 2020;135(3):e80–97.

20. Mercer BM. Preterm premature rupture of the membranes. Obstet Gynecol 2003; 101(1):178–93.

21. Garite TJ, Freeman RK. Chorioamnionitis in the preterm gestation. Obstet Gynecol 1982;59(5):539–45.

22. Melamed N, Hadar E, Ben-Haroush A, et al. Factors affecting the duration of the latency period in preterm premature rupture of membranes. *J Matern Fetal Neonatal Med* Nov 2009;22(11):1051–6.

23. Obstetric Care Consensus No. 6 Summary: Periviable Birth. Obstet Gynecol 2017;130(4):926–8.

24. Kenyon S, Boulvain M, Neilson JP. Antibiotics for preterm rupture of membranes. Cochrane Database Syst Rev 2013;12:CD001058.

25. Lee J, Romero R, Kim SM, et al. A new antibiotic regimen treats and prevents intra-amniotic inflammation/infection in patients with preterm PROM. J Matern Fetal Neonatal Med 2016;29(17):2727–37.

26. Operative Vaginal Birth: ACOG Practice Bulletin, Number 219. Obstet Gynecol 2020;135(4):e149–59.

27. Liabsuetrakul T, Choobun T, Peeyananjarassri K, et al. Antibiotic prophylaxis for operative vaginal delivery. Cochrane Database Syst Rev 2020;3:CD004455.

28. Mohamed-Ahmed O, Hinshaw K, Knight M. Operative vaginal delivery and postpartum infection. Best Pract Res Clin Obstet Gynaecol 2019;56:93–106.
29. Murphy DJ, Strachan BK, Bahl R, et al. Assisted Vaginal Birth: Green-top Guideline No. 26. BJOG 2020;127(9):e70–112.
30. Knight M, Chiocchia V, Partlett C, et al. Prophylactic antibiotics in the prevention of infection after operative vaginal delivery (ANODE): a multicentre randomised controlled trial. Lancet 2019;393(10189):2395–403.
31. Smaill FM, Grivell RM. Antibiotic prophylaxis versus no prophylaxis for preventing infection after cesarean section. Cochrane Database Syst Rev 2014;10: CD007482.
32. Kawakita T, Landy HJ. Surgical site infections after cesarean delivery: epidemiology, prevention and treatment. Matern Health Neonatol Perinatol 2017;3:12.
33. Curtin SC, Gregory KD, Korst LM, et al. Maternal Morbidity for Vaginal and Cesarean Deliveries, According to Previous Cesarean History: New Data From the Birth Certificate, 2013. Natl Vital Stat Rep 2015;64(4):1–13, back cover.
34. Bollag L, Lim G, Sultan P, et al. Society for Obstetric Anesthesia and Perinatology: Consensus Statement and Recommendations for Enhanced Recovery After Cesarean. Anesth Analg 2021;132(5):1362–77.
35. Valent AM, DeArmond C, Houston JM, et al. Effect of Post-Cesarean Delivery Oral Cephalexin and Metronidazole on Surgical Site Infection Among Obese Women: A Randomized Clinical Trial. JAMA 2017;318(11):1026–34.
36. ACOG Practice Bulletin No. 198. Summary: Prevention and Management of Obstetric Lacerations at Vaginal Delivery. Obstet Gynecol 2018;132(3):795–7.
37. Hordnes K, Bergsjø P. Severe lacerations after childbirth. Acta Obstet Gynecol Scand 1993;72(6):413–22.
38. Ramar CN, Grimes WR. Perineal lacerations. StatPearls 2022.
39. Duggal N, Mercado C, Daniels K, et al. Antibiotic prophylaxis for prevention of postpartum perineal wound complications: a randomized controlled trial. Obstet Gynecol 2008;111(6):1268–73.
40. Committee Opinion No. 712. Intrapartum Management of Intraamniotic Infection. Obstet Gynecol 2017;130(2):e95–101.
41. Higgins RD, Saade G, Polin RA, et al. Evaluation and Management of Women and Newborns With a Maternal Diagnosis of Chorioamnionitis: Summary of a Workshop. Obstet Gynecol 2016;127(3):426–36.
42. WHO Recommendations for Prevention and Treatment of Maternal Peripartum Infections. 2015. WHO Guidelines Approved by the Guidelines Review Committee.
43. Hopkins L, Smaill F. Antibiotic regimens for management of intraamniotic infection. Cochrane Database Syst Rev 2002;3:CD003254.
44. Taylor M, Pillarisetty LS. Endometritis. StatPearls 2022.
45. Mackeen AD, Packard RE, Ota E, et al. Antibiotic regimens for postpartum endometritis. Cochrane Database Syst Rev 2015;2:CD001067.
46. Meaney-Delman D, Bartlett LA, Gravett MG, et al. Oral and intramuscular treatment options for early postpartum endometritis in low-resource settings: a systematic review. Obstet Gynecol 2015;125(4):789–800.
47. Habak PJ, Griggs JRP. Urinary tract infection in pregnancy. StatPearls 2022.
48. Gazmararian JA, Petersen R, Jamieson DJ, et al. Hospitalizations during pregnancy among managed care enrollees. Obstet Gynecol 2002;100(1):94–100.
49. Wing DA, Fassett MJ, Getahun D. Acute pyelonephritis in pregnancy: an 18-year retrospective analysis. Am J Obstet Gynecol 2014;210(3):219.e1–6.
50. Smaill FM, Vazquez JC. Antibiotics for asymptomatic bacteriuria in pregnancy. Cochrane Database Syst Rev 2019;11.

51. Delzell JE Jr, Lefevre ML. Urinary tract infections during pregnancy. Am Fam Physician 2000;61(3):713–21.
52. Epp A, Larochelle A. Recurrent urinary tract infection. J Obstet Gynaecol Can 2010;32(11):1082–90.
53. Vazquez JC, Abalos E. Treatments for symptomatic urinary tract infections during pregnancy. Cochrane Database Syst Rev 2011;1.
54. Ibrahim AM, Siddique MS. Subacute bacterial endocarditis prophylaxis. StatPearls 2022.
55. Dajani AS, Taubert KA, Wilson W, et al. Prevention of bacterial endocarditis. Recommendations by the American Heart Association. JAMA 1997;277(22):1794–801.
56. Habib G, Lancellotti P, Antunes MJ, et al. ESC Guidelines for the management of infective endocarditis: The Task Force for the Management of Infective Endocarditis of the European Society of Cardiology (ESC). Endorsed by: European Association for Cardio-Thoracic Surgery (EACTS), the European Association of Nuclear Medicine (EANM). Eur Heart J 2015;36(44):3075–128.

Analgesia in Pregnancy

Leslie Matthews, MD, PharmD[a],*, Grace Lim, MD, MS[a,b]

KEYWORDS

- Labor analgesia • Physiology of pregnancy • Pain management
- Anesthetic complications

KEY POINTS

- Pain during labor and delivery has unique characteristics that differ from other acute pain scenarios.
- Pain management during labor and delivery, as well as in the postpartum period, must address the safety of both the pregnant patient and the fetus/newborn.
- An individualized approach with considerations for each patient's psychological, physiologic, and pharmacokinetic parameters is essential to providing safe and effective care during labor and delivery.

INTRODUCTION

Labor and delivery is a painful experience due to complex interactions between physiologic and psychological mechanisms. Many of these mechanisms are similar to those with acute pain from other causes, but labor pain also is unique. Given the physiologic changes of pregnancy and exposure of both the patient and fetus to pain interventions, additional considerations are required to ensure safe and effective pain management while minimizing toxicity to both mother and child during labor, delivery, and postpartum.[1]

Funding: Supported by the Department of Anesthesiology & Perioperative Medicine, University of Pittsburgh School of Medicine.
Disclosures/Conflicts of Interest: None.
Author attestations: L. Matthews wrote manuscript, approved the final manuscript. G. Lim wrote manuscript, approved the final manuscript.
[a] Department of Anesthesiology & Perioperative Medicine, Division of Obstetric & Women's Anesthesiology, University of Pittsburgh School of Medicine, 300 Halket Street Suite 3510, Pittsburgh, PA 15215, USA; [b] Department of Obstetrics Gynecology and Reproductive Sciences University of Pittsburgh School of Medicine, 300 Halket Street Suite 3510, Pittsburgh, PA 15215, USA
* Corresponding author. Department of Anesthesiology & Perioperative Medicine, Division of Obstetric & Women's Anesthesiology, 300 Halket Street Suite 3510, Pittsburgh, PA 15215.
E-mail address: matthewslj@upmc.edu

Obstet Gynecol Clin N Am 50 (2023) 151–161
https://doi.org/10.1016/j.ogc.2022.10.016
0889-8545/23/© 2022 Elsevier Inc. All rights reserved.

obgyn.theclinics.com

PATHOPHYSIOLOGY OF PAIN

All pain, including labor pain, is mediated by sensory pathways that transmit signals from the periphery to the cerebral cortex. Receptors in the skin, muscles, or viscera are activated by noxious stimuli, which transmit signals along afferent neurons to the dorsal horn of the spinal cord. Pain signals then ascend via the spinothalamic tract to the thalamus, where second-order neurons synapse and transmit pain signals via third-order neurons through the internal capsule to the corresponding cortical regions of the brain.[1]

The skin contains several subtypes of nociceptors that sense and transmit signals for different types of pain. Sharp painful stimuli generate signals along A-delta pain fibers. A-delta fibers are myelinated and transmit quickly, resulting in a well-localized response. Dull, generalized pain with a gradual onset is transmitted by C fibers, which are unmyelinated and transmit slower. C fibers mediate pain induced by visceral stretch and pressure (**Fig. 1**). Labor pain, as well as surgical pain from cesarean delivery, result from stimulation of both mechanisms.[1] Because C fibers are small and unmyelinated, blockade with local anesthetics is more challenging, and patients with functional anesthesia or analgesia will still feel pressure and dull stretch sensations.

Labor pain correlates with the stages of labor. Uterine contractions and cervical dilation cause pain during the first stage of labor. It was previously thought that signals from the uterine body produced most of the pain in this stage; however, it is now accepted that pain signals from the lower uterine segment and cervix are responsible for most of the pain in the first stage of labor. The cervix is innervated by 2 sources, which result in different manifestations of pain in both the first and second stages of labor. In the first stage, cervical dilation activates primarily C fiber afferent fibers that enter the spinal cord at lower thoracic levels, specifically from T10 to L1 dorsal root ganglia. These afferent fibers originate in the paracervical region and ascend through the hypogastric plexus and along the lumbar

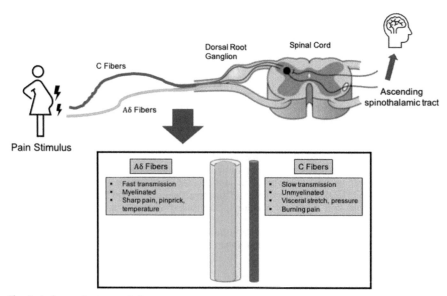

Fig. 1. Labor pain transmission.

sympathetic chain before spinothalamic tract potentiation. For this reason, optimization of analgesia during the first stage of labor should address this pathway, and neuraxial analgesia during the first stage should target the T10 to L1 levels specifically.[2]

Pain during the second stage of labor is a mix of continued cervical pain plus traction and stretch of the pelvic floor and perineum as the infant descends through the pelvis and vaginal canal. Second-stage labor pain signals originate from the pudendal nerve and sacral nerve roots at S2 to S4. A-delta pain fibers transmit sharp, fast pain signals during this stage of labor.[1] The distinct shift in pain physiology during the second stage explains why some patients may have well-controlled pain during the earlier stage of labor and then have different pain sensation in the second stage. It is not uncommon for obstetric anesthesiologists to adjust medications, doses, or adjuvants to address pain in the second-stage of labor, as it is physiologically very different from the pain experienced in the first stage.

NEURAXIAL ANALGESIA

Neuraxial analgesia is the most effective strategy to manage labor pain. Neuraxial techniques for labor and delivery commonly include spinal, epidural, and combined spinal-epidural analgesia. Spinal analgesia involves administering medications, usually a local anesthetic with or without a lipophilic opioid (eg, fentanyl, sufentanil) into the intrathecal space. The advantage of spinal analgesia is that the location is verified at the time of placement, with return of cerebrospinal fluid through the needle before injecting medication. The onset of analgesia is rapid and is less likely to be patchy or unilateral compared with epidural analgesia. A major disadvantage to spinal analgesia and anesthesia, which limits its use during labor, is that the procedure introduces a single dose of medication with a short duration of action. No catheter is left in place to allow for continued pain relief over many hours. For this reason, single-dose spinal anesthesia has been largely abandoned for labor analgesia and is typically reserved for scenarios when a predictable, short duration of analgesia is required, such as cesarean delivery or postpartum sterilization. The predicted effect and duration of a spinal anesthetic depends on the dose and choice of specific local anesthetic and the adjuvants included in the injection.

Epidural analgesia is the most effective technique for managing labor pain. Insertion of an epidural catheter is performed by advancing a needle through the skin and ligaments between the spinous processes (**Fig. 2**). As the needle is advanced, the proceduralist can feel the change in tissue layers while gentle resistance is applied to a syringe attached to a large-bore needle. When the epidural space is encountered, the contents of the syringe fill the epidural space, and the plunger of the syringe collapses; this is called the "loss of resistance" technique and is the most used technique for epidural placement. Although the end of the large-bore needle is within the epidural space, a catheter is threaded through the needle and left in place. Medications can be administered by continuous infusion or intermittent boluses to provide a desired anesthetic effect depending on the location of the catheter and the medications selected. To treat first- and second-stage labor pain, epidural analgesia ideally covers dermatomal levels from T10 superiorly to the sacral nerve roots of the perineum. Functional epidural analgesia achieves excellent pain intensity reduction, minimizes motor block with modern dosing strategies, and results in minimal systemic medication exposure and thus fewer undesirable maternal and fetal side effects. The presence of a functional epidural catheter also allows for conversion to cesarean delivery without general anesthesia.[3]

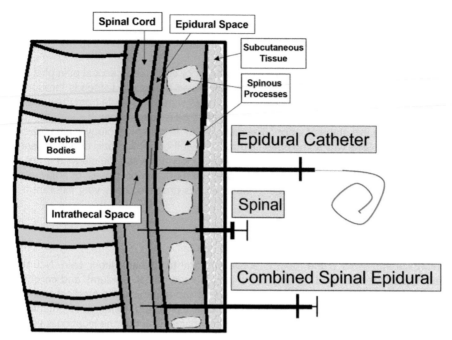

Fig. 2. Comparison of neuraxial techniques.

Clinical Scenario

A 25-year-old G1P0 at 37w2d presents with rupture of membranes and painful contractions. She has been taking prophylactic enoxaparin twice daily for a history of deep venous thrombosis and factor V Leiden. Her last dose of enoxaparin was 4 hours ago. What options are available for labor analgesia for this patient?

Scenario Considerations

Because this patient is anticoagulated, neuraxial procedures are contraindicated due to the risk of bleeding and neurologic injury (specifically, spinal or epidural hematoma that can lead to permanent loss of neurologic function). This patient is on prophylactic twice-daily enoxaparin, which should be held for a period of 12 hours before neuraxial procedures. Full-dose therapeutic enoxaparin should be held for 24 hours before neuraxial procedures. In patients presenting in spontaneous labor, therapeutic anticoagulation may preclude spinal or epidural procedures and confer elevated risk for additional bleeding and hemorrhage. Therefore, planned deliveries are desirable in patients who require anticoagulation. Anticoagulation should be held before hospital admission, with the recommended duration of cessation depending on which agent is used for chemoprophylaxis.[4] Inhaled nitrous oxide and intravenous medications are alternative pharmacologic options in patients with a contraindication to neuraxial anesthesia.

PARENTERAL (INTRAVENOUS, INTRAMUSCULAR, SUBCUTANEOUS) ANALGESICS

Parenteral opioids are some of the most common agents used for analgesia during labor but they have distinct disadvantages that limit their utility in this setting. Most opioids can be administered by multiple routes, such as intramuscularly or subcutaneously, when intravenous access is not available. Opioid effects can be variable and are associated with adverse effects, of which sedation, respiratory depression, nausea, and vomiting are the most common.[5] Opioids are lipid soluble and have low molecular weight, and therefore can cross the placenta, causing fetal bradycardia and respiratory depression if administered near delivery, or redistributed after accumulation in fatty tissues throughout labor and delivery.[6]

Patient-controlled analgesia (PCA) with remifentanil or fentanyl has recently emerged as a strategy for labor analgesia in patients who have contraindications to neuraxial analgesia. In the RESPITE trial, remifentanil was found to have superior analgesia to pethidine, the standard parenteral analgesic for laboring patients.[7] Advantages to PCA are that the patient remains in control of the timing of medication, and the PCA settings can be titrated to each patient's needs, which may improve patient satisfaction. Fentanyl and remifentanil are desirable for PCA during labor because their onset of action is fast and duration of action is short, allowing patients to achieve benefit quickly, without prolonged effects that could impair maternal or fetal status. Remifentanil is an ultra-short-acting opioid that undergoes metabolism by plasma esterases both in maternal and fetal circulation and is unaffected by renal or hepatic impairment. Its duration of activity is only 3 minutes, and the drug does not accumulate after prolonged infusion. One study by Kan and colleagues showed that remifentanil readily crosses the placenta, but it is also rapidly cleared in the fetus and thus has fewer detrimental effects than other opioids.[8] However, PCA still is less effective than neuraxial analgesia for labor pain and comes with increased risk of respiratory depression and somnolence.[9] When comparing fentanyl with remifentanil PCA for labor analgesia, maternal and fetal effects contrast. Fentanyl PCA is associated with less risk for maternal respiratory depression but higher risk of neonatal respiratory depression requiring intervention at delivery. In contrast, remifentanil PCA is associated with higher risk of maternal sedation and respiratory depression but lower risk of neonatal respiratory depression requiring intervention at delivery.[10]

NITROUS OXIDE

Nitrous oxide was first described for labor analgesia in the late 1800s and remains the most used inhalational agent for labor across the world. In the United States, nitrous oxide is administered as a mixture of 50% nitrous oxide with 50% oxygen using blending equipment, either attached to the labor suite wall supply or via portable tanks. The gas is odorless, tasteless, and can be self-administered to provide a degree of analgesia that has a very rapid onset of action and a very short duration of action. Patients have control over the timing of anesthetic delivery, with effects that quickly dissipate and allow for baseline mental status between contractions and minimal adverse effects.

The exact mechanism by which nitrous oxide provides analgesia is not clear, but models have proposed that it may stimulate the release of endogenous opioids, which affects spinal cord pain pathways.[11] It is typically used in the general anesthesia setting to augment the kinetics of other volatile anesthetics and in outpatient clinic settings as a solitary inhaled anesthetic agent to provide procedural anxiolysis and mild analgesia. In cesarean deliveries under general anesthesia, nitrous oxide may be used to enhance the depth of anesthesia without exacerbating uterine atony. Nitrous oxide does have disadvantageous properties such as nausea and vomiting, reported in 45% of patients in one study, and environmental pollution from unscavenged gas.[12] It has not been shown to have detrimental effects on the fetus, as the gas is cleared rapidly from fetal circulation as well. However, high-quality clinical trial data are lacking on the effects of nitrous oxide on fetal-neonatal neurotoxicity or other important developmental outcomes.[12]

Although nitrous oxide is a less effective analgesic during labor, patient satisfaction scores are high. Even in patients who report poor analgesia during labor, those who used nitrous oxide were more likely to be satisfied with the anesthetic care during their delivery than those who received neuraxial analgesia. These findings highlight the importance of patient autonomy in clinical care and the ability to maintain control over one's labor experience, features that nitrous oxide can afford.[13] Nitrous oxide, despite having minimal analgesic properties itself, fills a role in addressing the more intangible aspects of the labor pain experience such as agency, choice, and therapeutic alliances with caregivers.[14,15]

Clinical Scenario

A 32-year-old G4P1112 at 36w4d with placenta previa presents with painful contractions and vaginal bleeding. Her obstetric history is notable for an emergent cesarean delivery at 27w1d in her G1 pregnancy for preeclampsia with severe features. She is hemodynamically stable, last ate 2 hours before presentation, and is becoming increasingly uncomfortable. An urgent cesarean delivery is planned. What anesthetic options are available for her delivery?

Scenario Considerations

When considering the anesthetic plan for an obstetric patient, one of the first decision points is whether neuraxial anesthesia is an option or whether the patient must undergo general anesthesia. Neuraxial anesthesia is universally preferred when there are no contraindications, as it minimizes fetal exposure to anesthetic medications, has little effect on uterine tone, and reduces the risk to the parturient by minimizing aspiration risk and eliminating the need for airway manipulation. In urgent and emergent settings, spinal anesthesia is preferred over epidural anesthesia, given the ability to perform the procedure and achieve surgical anesthesia rapidly.

UNPLANNED CESAREAN DELIVERY

The primary goal of the unplanned cesarean delivery is to deliver the fetus as quickly and safely as possible. The anesthetic plan must support this goal while also considering maternal comorbidities and risks.

General Anesthesia

General anesthesia is the fastest way to achieve surgical anesthesia and delivery of the fetus but confers the highest anesthetic risks to both mother and fetus. Airway management becomes challenging throughout pregnancy due to oropharyngeal tissue edema, difficulty achieving optimal intubating position, and increased aspiration risk. The most common causes of anesthesia-related deaths in the obstetric population are related to airway complications such as failed intubation and aspiration.[16,17] Neonatal outcomes were also more likely to be worse in deliveries under general anesthesia, with lower Apgar scores and higher rates of neonatal intensive care admissions,[18] although the correlation versus causation of the general anesthesia exposure to these outcomes is debatable. Despite achieving the shortest time-to-incision interval, the risks of maternal and fetal complications following general anesthesia remain significant, and thus general anesthesia for cesarean delivery should be avoided whenever possible.[19]

Spinal Anesthesia

Spinal anesthesia is typically the most quickly performed neuraxial technique and produces rapid anesthesia for surgical incision in approximately 3 to 5 minutes, with peak effect within 5 to 10 minutes. Spinal anesthesia involves injection of medication directly into the intrathecal space, allowing for small doses of local anesthetic (1–2 mL of 0.75% bupivacaine, for example) and opioids (such as 10 mcg fentanyl) to achieve surgical anesthesia, thus minimizing both maternal and fetal systemic effects. Adequate surgical anesthesia may be produced with local anesthetic alone, but addition of adjuvants such as fentanyl, clonidine, or epinephrine can extend the duration of anesthesia up to approximately 2 hours for longer procedures. A small dose of morphine (0.1–0.2 mg) can also be added to the intrathecal injection to provide 24 hours of postoperative analgesia. Surgical anesthesia for cesarean delivery is targeted to the level of T4-T6, providing analgesia of the entire peritoneal cavity without interrupting the respiratory drive from the cervical nerve roots. Patients remain awake, interactive, and involved in the delivery process, which confers safety and patient satisfaction.[20]

In emergent settings involving massive hemorrhage with potential coagulopathy, the anesthesiologist must consider whether the patient is at high risk for bleeding or hemodynamic instability, which can make spinal anesthesia unsafe. Severe thrombocytopenia and other coagulopathies can increase the risk of spinal or epidural hematoma formation and devastating neurologic injury, although these risks remain low overall. A large meta-analysis of 7476 neuraxial procedures demonstrated an inflection point with an increased risk of epidural hematoma formation with a platelet count of less than $75,000/mm^3$.[21] In patients with platelet count greater than $70,000/mm^3$, the risk of hematoma formation is less than 0.5%.[22]

Spinal anesthesia also induces rapid vasodilation, which can lead to profound maternal hypotension and fetal compromise, or in the worst cases of patients with depleted intravascular volume, can induce a cardiac arrest. Therefore, anesthesiologists must be proactive in managing volume status and administering vasoactive medications to maintain systemic vascular resistance and cardiac output, regardless of anesthetic choice.

Epidural Anesthesia

Epidural anesthesia is also acceptable in unplanned cesarean delivery and is typically used for intrapartum cesarean deliveries in patients with existing labor epidural catheters in place. Obstetric anesthesiology practice has evolved so that labor epidural analgesia functions well using dilute local anesthetics with adjuncts to maintain motor function and attenuate hypotension. For surgical anesthesia, higher concentration solutions are typically used to increase the quality of the sensory block before surgical incision. Labor epidural catheters may be bolused with more concentrated local anesthetic, such as 2% lidocaine or 3% chloroprocaine, 15 to 20 mL, to convert a labor epidural anesthesia into a surgical anesthesia. Adjuvants such as epinephrine or fentanyl can be added to the local anesthetic bolus to improve onset or density of the block. Depending on the local anesthetic and concentration selected, the time required to achieve a surgical block varies from 10 minutes to 20 minutes or more. For this reason, conversion of labor analgesia to surgical anesthesia via epidural routes may not be feasible in the most time-sensitive emergencies. Good communication and supporting systems that allow anesthesiology teams to dose medications early can avoid the risk of unsuccessful conversion of epidural analgesia to anesthesia.

POSTDELIVERY CONSIDERATIONS

The Society for Obstetric Anesthesia and Perinatology has released a consensus statement regarding enhanced recovery after cesarean delivery, part of which addresses postdelivery analgesia in both emergent and nonemergent settings. This statement supports the primary goals after cesarean delivery of maternal and infant attachment, prevention of venous thromboembolism by encouraging mobility, and facilitating care of the infant by optimizing postdelivery pain control and minimizing adverse medication effects. Most patients have adequate pain control with acetaminophen and nonsteroidal antiinflammatory drug (NSAID) medications following uncomplicated vaginal deliveries. Unsurprisingly, pain control following cesarean delivery is more multifaceted.[23]

Postoperative pain control is more challenging when general anesthesia is used for cesarean delivery because long-acting opioid analgesics (ie, morphine) are not administered via the spinal or epidural route. Recent regional and obstetric anesthesia literature have described fascial plane blocks to improve postoperative analgesia in patients who undergo general anesthesia for cesarean delivery and may help minimize opioid requirement. Transversus abdominus plane (TAP), quadratus lumborum (QL), and erector spinae plane blocks are all performed under ultrasound guidance and can be used after conclusion of the cesarean section before emergence from anesthesia or in the postanesthesia recovery phase. TAP and QL produce equivalent postcesarean delivery analgesia and neither add benefit in the presence of neuraxial morphine.[24–26]

Short-term use of low-dose opioids for acute pain management is not considered to be harmful for a breastfeeding infant, and the benefits of breastfeeding still outweigh these nominal risks. Nevertheless, minimizing opioid use while breastfeeding is important. Most opioids have a relatively low relative infant dose when exposure is via breastmilk, but adverse effects are possible in large doses or in long-term use. Neonatal metabolism and excretion pathways are immature, thus reducing drug clearance and allowing for accumulation and toxicity.

Some medications, such as codeine and tramadol, are not recommended for use during breastfeeding. Codeine has been implicated as particularly risky in breastfeeding, given its known variability in metabolism related to CYP2D6 polymorphisms. Codeine requires metabolic conversion by CYP2D6 to morphine, its active form. Codeine can be ineffective for poor metabolizers, as the drug is not readily converted into its active form. In patients who may be ultrarapid metabolizers, excess codeine may be metabolized into morphine, which may increase the risk for adverse effects and affect the neonate. Metabolism of morphine may be impaired in newborns with developing hepatic and renal function, putting these infants at greater risk for adverse events, respiratory depression, and even death. However, there is a lack of clear pharmacokinetic data describing codeine metabolism and extent of transfer to breastmilk, so it is generally recommended that breastfeeding patients avoid codeine use altogether, or the infant should be monitored closely for adverse events during the period of maternal codeine use.[27]

Clinical Scenario

A 33-year-old G3P3003 who is 24 hours postvaginal delivery with epidural analgesia complains of a severe bilateral headache unrelieved by acetaminophen with neck stiffness and nausea. She has been having difficulty breastfeeding her infant because her headache is more severe when sitting up with the lights on in her room. She gets relief only when lying in bed in a completely dark and quiet room.

Scenario Considerations

Regardless of method of delivery, patients who have had spinal or epidural anesthesia are at risk for postdural puncture headache (PDPH), which is a known complication of these procedures and occurs in approximately 1% of cases. PDPH is caused by intracranial hypotension secondary to leakage of cerebrospinal fluid through a defect in the dura created intentionally or inadvertently during neuraxial procedures. This intracranial hypotension leads to cerebral vasodilation and irritation of the meninges. The most common presenting symptom of PDPH is postural headache that improves when laying supine and can also be associated with tinnitus, blurred vision, photophobia, and neck pain or stiffness. PDPH symptoms can overlap with other postpartum conditions including preeclampsia, venous sinus thrombosis, migraine headache, or simple nonspecific headache. PDPH may occur in patients whose neuraxial procedures were uncomplicated and without known dural puncture, so it is important to perform a thorough evaluation of a patient with postpartum headache and consult anesthesiology if concerned for this condition. Early management of PDPH can both improve acute symptoms and minimize complications such as chronic headache, chronic back pain, postpartum depression, and difficulty breastfeeding.[28,29]

Management of PDPH varies, as studies have not shown proven benefit with noninvasive interventions. Intravenous hydration, rest, acetaminophen, and NSAIDs are typically encouraged, as most PDPH resolve within 7 days. Historically, oral or intravenous caffeine has been suggested as an effective treatment option, as caffeine has been shown to both vasoconstrict dilated cerebral vessels and increase cerebrospinal fluid production, but studies have failed to show a definitive benefit. Intravenous adrenocorticotropic hormone has also been used to stimulate cerebrospinal fluid production, but data are also limited.[30]

In cases refractory to these treatments, epidural blood patch (EBP) is the gold standard in treatment of PDPH. During this procedure, sterile peripheral blood is injected into the epidural space, which is accessed in a similar fashion as placement of an epidural catheter. Sterile technique during this procedure is critical to prevent infectious complications. EBP is thought to work by immediate correction of intracranial hypotension followed by formation of fibrin cross-linking at the level of the dural hole, which accelerates healing. EBP is contraindicated in patients with malignancy, systemic or local infection, and coagulopathies. Many patients obtain relief almost immediately following the procedure, with the most common adverse effect being mild back pain or soreness, which usually resolves without further intervention. Because EBP is at least partially effective in up to 75% of patients,[30] early evaluation and treatment by an anesthesiologist is important. Professional organizations continue to evaluate existing data and develop official recommendations for the management of this complication.

SUMMARY

Obstetric anesthesia is a unique practice in which close communication by a multidisciplinary team can have significant benefits for patient safety and effective care. Labor and delivery is a highly emotional and meaningful experience for patients, so it is critical that a holistic approach be taken to improve not only the physical aspects of care but also the psychosocial aspects. Pain control is an important component of labor and delivery that can critically affect the patient's overall experience. Engaging all members of the care team and using a patient-centered approach can greatly improve achievement of a safe and effective outcome.

CLINICS CARE POINTS

- Analgesia during pregnancy, labor, and delivery must address not only efficacy, but safety of both the pregnant patient and fetus.
- Neuraxial analgesia is the most effective method of pain management during labor and delivery, but there are alternative options available to patients who desire other methods or who have contraindications to neuraxial procedures.
- Post dural puncture headache is a common complication of neuraxial procedures even when performed correctly. Prompt assessment and treatment can alleviate symptoms and allow for a more functional postpartum recovery.

REFERENCES

1. Rowlands S, Permezel M. Physiology of pain in labour. Baillieres Clin Obstet Gynaecol 1998;12(3):347–62.
2. Wong CA. Epidural and spinal analgesia: Anesthesia for labor and vaginal delivery. In: Chestnut D, Wong C, Tsen LC, et al, editors. Chestnut's Obstet Anesth Principles Pract23, 6th edition. Philadelphia: Elsevier; 2020. p. 474–539.
3. Nanji JA, Carvalho B. Pain management during labor and vaginal birth. Best Pract Res Clin Obstet Gynaecol 2020;67:100–12.
4. Horlocker TT, Vandermeuelen E, Kopp SL, et al. Regional anesthesia in the patient receiving antithrombotic or thrombolytic therapy: American Society of Regional Anesthesia and Pain Medicine evidence-based guidelines (fourth edition). Reg Anesth Pain Med 2018;43(3):263–309.
5. Jones L, Othman M, Dowswell T, et al. Pain management for women in labour: an overview of systematic reviews. Cochrane Database Syst Rev 2012;2012(3): CD009234.
6. Reynolds F. The effects of maternal labour analgesia on the fetus. Best Pract Res Clin Obstet Gynaecol 2020;(24):289–302.
7. Wilson MJA, MacArthur C, Hewitt CA, et al. Intravenous remifentanil patient-controlled analgesia versus intramuscular pethidine for pain relief in labour (RESPITE): an open-label, multicentre, randomized controlled trial. Lancet 2018;392(10148):662–72.
8. Kan RE, Hughes SC, Rosen MA, et al. Intravenous remifentanil: placental transfer, maternal and neonatal effects. Anesthesiology 1998;88(6):1467–74.
9. Van de Velde M, Carvalho B. Remifentanil for labor analgesia: an evidence-based narrative review. Int J Obstet Aneesth 2016;25:66–74.
10. Marwah R, Hassan S, Carvalho J, et al. Remifentanil vs fentanyl for intravenous patient-controlled labor analgesia: an observational study. Can J Anaesth 2012; 59(3):246–54.
11. Setty T, Fernando R. Systemic analgesia: Parenteral and inhalational agents. In: Chestnut D, Wong C, Tsen LC, et al, editors. Chestnut's Obstet Anesth Principles Pract22, 6th edition. Philadelphia: Elsevier; 2020. p. 453–73.
12. Likis FE, Andrews JC, Collins MR, et al. Nitrous oxide for the management of labor pain: A systematic review. Anesth Analg 2014;(118):153–67.
13. Richardson MG, Lopez BM, Baysinger CL, et al. Nitrous oxide during labor: Maternal satisfaction does not depend exclusively on analgesic effectiveness. Anesth Analg 2017;124(2):548–53.

14. Hodnett ED. Pain and women's satisfaction with the experience of childbirth: a systematic review. Am J Obstet Gynecol 2002;186:S160S172.
15. Camann W. Pain, pain relief, satisfaction, and excellence in obstetric anesthesia: A surprisingly complex relationship. Anesth Analg 2017;124(2):383–5.
16. Creanga AA, Syverson C, Seed K, et al. Pregnancy-related mortality in the United States, 2011-2013. Obstet Gynecol 2017;130:366–73.
17. Sobhy S, Zamora J, Dharmarajah K, et al. Anaesthesia-related maternal mortality in low-income and middle-income countries: A systematic review and meta-analysis. Lancet Glob Health 2016;4:e320–7.
18. Ring L, Landau R, Delgado C. The current role of general anesthesia for cesarean delivery. Curr Anesthesiol Rep 2021;11(1):18–27.
19. Carvalho B, Mhyre JM. Centers of excellence for anesthesia care of obstetric patients. Anesth Analg 2019;124(5):844–6.
20. Tsen LC, Bateman BT. Anesthesia for cesarean delivery. In: Chestnut D, Wong C, Tsen LC, et al, editors. Chestnut's Obstet Anesth Principles Pract26, 6th edition. Philadelphia: Elsevier; 2020. p. 568–626.
21. Bauer ME, Toledano RD, Houle T, et al. Lumbar neuraxial procedures in thrombocytopenic patients across populations: A systematic review and meta-analysis. J Clin Anesth 2020;61:109666.
22. Lee LO, Bateman BT, Kheterpal S, et al. Risk of epidural hematoma after neuraxial techniques in thrombocytopenic parturients: a report from the multicenter perioperative outcomes group. Anesthesiology 2017;126(6):1053–63.
23. Bollag L, Lim G, Sultan P, et al. Society for Obstetric Anesthesia and Perinatology: Consensus statement and recommendations for enhanced recovery after cesarean. Anesth Analg 2021;132:1362–77.
24. Blanco R, Ansari T, Girgis E. Quadratus lumborum block for postoperative pain after caesarean section: A randomised controlled trial. Eur J Anaesthesiol 2015;32:812–8.
25. Hamed MA, Yassin HM, Botros JM, et al. Analgesic efficacy of erector spinae plane block compared with intrathecal morphine after elective cesarean section: a prospective randomized controlled study. J Pain Res 2020;13:597–604.
26. Mishriky BM, George RB, Habib AS. Transversus abdominis plane block for analgesia after Cesarean delivery: a systematic review and meta-analysis. Can J Anaesth 2012;59:766–78.
27. Ito S. Opioids in breast milk: Pharmacokinetic principles and clinical implications. J Clin Pharm 2018;58(S10):S151–63.
28. Vallejo MC, Zakowski MI. Post-dural puncture headache diagnosis and management. Best Pract Res Clin Anaesthesiol 2022;36(1):179–89.
29. Ranganathan P, Golfeiz C, Phelps AL, et al. Chronic headache and backache are long-term sequelae of unintentional dural puncture in the obstetric population. J Clin Anesth 2015;27:201–6.
30. Patel R, Urits I, Orhurhu V, et al. A comprehensive update on the treatment and management of postdural puncture headache. Curr Pain Headache Rep 2020;24(6):24.

COVID-19 Therapeutics and Considerations for Pregnancy

Naima T. Joseph, MD, MPH[a,b,*], Ai-Ris Y. Collier, MD[a,b]

KEYWORDS

- COVID-19 • Pregnancy • Therapeutics • Vaccines

KEY POINTS

- COVID-19 is associated with heightened risk for worsened disease severity and poor obstetric outcomes.
- Although COVID-19 therapeutics have not been adequately studied in pregnancy, safe options exist for the pharmacologic treatment of mild, moderate, or severe disease in pregnancy.
- Vaccination in pregnancy is safe and associated with both maternal and neonatal protection against severe disease.

INTRODUCTION

The unprecedented impact of the novel Coronavirus Disease 2019 (COVID-19) pandemic has been met with equally unprecedented scientific innovation. More than 3000 vaccine and drug clinical trials are underway or completed,[1] yet 80% excluded pregnant patients,[2] resulting in administration to pregnant patients without research protocol safeguards or delay in the receipt of life-saving interventions. Considerations for the clinical management of COVID-19 disease in pregnancy have been published, and basic tenets remain mostly unchanged.[3,4] However, the data supporting the use of vaccines and therapeutics have evolved and warrant pregnancy-specific consideration.

Perinatal Implications

Multiple studies demonstrate that pregnancy is associated with a higher risk for severe COVID-19 disease, defined by intensive care unit (ICU) admission, mechanical

[a] Division of Maternal Fetal Medicine, Department of Obstetrics and Gynecology, Beth Israel Deaconess Medical Center, 330 Brookline Avenue, Kirstein 3rd Floor, Boston, MA 02215, USA;
[b] Department of Obstetrics, Gynecology and Reproductive Biology, Harvard Medical School, Boston, MA, USA
* Corresponding author. 330 Brookline Avenue, Kirstein, 3rd Floor, Boston, MA 02215.
E-mail address: Njoseph5@bidmc.harvard.edu

Obstet Gynecol Clin N Am 50 (2023) 163–182
https://doi.org/10.1016/j.ogc.2022.10.018
0889-8545/23/© 2022 Elsevier Inc. All rights reserved.

ventilation, extracorporeal membrane oxygenation (ECMO), and death, compared with nonpregnant persons.[5,6] Compared with unaffected pregnancies, COVID-19 disease in pregnancy is associated with increased risk for preeclampsia,[7,8] cesarean delivery, and severe maternal morbidity from direct obstetric causes.[8] A systematic review including 42 studies comparing fetal and neonatal outcomes in pregnant patients with and without confirmed SARS-CoV-2 infection demonstrated 2-fold increased risk for stillbirth, low birth weight, and prematurity.[7] Whether there is increased risk for other neonatal complications, such as neonatal ICU admission, respiratory disorders, and hyperbilirubinemia, is controversial and may be mediated by disease severity.[9] Congenital infection does occur in 1% to 3%.[10–12] There are insufficient data to describe a congenital viral syndrome or to clarify disease severity in infants born with infection. There is a global registry to better understand long-term childhood and adult outcomes following prenatal exposure to SARS-CoV-2 infection.[13]

COVID-19 Drug Treatments

COVID-19 therapeutics affect the 2 main pathophysiologic processes implicated in disease progression. The early phase is driven by SARS-CoV-2 viral replication, whereas progression to multiorgan involvement in the later phase is driven by cytokine release syndrome. Therefore, therapies that directly target and limit viral replication have the greatest efficacy early in the disease course, whereas immunosuppressive/antiinflammatory therapies are more beneficial in later stages of the disease.

Outpatient Treatments

High-risk, nonhospitalized patients with mild or moderate COVID-19[14] may be offered secondary preventive therapeutics to reduce the risk of severe disease and death. Pregnant or recently pregnant individuals are included in the "high-risk" criteria, which also includes age greater than or equal to 65 years, Hispanic, non-Hispanic Black, American Indian or Alaska Natives race/ethnicity, and certain medical conditions (eg, active malignancy; chronic lung, liver, or kidney disease; cystic fibrosis; insulin-dependent diabetes mellitus; cardiac conditions; disabilities; primary and secondary immunodeficiency; use of corticosteroids or other immunosuppressive medications). Available antivirals include bebtelovimab, remdesivir, nirmatrelvir/ritonavir, and molnupiravir (**Table 1**).

Bebtelovimab

Bebtelovimab is a monoclonal antibody (MAb) targeting the highly antigenic and immunogenic surface spike glycoprotein of the SARS-CoV-2 virus. As a drug class, MAbs have low potential for adverse effects (hypersensitivity reaction in < 1%) or significant drug interactions (not metabolized by cytochrome P450 enzymes). MAbs readily cross the placenta; the degree of fetal transfer is variable and depends on specific drug structure, drug half-life, dose, and the timing of the last dose in relation to the gestational age.[26] Transfer is minimal during the first trimester and occurs by simple diffusion. By 20 weeks, MAbs are actively transferred in increasing amounts across the placenta, with the highest rate occurring after 36 weeks. Although not empirically studied, this may have added benefit of protecting infants younger than 6 months from severe COVID-19. Nonclinical and observational data have not demonstrated increased risk for birth defects in exposed infants.[27]

Bebtelovimab is currently recommended because it retains activity against Omicron. Although not studied in phase 3 clinical trials, MAbs used before widespread circulation of Omicron were associated with 70% relative reduction in COVID-19–related

Table 1
Outpatient therapeutics and considerations in pregnancy

Agent	Remdesivir	Nirmatrelvir/Ritonavir	Molnupiravir	Bebtelovimab	Tixagevimab/Cilgavimab
Drug class	Antiviral agent RNA polymerase inhibitor	Antiviral agent SARS-CoV-2 main protease inhibitor (Mpro) HIV-1 protease inhibitor and Mpro concentration booster	Antiviral agent < nucleoside inhibitor	Antiviral agent < monoclonal antibody	Antiviral agent < monoclonal antibody
Dose	Day 1: 200 mg Day 2 and 3: 100 mg	Nirmatrelvir 300 mg (two 150 mg tablets) with ritonavir 100 mg TWICE daily for 5 days	800 mg twice daily for 5 d (four 200 mg capsules)	175 mg once	Tixagevimab 150 mg and cilgavimab 150 mg administered every 6 mo while SARS-CoV-2 in circulation
Route of administration	Intravenous infusion over 30–120 min	Oral (do not crush)	Oral (do not crush)	Intravenous infusion over 30 s	2 separate intramuscular injections in separate sites
Dose adjustments	Renal: • eGFR < 30 mL/min: theoretic risk SBECD accumulation in kidneys, manufacturer labeling does not recommend, however significant toxicity with 5–10 d	Renal: • eGFR ≥ 30 to < 60 mL/ min nirmatrelvir 150 mg with ritonavir 100 mg TWICE daily for 5 d • eGFR < 30 mL/min: not recommended Hepatic:	None	None	None

(continued on next page)

Table 1
(continued)

Agent	Remdesivir	Nirmatrelvir/Ritonavir	Molnupiravir	Bebtelovimab	Tixagevimab/Cilgavimab
	treatment unlikely, multiple studies have not shown adverse events. Discuss risk/benefit with patient Hepatic: • ALT >10 times upper limit, consider discontinuation	• Child-Pugh C: not recommended			
Drug-drug interactions	Chloroquine, hydroxychloroquine, CYP3A inducers	Significant CYP3A interactions; review patient's other medications for possible temporary discontinuation	Cladribine	None	None
Indication	Mild to moderate COVID-19 or positive direct SARS-CoV-2 viral test <and at high risk for progression to severe disease				Preexposure prophylaxis
Time frame from symptom onset	≤ 7 d	≤ 5 d	≤ 3–5 d	≤ 7 d	—
Contraindications and considerations	• Hypersensitivity • Chloroquine or hydroxychloroquine may diminish therapeutic effect of RDV	• eGFR < 30 mL/min • Severe hepatic impairment (Child-Pugh class C) • CYP3A induce=rs may reduce nirmatrelvir or ritonavir plasma concentrations,	• May diminish therapeutic effect of cladribine • Evaluate and verify pregnancy status • Use when preferred treatment options unavailable	• Consider local prevalence of SARS-CoV-2 variants and available susceptibility data	• May diminish effect of COVID-19 vaccines • Suggest at least 2 wk interval from receipt of COVID-19 vaccine before administration

• CYP3A inducers may decrease serum concentration RDV	• leading to loss of virologic response and resistance • CYP3A substrates where elevated concentrations are associated with serious/life-threatening reactions (ie, methergine, statins) • HIV screening if untested and resistance testing among untreated or nonvirally suppressed patients • Hypersensitivity • Switch to nonhormonal contraceptive			• Use when preferred treatment options unavailable
EUA documentation Requirement No Patient Fact Sheet[15] Submit FDA Form 3500 to report adverse events[20]	Yes Patient EUA Form[16]	Yes Patient Fact Sheet[17]	Yes Patient Fact Sheet[18]	Yes Patient Fact Sheet[19]
Evidence				
Primary Trial PINETREE[21]	EPIC-HR[22]	MOVE-OUT[14]		PROVENT[23]
Population studied Double-blind, randomized, placebo-controlled trial in symptomatic, unvaccinated, nonhospitalized adults at high risk for	Phase 2–3 double-blind, randomized, placebo-controlled trial in symptomatic, unvaccinated, nonhospitalized adults at high risk for	Phase 3 double-blind, randomized, placebo-controlled trial in symptomatic, unvaccinated, nonhospitalized adults at high risk for	No phase 3 clinical efficacy data, based on in vitro data showing activity against all circulating Omicron subvariants and clinical efficacy	Phase 3 randomized, placebo-controlled trial in adults with increased risk of inadequate response to vaccination

(continued on next page)

Table 1
(continued)

Agent	Remdesivir	Nirmatrelvir/Ritonavir	Molnupiravir	Bebtelovimab	Tixagevimab/Cilgavimab
	progression to severe disease (n = 562)	progression to severe disease (n = 1379)	progression to severe disease (n = 1433)	data from phase 2 clinical trial in an era when Omicron was not dominant[24]	followed to 6–7 mo (n = 5197)
Relative risk reduction (RRR)	87%	88.9%	31% (hazard ratio [HR] 0.69, 95% CI 0.48–1.01)	Not known for bebtelovimab, 85% for sotrovimab	77% (HR 0.23, 95% CI 0.10–0.54)
Number needed to prevent hospitalization or death	21.7	16	14.7	Not known for bebtelovimab. 17% for sotrovimab	66.7
Adverse events	Any 42.3%, serious 5% (vs 46.3% and 5% in placebo, respectively); nausea, headache, cough, ↑ALT, ↓creatinine clearance, severe bradycardia, heart failure, acute liver failure	Any 22.6%, serious 2.1% (vs 23.9% and 4.1% in placebo, respectively); treatment discontinuation, dysgeusia, diarrhea, hypertension, ↑ALT, ↓creatinine clearance, angioedema	30.4% vs 33.0% in placebo; diarrhea, nausea, dizziness, urticaria, anaphylaxis, angioedema	22% vs 23% in placebo; diarrhea, headache, nausea, pruritis, rash, vasovagal reaction, hypersensitivity	Any 35.3%, serious 1.4% in both groups; injection site reaction
Inpatient use	Can continue in the inpatient setting to complete 5 consecutive days of treatment if admitted	Continuation of outpatient therapy allowed if admitted for reasons other than COVID-19	If hospitalization required, complete at provider discretion	Discontinue if hospitalization for disease progression required	N/A

	for reasons other than COVID-19	without severe or critical illness			
Pregnancy data					
DART	No adverse effect on embryo/fetal development	Nirmatrelvir: reduced fetal body weights Ritonavir: no adverse developmental outcomes	Increased risk of miscarriage; malformation of eye, kidney, axial skeleton, and ribs; delayed ossification; decreased fetal birthweight	None	None
Human data	Observational study of 67 pregnant people: no adverse pregnancy outcomes. Insufficient data to identify drug-associated risk of birth defects or miscarriage[25]	Nirmatrelvir: none Ritonavir: observational studies have not identified an increase in risk of major birth defects and are insufficient to identify a drug-associated risk of miscarriage	None	None	None

High risk factors include age > 60 years, obesity (BMI > 30 kg/m^2), patient with immunocompromising conditions (B-cell depleting therapies, ie, rituximab, patients receiving tyrosine kinase inhibitors, chimeric antigen receptor T-cell recipients, posthematopoietic cell transplant recipients, active malignancy, lung and solid organ transplant recipients, patients with severe combined primary immunodeficiencies, patients with untreated HIV and CD4 T lymphocyte cell counts < 500 cells/mm^3), unvaccinated individuals, cardiovascular conditions (eg, hypertension, myocardial infarct, stroke), diabetes, liver disease, kidney disease.

Abbreviations: ALT, alanine transaminase; CYP, cytochrome P450; DART, Development and Reproductive Toxicity; eGFR, estimated glomerular filtration rate; EUA, emergency use authorization; FDA, Food and Drug Administration; RDV, remdesivir; SARS-CoV-2, severe acute respiratory syndrome coronavirus 2; SBECD, sulfobutylether-beta-cyclodextrin.

Therapeutics can be located at https://healthdata.gov/Health/COVID-19-Public-Therapeutic-Locator/rxn6-qnx8/data. Clinicians are encouraged to refer to most recent https://www.covid19treatmentguidelines.nih.gov/management/clinical-management/nonhospitalized-adults–therapeutic-management/for recommendations.

hospitalization or death from any cause, including in pregnant patients.[28–30] It may be offered to high-risk patients who present more than 5 days from symptom onset or positive viral test when first-line antivirals are not available.[31]

Tixagevimab/cilgavimab reduces the risk of symptomatic COVID-19 by 77% and is the only currently available antiviral for preexposure prophylaxis. It can be offered to uninfected individuals with moderate to severe immune compromise who are unlikely to mount an adequate immune response to COVID-19 vaccination or for whom COVID-19 vaccine is not recommended.[19,32] Pregnancy-specific effectiveness data are not available.

Ritonavir-Boosted Nirmatrelvir

Nirmatrelvir, which is metabolized by CYP3A enzyme, inhibits viral replication through direct inhibition of the SARS-CoV-2 main protease. Ritonavir is an HIV-1 protease inhibitor, has no activity against SARS-CoV-2, but functions to boost nirmatrelvir plasma levels by inhibition of the CYP3A enzyme. These medications are co-packaged and sold under the commercial name Paxlovid. Paxlovid is 89.1% effective in reducing the incidence of COVID-19–related hospitalization or death in patients treated within 5 days of symptom onset.[22] Preliminary data suggest it retains effectiveness in vaccinated individuals.[33]

Paxlovid is currently the preferred treatment of mild COVID-19 in high-risk individuals and ideally is administered within 5 days of positive test or symptom onset. There are no available human data on the use of nirmatrelvir during pregnancy to evaluate drug-associated risks of major birth defects, miscarriage, adverse maternal or fetal outcomes, or its pharmacokinetics, given the known increase in CYP3A activity in pregnancy. Published observational studies on ritonavir use in pregnant women have not identified an increase in the risk of major birth defects.[34] Although placental transfer of ritonavir occurs, fetal ritonavir concentrations are low.

Remdesivir

Remdesivir is an antiviral initially indicated for treatment in hospitalized patients until the PINETREE trial demonstrated that the highest mortality benefit occurred in patients whose treatment was initiated early in the disease course.[21] It is administered as a 3-day infusion and is resource intensive, which limits its use. Remdesivir has not been approved specifically for use in pregnancy. Data suggest a low (16%) rate of serious adverse events and high tolerablity,[25] yet efficacy, and pharmacokinetic data are lacking. The International Maternal Pediatric Adolescent AIDS Clinical Trials (IMPAACT) Network is currently comparing remdesivir pharmacokinetics in pregnant and nonpregnant women of reproductive age who are hospitalized with COVID-19 to assess pregnancy-specific adverse events.[35]

Molnupiravir

Molnupiravir is a nucleoside analogue (NA) antiviral that acts by causing chain termination of nascent viral DNA. NAs are currently used to treat viral infections, rheumatologic disorders, and cancer.[36] Despite being named after Mjölnir, the hammer of the god Thor, the observed effect showed that it was only 30% effective in reducing the risk of hospitalization of death, compared with untreated patients.[14] In addition to its reduced efficacy, there are several concerns that limit use in pregnancy. First, the greatest benefit was observed in patients who initiated therapy within 72 hours of symptom onset; however, a readily available diagnostic test is unavailable. Second, mutagenic and carcinogenic toxicity have been demonstrated in mammalian hamster models, but in vivo risk is under debate.[37,38] Finally, although there are no human pregnancy data, animal data reported in the Food and Drug Administration's Emergency Use Authorization suggested risk for embryo toxicity, lethality, mutagenicity, and low birth weight.[17] Nonetheless, as 1 of 2 orally bioavailable therapies for COVID-19, it retains a role in the arsenal. Molnupiravir is recommended when nirmatrelvir or remdesivir are not available or not appropriate, often because of potential drug interactions with ritonavir, and should only be offered to pregnant individuals after consideration of alternative therapies, risk for severe disease, and fetal risk.

Inpatient Treatments

Therapeutic management of adults hospitalized for COVID-19 is based on disease severity and includes the use of systemic corticosteroids and antiviral and immunomodulatory therapy (**Table 2**).[40]

Corticosteroids

Corticosteroids are currently the standard-of-care treatments of severe disease for both pregnant and nonpregnant people. Dexamethasone was the first trial-proven beneficial treatment of COVID-19. In the RECOVERY randomized controlled trial, dexamethasone reduced the risk of all-cause mortality in patients requiring invasive mechanical ventilation by 36% compared with placebo.[41] It is administered as a once daily oral or intravenous dose of 6 mg for up to 10 days.

Dexamethasone (and betamethasone) is preferentially administered to women at high risk for preterm birth within 7 days. Unlike other steroids, which are extensively metabolized by placental 11-b-hydroxlase steroid dehydrogenase-2, dexamethasone and betamethasone have high rates of placental transfer and have been shown to reduce the rates of pulmonary, neurologic, and infectious morbidity and mortality associated with prematurity. However, repeated courses have been associated with deleterious effects, such as decreased fetal head circumference, fetal growth restriction, and impaired neurodevelopment.[42] After the RECOVERY trial was published, debate ensued regarding how to manage critically ill pregnant patients, as dexamethasone was the only proven treatment with mortality benefit, yet repeated doses were associated with significant fetal or neonatal adverse outcomes.[39] However, a landmark meta-analysis evaluating dexamethasone, hydrocortisone, and methylprednisolone demonstrated the mortality benefit as a class effect of corticosteroids.[43] Given concerns regarding impact of repeated prenatal steroid exposure on long-term neurodevelopment and the presence of reassuring effectiveness data for other steroids, hydrocortisone or methylprednisolone, rather than dexamethasone, should be administered to pregnant patients with severe COVID-19 meeting criteria. If there is a high likelihood of preterm delivery, clinicians should first administer intravenous dexamethasone or betamethasone, dosed for fetal lung maturity, then complete the steroid course using hydrocortisone or methylprednisolone.

Remdesivir

The effectiveness of remdesivir for inpatient adults with severe COVID-19 has been mixed.[24,44] The Adaptive Covid-19 Treatment Trial showed that remdesivir led to a shorter median time from randomization to recovery (10 days vs 15 days with placebo) and may have reduced the time to hospital discharge (12 days vs 17 days), yet no mortality benefit in mechanically ventilated patients.[45] However, the Solidarity Trial meta-analysis showed a modest mortality benefit (remdesivir 14.6% vs control 16.3%; risk ratio [RR] 0.87, 95% confidence interval [CI] 0.76–0.99, $P = .03$) and a reduction in need for mechanical ventilation (23.7% vs 27.1%; RR 0.83, 95% CI 0.75–0.93, $P = .001$).[46] Remdesivir is recommended for hospitalized patients with moderate or

Table 2
Inpatient therapeutics and considerations in pregnancy

Agent	Dexamethasone	Remdesivir	Tocilizumab	Baricitinib
Drug class	Systemic corticosteroid, antiinflammatory	Antiviral, RNA polymerase inhibitor	Recombinant human monoclonal antibody Interleukin-6 receptor antagonist	Janus kinase 1 and 2 inhibitors, reduces cytokine and growth factor stimulation
Dose	6 mg daily for 7 d or until discharge	Day 1: 200 mg Day 2–10: 100 mg	Weight > 30 kg: 8 mg/kg Weight < 30 kg: 12 mg/kg Max dose 800 mg/infusion Single dose, second dose administered if clinical symptoms worsen or do not improve	4 mg daily for 14 d
Route of administration	Intravenous or oral	Intravenous	Intravenous	Oral Oral dispersion
Dose adjustments	None	None, monitor transaminase levels	Renal: • None Hepatic: • Not recommended for patients with ALT or AST >10 times upper limit	Renal: • eGFR < 15 mL/min: not recommended Hepatic: • Treatment interruption if increasing LFTs to exclude diagnosis of drug-induced liver injury
Drug-drug interactions	Multiple considerations CYA3A4 substrate and weak inducer	See Table 1	Uncertain CYP450 metabolism in the setting of severe disease and pregnancy; therefore close drug monitoring recommended Should not be used with other immunomodulators	Increased levels when co-administered with strong OAT3 inhibitors (ie, probenecid) Should not be used with other immunomodulators

Indication	Hospitalized patients with severe or critical COVID-19 disease requiring oxygen support	Hospitalized patients who require noninvasive oxygen support • Given alone in patients requiring supplemental oxygen • Given with dexamethasone in patients requiring noninvasive oxygen therapy	Severe or critical COVID-19 receiving systemic corticosteroids and requiring supplemental oxygen, mechanical ventilation, and/or ECMO	Severe or critical COVID-19 receiving systemic corticosteroids and requiring supplemental oxygen, mechanical ventilation, and/or ECMO Considered case-by-case basis in patients with rapidly increasing oxygen requirements and evidence of systemic inflammation
Contraindications and considerations	Monitor adverse effects including hyperglycemia, fungal, bacterial, or *Strongyloides* infections (especially if using with baricitinib or tocilizumab), and diffuse multiorgan toxicity	See **Table 1**	• Known hypersensitivity • Any non-COVID concurrent active infection, including localized infection • Absolute neutrophil count < 1000 per mm^3, platelet count < 50,000 per mm^3, or ALT/AST > 10x upper limit	• None known • Consider treatment interruption if absolute lymphocyte count < 200 cells/per mm^3 or absolute neutrophil count < 500 per mm^3
Adverse events	• Multiple cardiac, dermatologic, endocrine, metabolic, gastrointestinal, hepatic, and psychiatric effects • Hyperglycemia, pulmonary edema, poor wound healing frequent	See **Table 1**	• Adverse effects (3%): constipation, anxiety, diarrhea, insomnia, hypertension, nausea • High risk for serious and fatal infections due to bacterial, mycobacterial, invasive fungal, viral, protozoal, or other opportunistic pathogens • GI perforation • Hepatotoxicity	• Transaminitis (18%) • Neutropenia (2.2%) • Venous thromboembolism (1.5%) • Serious opportunistic infections (0.9%)

(continued on next page)

Table 2
(continued)

Agent	Dexamethasone	Remdesivir	Tocilizumab	Baricitinib
Evidence				
Effectiveness in general population	Reduction in all cause 28-d mortality[39]	• Modest mortality benefit in nonmechanically ventilated patients • Shorter median time to recovery • Reduced need for mechanical ventilation	• Reduced all-cause mortality at 28 d • Reduced risk of progression to mechanical ventilation or death • Reduced risk of hemodialysis or hemofiltration • Greater probability of discharge alive at 28 d	• Reduced progression to mechanical ventilation or death • Most pronounced in patients receiving high flow oxygen or noninvasive ventilation
Pregnancy considerations	Concern for small head circumference, low birthweight, long-term mental and neurocognitive disorders Alternates: • IV or oral hydrocortisone 5160 mg in divided doses for 7 d or until discharge • IV or oral methylprednisolone 32 mg daily in divided doses for 7 d or until discharge	See **Table 1** Report of 67 pregnant women treated demonstrated similar recovery rates to nonpregnant and low rate of adverse events[25]	Human data insufficient to determine drug associated risk for major birth defects and miscarriages Risk for miscarriage at 1.25 times maximum recommended human dose in animal studies May interfere with parturition	Human data insufficient to determine drug associated risk for major birth defects and miscarriages Increased risk of skeletal anomalies and pregnancy loss in animal data

Abbreviations: ALT, alanine transaminase; AST, aspartate transaminase; CYP, cytochrome P450; DART, Development and Reproductive Toxicity; ECMO, extracorporeal membrane oxygenation; eGFR, estimated glomerular filtration rate; EUA, emergency use authorization; FDA, Food and Drug Administration; OAT, ornithine aminotransferase; RDV, remdesivir; SARS-CoV-2, severe acute respiratory syndrome coronavirus 2.

severe disease, not requiring invasive ventilation or ECMO. An intravenous 200 mg loading dose is administered on day 1, followed by 100 mg intravenously from day 2. For patients who require minimal oxygen supplementation, the recommended treatment duration is 5 days. For patients requiring escalating oxygen support, the recommended treatment duration is 10 days.[46] Although efficacy data in pregnant patients are lacking, remdesivir should be offered to pregnant patients who meet clinical criteria.

Interleukin-6 Inhibitors

Hyperactivation of the immune response, including release of proinflammatory cytokines such as interleukin-6 (IL-6) is implicated in pathophysiology of severe illness. Tocilizumab is a recombinant humanized MAb that inhibits binding of IL-6 to its receptors.[47]

Tocilizumab has been associated with a 15% to 44% reduction in need for mechanical ventilation and a 15% reduction in all-cause mortality, when given in combination with steroids or remdesivir.[48,49] It is currently recommended as adjunctive treatment of severe or critically ill patients. The available pregnancy data for tocilizumab are not sufficient to determine whether there is a drug-associated risk for major birth defects and miscarriage with exposure. The Developmental and Reproductive Toxicity (DART) data show embryo-fetal lethality at concentrations 1.25 times higher than the maximum recommended human dose.[50] IL-6 inhibition may theoretically delay parturition through interference with cervical ripening and dilation.

Janus Kinase Inhibitors

Janus kinase (JAK) inhibitors reduce cytokine and growth factor stimulation, leading to reduced immune cell function. Baricitinib is currently available on a case-by-case basis in patients with rapidly increasing oxygen requirements and evidence of systemic inflammation. It is orally administered and only given in combination with dexamethasone or another corticosteroid.[51]

The data on effectiveness of JAK inhibitors are inconclusive. The COV-BARRIER trial did not find a statistically significant benefit for baricitinib in patients on low-flow oxygen; however, patients were also receiving remdesivir and steroids.[52]

An increased risk of serious infection (eg, *Strongyloides*, herpes zoster, tuberculosis, protozoal), gastrointestinal perforations, and venous thromboembolism (VTE) has been described in patients receiving either JAK or IL-6 inhibitors. Embryo-fetal toxicities including skeletal anomalies have been observed in animal studies; however, the limited data on use of baricitinib in pregnancy are not sufficient to inform a drug-associated risk for major birth defects or miscarriage.[50]

Anticoagulation

Severe and critical COVID-19 is associated with an inflammatory and hypercoagulable state characterized by increased D-dimers, fibrin, fibrin degradation products, and fibrinogen. Yet trials evaluating the efficacy and safety of different antithrombotic regimens in patients with COVID-19 have found little benefit of therapeutic anticoagulation in the treatment of mild, moderate, or severe disease. In addition, a clinically significant increased risk of major bleeding events in patients receiving therapeutic dose anticoagulation has been consistent across all trials.[53–56] In mild disease, neither aspirin, prophylactic, or therapeutic coagulation has demonstrated any benefit against risk for symptomatic venous or arterial VTE, myocardial infarction, stroke, or hospitalization for cardiovascular or pulmonary cause.[57]

The failure of anticoagulation to demonstrate a benefit suggests that COVID-19 thrombosis is immunologically mediated, rather than through the conventional VTE pathway.

Pregnant patients were excluded from these trials, and pregnancy is known to confer additional increased risk for VTE. The only available data evaluating the combined risks of COVID-19, pregnancy, and venous or arterial thromboembolisms are limited by their retrospective nature and lack of appropriate controls.[58] Based on the available data, there does not seem to be a role for prophylactic anticoagulation in the outpatient setting. Prophylactic anticoagulation should be administered to all hospitalized pregnant patients. The choice to use intermediate dosing should be guided by disease severity, patient mobility, and patient risk factors (ie, body mass index > 30 kg/m^2, multifetal gestation, personal history of thrombophilia disorder). Therapeutic anticoagulation should be reserved for patients with active VTE.

Vaccination

Vaccination is the primary mode of protection against SARS-CoV-2. It is currently recommended that pregnant people receive either of the 2 available mRNA vaccines (Pfizer-BioNTech's BNT162b2[59] or Moderna/NIAID's mRNA-1273[60]). Both vaccines instruct cells to make large amounts of spike protein antigen, mimicking natural infection, but induce a rapid, robust humoral immune response.[61] Other COVID-19 vaccines are available in the United States; however, the COVID-19 protein subunit and adenovirus vector vaccines are not preferred for use in pregnancy.

Initial vaccine data for use in pregnancy were derived from inadvertent inclusion of pregnant persons in clinical trials that demonstrated no increased rates of adverse effects.[62] Subsequently, a report of 3958 participants enrolled in the Centers for Disease Control and Prevention's V-safe Surveillance System and Pregnancy Registry demonstrated pregnancy outcomes such as miscarriage, stillbirth, congenital anomalies, small for gestational age, and preterm birth did not differ significantly in vaccinated patients when compared against historic controls.[63] In addition, reactogenicity and immunogenicity data were reassuring. The most common events, injection-site pain, fatigue, headache, myalgia, and fever, were more prevalent following the second dose and occurred much less frequently in pregnant, compared with nonpregnant women.[64] Multiple other epidemiologic studies have failed to identify an association of COVID-19 vaccination with adverse fetal/neonatal outcomes such a stillbirth, prematurity, or congenital anomalies.[63,65,66]

COVID-19 mRNA vaccines elicit similar immune responses in pregnant and nonpregnant adults. A prospective study enrolled 103 women, 30 of whom were pregnant and 16 lactating. Binding, neutralizing, and functional nonneutralizing antibody responses as well as CD4 and CD8 T cell responses in pregnant, lactating, and nonpregnant women following vaccination were present in equal amounts and higher than immune response following natural infection.[67,68] Binding and neutralizing antibodies were also observed in infant cord blood and breast milk.

Vaccination is equally effective in protection against severe disease and averting COVID-19–related pregnancy complications. An observational cohort of 10,861 vaccinated pregnant patients matched to 10,861 unvaccinated pregnant without prior history of infection showed 89% effectiveness against hospitalization and severe disease 7 to 77 days after the second dose.[69] Another study demonstrating protection from adverse pregnancy outcomes included 1332 vaccinated patients and 8760 incompletely vaccinated or unvaccinated patients and found a higher association with stillbirth in unvaccinated patients with infection versus vaccinated patients with breakthrough infection.[70]

Finally, maternal vaccination is associated with neonatal benefit through passive immunity. Infants younger than 6 months are especially vulnerable given dampened immunity. Transplacental antibody transfer is an important source of protection from COVID-19 in this group. Studies have demonstrated that infant concentrations are increased and more persistent following maternal vaccination compared with maternal infection, especially when delivery occurs at least 1 week following the second mRNA dose.[67,71,72] A large, multicenter, case-controlled trial of 1000 mother-infant pairs, half of whom had received COVID-19 vaccination during pregnancy, demonstrated that maternal vaccine effectiveness against COVID-19–associated hospitalization among infants was 52% and against ICU admission for infants was 70%.[73] These data support current recommendations for COVID-19 vaccination for all persons who are pregnant or considering pregnancy or lactating.[2,74]

The current immunization schedule for persons 18 years of age or older include a 2-dose primary series with either monovalent mRNA COVID-19 vaccine or the monovalent protein subunit vaccine, given 4 to 8 weeks or 3 weeks apart, respectively. A single-dose mRNA bivalent booster vaccine should be given 8 weeks following.[75] Vaccination is also recommended in previously infected individuals.[76]

SUMMARY

Despite substantial research and therapeutic developments arising out of necessity during the global pandemic, there are still many unanswered questions. Data on how pregnancy affects the pharmacokinetics or effectiveness of current interventions are limited. It is unclear how in utero exposure to SARS-CoV-2 versus treatments affect long-term child development.

Clinicians must therefore be prepared to discuss the evidence for safety, effectiveness, maternal and fetal risks with nontreatment, and potential for harms with treatment options during pregnancy. In addition, clinicians should be empowered to advocate for inclusion and access to live-saving interventions for their pregnant patients.

CLINICS CARE POINTS

- Most pregnant patients with COVID-19 will require supportive care, yet disease in pregnancy is associated with worsened maternal, fetal, and obstetric outcomes.
- COVID-19 mRNA vaccines are safe and recomended in pregnancy.
- For pregnant patients with COVID-19 with moderate disease or at risk for moderate - severe disease, treatment with Paxlovid is preferred in the absence of medical or pharmacologic contraindications, followed by remdesivir. Patients should be counseled regarding the lack of pregnancy-specific data and low theoretical risk of harm.
- For patients with moderate-severe disaese regarding inpatient management, first line treatment with steroids is recommended. To reduce unintended adverse fetal exposure, prednisone or methylprednisolone should be considered over dexamethasone.

REFERENCES

1. COVID-19 views - clinicaltrials.gov. Available at: https://clinicaltrials.gov/ct2/covid_view. Accessed October 5, 2022.
2. COVID Clinical | SMFM.org - The society of maternal-fetal medicine. Available at: https://www.smfm.org/covidclinical. Accessed October 5, 2022.

3. Joseph NT, Miller ES. Obstetric outpatient management during the COVID-19 pandemic: prevention, treatment of mild disease, and vaccination. Clin Obstet Gynecol 2022;65(1):161–78.

4. Vaught AJ. Inpatient management and OBICU care for pregnant patients with severe COVID-19 disease. Clin Obstet Gynecol 2022;65(1):189–94.

5. Zambrano LD, Ellington S, Strid P, et al. Update: characteristics of symptomatic women of reproductive age with laboratory-confirmed SARS-CoV-2 infection by pregnancy status — United States, January 22–October 3, 2020. MMWR Morb Mortal Wkly Rep 2020;69(44):1641–7.

6. Galang RR, Newton SM, Woodworth KR, et al. Risk factors for illness severity among pregnant women with confirmed severe acute respiratory syndrome coronavirus 2 infection-surveillance for emerging threats to mothers and babies network, 22 state, local, and territorial health departments, 29 march 2020-5 march 2021. Clin Infect Dis 2021;73(Suppl 1):S17–23.

7. Wei SQ, Bilodeau-Bertrand M, Liu S, et al. The impact of COVID-19 on pregnancy outcomes: a systematic review and meta-analysis. CMAJ 2021;193(16):E540–8.

8. Metz TD, Clifton RG, Hughes BL, et al. Association of SARS-CoV-2 infection with serious maternal morbidity and mortality from obstetric complications. JAMA 2022;327(8):748–59.

9. Norman M, Navér L, Söderling J, et al. Association of maternal SARS-CoV-2 infection in pregnancy with neonatal outcomes. JAMA 2021;325(20):2076–86.

10. Zhang H, Zhang H. Entry, egress and vertical transmission of SARS-CoV-2. J Mol Cell Biol 2021;13(3):168–74.

11. Gale C, Quigley MA, Placzek A, et al. Characteristics and outcomes of neonatal SARS-CoV-2 infection in the UK: a prospective national cohort study using active surveillance. Lancet Child Adolesc Health 2021;5(2):113–21.

12. Shook LL, Collier AY, Goldfarb IT, et al. Vertical transmission of SARS-CoV-2: consider the denominator. Am J Obstet Gynecol MFM 2021;3(4):100386.

13. Banerjee J, Mullins E, Townson J, et al. Pregnancy and neonatal outcomes in COVID-19: study protocol for a global registry of women with suspected or confirmed SARS-CoV-2 infection in pregnancy and their neonates, understanding natural history to guide treatment and prevention. BMJ Open 2021;11(1): e041247.

14. Jayk Bernal A, Gomes da Silva MM, Musungaie DB, et al. Molnupiravir for oral treatment of covid-19 in nonhospitalized patients. N Engl J Med 2022;386(6): 509–20.

15. VEKLURY® (remdesivir) | approved treatment for COVID-19. Available at: https://www.veklury.com/. Accessed October 8, 2022.

16. FDA paxlovid fact sheet for patients. Available at: https://www.fda.gov/media/155051/download. Accessed October 8, 2022.

17. Fact sheet for healthcare providers. emergency use authorization for lagevrio (molnupiravir) capsules. Available at: https://www.fda.gov/media/155054/download. Accessed October 5, 2022.

18. Fact sheet for patients, parents, and caregivers emergency use authorization (EUA) of bebtelovimab. Available at: https://www.fda.gov/media/156153/download. Accessed October 8, 2022.

19. Fact sheet for healthcare providers: emergency use authorization for evusheld. Available at: https://www.fda.gov/media/154701/download. Accessed October 5, 2022.

20. MedWatch online voluntary reporting form. Available at: https://www.accessdata.fda.gov/scripts/medwatch/index.cfm. Accessed October 8, 2022.

21. Gottlieb RL, Vaca CE, Paredes R, et al. Early remdesivir to prevent progression to severe covid-19 in outpatients. N Engl J Med 2022;386(4):305–15.
22. Hammond J, Leister-Tebbe H, Gardner A, et al. Oral nirmatrelvir for high-risk, nonhospitalized adults with covid-19. N Engl J Med 2022;386(15):1397–408.
23. Levin MJ, Ustianowski A, De Wit S, et al. Intramuscular AZD7442 (Tixagevimab–Cilgavimab) for Prevention of Covid-19. N Engl J Med 2022;386(23):2188–200.
24. Spinner CD, Gottlieb RL, Criner GJ, et al. Effect of remdesivir vs standard care on clinical status at 11 days in patients with moderate COVID-19: a randomized clinical trial. JAMA 2020;324(11):1048–57.
25. Burwick RM, Yawetz S, Stephenson KE, et al. Compassionate use of remdesivir in pregnant women with severe coronavirus disease 2019. Clin Infect Dis 2020; 73(11):e3996–4004. Published online October.
26. Pham-Huy A, Sadarangani M, Huang V, et al. From mother to baby: antenatal exposure to monoclonal antibody biologics. Expert Rev Clin Immunol 2019; 15(3):221–9.
27. Pham-Huy A, Top KA, Constantinescu C, et al. The use and impact of monoclonal antibody biologics during pregnancy. CMAJ Can Med Assoc J J Assoc Medicale Can 2021;193(29):E1129–36.
28. Chen P, Nirula A, Heller B, et al. SARS-CoV-2 neutralizing antibody LY-CoV555 in outpatients with Covid-19. N Engl J Med 2021;384(3):229–37.
29. Weinreich DM, Sivapalasingam S, Norton T, et al. REGN-COV2, a neutralizing antibody cocktail, in outpatients with Covid-19. N Engl J Med 2021;384(3): 238–51.
30. Gottlieb RL, Nirula A, Chen P, et al. Effect of bamlanivimab as monotherapy or in combination with etesevimab on viral load in patients with mild to moderate COVID-19: a randomized clinical trial. JAMA 2021;325(7):632–44.
31. Westendorf K, Žentelis S, Wang L, et al. LY-CoV1404 (bebtelovimab) potently neutralizes SARS-CoV-2 variants. Cell Rep 2022;39(7):110812.
32. Tixagevimab and cilgavimab (evusheld) for pre-exposure prophylaxis of COVID-19. JAMA 2022;327(4):384–5.
33. Wong CKH, Au ICH, Lau KTK, et al. Real-world effectiveness of early molnupiravir or nirmatrelvir-ritonavir in hospitalised patients with COVID-19 without supplemental oxygen requirement on admission during Hong Kong's omicron BA.2 wave: a retrospective cohort study. Lancet Infect Dis 2022;S1473-3099(22): 00507–12. Published online August 24.
34. Roberts SS, Martinez M, Covington DL, et al. Lopinavir/ritonavir in pregnancy. J Acquir Immune Defic Syndr 1999 2009;51(4):456–61.
35. National Institute of Allergy and Infectious Diseases (NIAID). Pharmacokinetics and Safety of Remdesivir for Treatment of COVID-19 in Pregnant and Non-Pregnant Women in the United States. Clinicaltrials.gov 2022. Available at: https://clinicaltrials.gov/ct2/show/NCT04582266. Accessed October 4, 2022.
36. Nucleoside analogues. In: LiverTox: clinical and research information on drug-induced liver injury. National Institute of Diabetes and Digestive and Kidney Diseases; 2012. Available at: http://www.ncbi.nlm.nih.gov/books/NBK548938/. Accessed October 5, 2022.
37. Zhou S, Hill CS, Sarkar S, et al. β-d-N4-hydroxycytidine inhibits SARS-CoV-2 through lethal mutagenesis but is also mutagenic to mammalian cells. J Infect Dis 2021;224(3):415–9.
38. Troth S, Butterton J, DeAnda CS, et al. Letter to the editor in response to Zhou et al. J Infect Dis 2021;224(8):1442–3.

39. Saad AF, Chappell L, Saade GR, et al. Corticosteroids in the management of pregnant patients with coronavirus disease (COVID-19). Obstet Gynecol 2020; 136(4):823–6.

40. Hospitalized Adults: Therapeutic Management. COVID-19 Treatment Guidelines. Available at: https://www.covid19treatmentguidelines.nih.gov/management/clinical-management-of-adults/hospitalized-adults–therapeutic-management/. Accessed October 5, 2022.

41. Dexamethasone in hospitalized patients with covid-19. N Engl J Med 2021; 384(8):693–704.

42. Ninan K, Liyanage SK, Murphy KE, et al. Evaluation of long-term outcomes associated with preterm exposure to antenatal corticosteroids: a systematic review and meta-analysis. JAMA Pediatr 2022;176(6):e220483.

43. WHO Rapid Evidence Appraisal for COVID-19 Therapies (REACT) Working Group, Sterne JAC, Murthy S, et al. Association between administration of systemic corticosteroids and mortality among critically Ill patients with COVID-19: a meta-analysis. JAMA 2020;324(13):1330–41.

44. Wang Y, Zhang D, Du G, et al. Remdesivir in adults with severe COVID-19: a randomised, double-blind, placebo-controlled, multicentre trial. Lancet Lond Engl 2020;395(10236):1569–78.

45. Beigel JH, Tomashek KM, Dodd LE, et al. Remdesivir for the treatment of covid-19 — final report. N Engl J Med 2020;383(19):1813–26.

46. Remdesivir and three other drugs for hospitalised patients with COVID-19: final results of the WHO Solidarity randomised trial and updated meta-analyses. Lancet 2022;399(10339):1941–53.

47. Gupta S, Leaf DE. Tocilizumab in COVID-19: some clarity amid controversy. Lancet Lond Engl 2021;397(10285):1599–601.

48. Salama C, Han J, Yau L, et al. Tocilizumab in patients hospitalized with Covid-19 pneumonia. N Engl J Med 2021;384(1):20–30.

49. Group RC. Tocilizumab in patients admitted to hospital with COVID-19 (RECOVERY): a randomised, controlled, open-label, platform trial. Lancet Lond Engl 2021;397(10285):1637–45.

50. Jorgensen SCJ, Lapinsky SE. Tocilizumab for coronavirus disease 2019 in pregnancy and lactation: a narrative review. Clin Microbiol Infect 2022;28(1):51–7.

51. Fact sheet for healthcare providers emergency use authorization (EUA) of baricitinib. Available at: https://www.fda.gov/media/143823/download. Accessed October 6, 2022.

52. Marconi VC, Ramanan AV, de Bono S, et al. Efficacy and safety of baricitinib for the treatment of hospitalised adults with COVID-19 (COV-BARRIER): a randomised, double-blind, parallel-group, placebo-controlled phase 3 trial. Lancet Respir Med 2021;9(12):1407–18.

53. Lopes RD, de Barros e Silva PGM, Furtado RHM, et al. Therapeutic versus prophylactic anticoagulation for patients admitted to hospital with COVID-19 and elevated D-dimer concentration (ACTION): an open-label, multicentre, randomised, controlled trial. Lancet Lond Engl 2021;397(10291):2253–63.

54. The ATTACC, ACTIV-4a, and REMAP-CAP Investigators. Therapeutic anticoagulation with heparin in noncritically Ill patients with covid-19. N Engl J Med 2021; 385(9):790–802.

55. Talasaz AH, Sadeghipour P, Kakavand H, et al. Recent Randomized trials of antithrombotic therapy for patients with COVID-19: JACC state-of-the-art review. J Am Coll Cardiol 2021;77(15):1903–21.

56. The REMAP-CAP, ACTIV-4a, and ATTACC Investigators. Therapeutic Anticoagulation with heparin in critically Ill patients with covid-19. N Engl J Med 2021; 385(9):777–89.
57. Connors JM, Brooks MM, Sciurba FC, et al. Effect of antithrombotic therapy on clinical outcomes in outpatients with clinically stable symptomatic COVID-19: the ACTIV-4B randomized clinical trial. JAMA 2021;326(17):1703–12.
58. Servante J, Swallow G, Thornton JG, et al. Haemostatic and thrombo-embolic complications in pregnant women with COVID-19: a systematic review and critical analysis. BMC Pregnancy Childbirth 2021;21(1):108.
59. Polack FP, Thomas SJ, Kitchin N, et al. Safety and efficacy of the BNT162b2 mRNA Covid-19 vaccine. N Engl J Med 2020;383(27):2603–15. NEJMoa2034577.
60. Baden LR, Sahly HME, Essink B, et al. Efficacy and safety of the mRNA-1273 SARS-CoV-2 vaccine. N Engl J Med 2021;384(5):403–16.
61. Collier A, Ris Y, Yu J, McMahan K, et al. Differential kinetics of immune responses elicited by covid-19 vaccines. N Engl J Med 2021;385(21):2010–2.
62. Vaccines and related biological products advisory committee december 17, 2020 MEETING announcement - 12/17/2020. FDA. Available at: https://www.fda.gov/advisory-committees/advisory-committee-calendar/vaccines-and-related-biological-products-advisory-committee-december-17-2020-meeting-announcement. Published September 27, 2022. Accessed October 6, 2022.
63. Zauche LH, Wallace B, Smoots AN, et al. Receipt of mRNA Covid-19 vaccines and risk of spontaneous abortion. N Engl J Med 2021;385(16):1533–5.
64. Shimabukuro TT, Kim SY, Myers TR, et al. Preliminary findings of mRNA Covid-19 vaccine safety in pregnant persons. N Engl J Med 2021;384(24):2273–82. Published online April.
65. COVID-19 vaccine weekly surveillance reports (weeks 39 to 40, 2021 to 2022). GOV.UK. Available at: https://www.gov.uk/government/publications/covid-19-vaccine-weekly-surveillance-reports. Accessed October 6, 2022.
66. Goldshtein I, Nevo D, Steinberg DM, et al. Association between BNT162b2 vaccination and incidence of SARS-CoV-2 infection in pregnant women. JAMA 2021; 326(8):728–35.
67. Collier A, Ris Y, McMahan K, Yu J, et al. Immunogenicity of COVID-19 mRNA Vaccines in Pregnant and Lactating Women. JAMA 2021;325(23):2370–80. Published online.
68. Gray KJ, Bordt EA, Atyeo C, et al. COVID-19 vaccine response in pregnant and lactating women: a cohort study. Am J Obstet Gynecol 2021;2021. Published online.
69. Dagan N, Barda N, Biron-Shental T, et al. Effectiveness of the BNT162b2 mRNA COVID-19 vaccine in pregnancy. Nat Med 2021;27(10):1693–5. Published online September.
70. Morgan JA, Biggio JR, Martin JK, et al. Maternal outcomes after severe acute respiratory syndrome coronavirus 2 (sars-cov-2) infection in vaccinated compared with unvaccinated pregnant patients. Obstet Gynecol 2022;139(1):107–9.
71. Prabhu M, Murphy EA, Sukhu AC, et al. Antibody response to coronavirus disease 2019 (covid-19) messenger rna vaccination in pregnant women and transplacental passage into cord blood. Obstet Gynecol 2021;138(2):278–80. Published online April.
72. Shook LL, Atyeo CG, Yonker LM, et al. Durability of anti-spike antibodies in infants after maternal COVID-19 vaccination or natural infection. JAMA 2022;327(11): 1087–9.

73. Halasa NB, Olson SM, Staat MA, et al. Maternal vaccination and risk of hospitalization for covid-19 among infants. N Engl J Med 2022;387(2):109–19.

74. Maternal immunization task force and partners urge that covid-19 vaccine be available to pregnant individuals. Available at: https://www.acog.org/en/news/news-releases/2021/02/maternal-immunization-task-force-and-partners-urge-that-covid-19-vaccine-be-available-to-pregnant-individuals. Accessed October 6, 2022.

75. Clinical Guidance for COVID-19 Vaccination | CDC. Available at: https://www.cdc.gov/vaccines/covid-19/clinical-considerations/interim-considerations-us.html. Published September 28, 2022. Accessed October 6, 2022.

76. Plumb ID, Feldstein LR, Barkley E, et al. Effectiveness of COVID-19 mRNA vaccination in preventing COVID-19-associated hospitalization among adults with previous SARS-CoV-2 infection - United States, June 2021-February 2022. MMWR Morb Mortal Wkly Rep 2022;71(15):549–55.

An Overview of Antiviral Treatments in Pregnancy

Naima T. Joseph, MD, MPH[a],*, Jaspreet Banga, MD, MPH[b], Martina L. Badell, MD[c]

KEYWORDS

- Viral infections • Pregnancy • Therapeutics • Antivirals

KEY POINTS

- Viral infections in pregnancy are associated with deleterious maternal, fetal, and neonatal outcomes.
- Understanding pregnancy-specific considerations for pharmacologic management of viral infections in pregnancy for both maternal and fetal treatment is important, given the increased frequency of viral epidemics.
- Antiviral agents such as nucleotide/nucleoside analogues are the mainstay of antiviral therapies, with observational data suggesting safety and efficacy in pregnancy.
- Pathogen-specific antibodies such as monoclonal antibody and hyperimmune globulin are increasingly used and safe adjuncts in pregnancy, yet therapeutic efficacy data and long-term infant data are lacking.
- Pregnancy-specific data to guide antiviral use are understudied, yet should be offered to mitigate poor outcomes after carefully considering safety, effectiveness, and teratogenic potential where available.

INTRODUCTION

Viral infections in pregnancy can be associated with increased risks of maternal morbidity and mortality, prematurity and cesarean delivery, and fetal congenital viral syndromes, growth restriction, and stillbirth. The recent global pandemics of SARS-CoV-2 and epidemics of Ebola and Zika have each uniquely demonstrated the enhanced impact of viral infections to pregnant people and their offspring. As the

Work supported by BIDMC Department of Obstetrics and Gynecology Young Investigator Grand and BIDMC Department of Obstetrics and Gynecology Eleanor and Miles Shore Grant.
[a] Division of Maternal Fetal Medicine, Department of Obstetrics and Gynecology, Beth Israel Deaconess Medical Center, Harvard Medical School, 330 Brookline Avenue Kirstein, 3rd Floor, Boston, MA 02215, USA; [b] Division of Infectious Disease, Department of Medicine, Beth Israel Deaconess Medical Center, Harvard Medical School, 110 Francis Street, Boston, MA 02215, USA; [c] Division of Maternal Fetal Medicine, Department of Gynecology and Obstetrics, Emory University School of Medicine, 550 Peachtree Street Northeast, Medical Office Tower, 15th Floor, Suite 1520, Atlanta, GA 30308, USA
* Corresponding author.
E-mail address: Njoseph5@bidmc.harvard.edu

Obstet Gynecol Clin N Am 50 (2023) 183–203
https://doi.org/10.1016/j.ogc.2022.10.017
obgyn.theclinics.com

frequency of epidemics caused by novel pathogens increases,[1] knowledge of pregnancy-specific treatments becomes critical for both obstetric and nonobstetric providers.

Pregnancy presents a unique challenge for viral therapeutics. Multiple physiologic changes occur in pregnancy that alter the pharmacokinetics and pharmacodynamics of drugs. Placental infection and inflammation may affect drug and immunoglobulin passage across the placenta with potential fetal consequences. In addition, some drugs may pose teratogenic risk. Selection of antivirals requires careful consideration of maternal, and fetal, risks and benefits. In this article, the authors discuss these challenges and provide an overview of the pharmacologic treatment of common and emerging viral infections in pregnancy. Disease-specific clinical manifestations and perinatal implications and treatment considerations are reviewed and expanded upon in **Table 1**. Although not discussed in detail, vaccination, when available, is the primary preventive strategy for many infections.

General Therapies and Principles of Antiviral Therapeutics

Most viral infections during pregnancy resolve with supportive care. Treatment with antivirals or pathogen-specific antibodies may be used empirically for primary prophylaxis, such as in herpes simplex; secondary prevention, for example, influenza; for primary maternal or fetal treatment, for example, hepatitis B; and/or for primary maternal benefit.

Antiviral medications

Antivirals are a class of medications used to combat viral infections. In 1999, 11 antivirals were available in the United States, which increased to 50 by 2022.[2] The arsenal of antivirals is complex.[2] Their mechanisms include improving cellular resistance to viral infection (eg, interferons), inhibition of viral synthesis of nucleic acids (eg, polymerase inhibitors), or inhibition of viral cell attachment and entry (eg, neuraminidase inhibitors). Despite the substantial physiologic changes that occur during pregnancy, which affect drug absorption, distribution, metabolism, and elimination, there is a paucity of pregnancy-specific data on the pharmacokinetics of antivirals.[3]

Pathogen-specific antibodies. The increase of multidrug-resistant pathogens has led to the proliferation of biologics, such as polyclonal and monoclonal antibodies, which target the host-pathogen interaction. Monoclonal antibodies (MAbs) are the most frequently used therapeutic immunoglobulins (Ig) due to their high affinity and selectivity to cell-surface antigens, plasma proteins, and Ig receptors, which enhances their therapeutic efficacy while minimizing side effects.[4] Because of their long circulating elimination half-lives and relative ease of production, all current clinically used MAbs are IgGs.[4] They must be administered parenterally (intravenous or subcutaneous) due to poor (<1%) oral bioavailability. MAbs do not carry the infectious risks associated with polyclonal antibody products; their most common adverse effects include infusion reactions and acute hypersensitivity reactions.[4]

In contrast, polyclonal antibody products, such as hyperimmune globulin therapy, are typically prepared from convalescent plasma. Similar to MAbs, polyclonal antibodies are parenterally administered. Adverse reactions are reported in 20% to 50% of individual receiving therapy and include immediate reactions such anaphylaxis, volume overload, and transfusion related lung injury, as well as delayed reactions such as thromboembolic events and acute renal failure.[5]

The use of biologics during pregnancy has expanded from primarily autoimmune conditions to now infectious conditions. However, safety and efficacy data have

Table 1
Viral features, diagnosis, and perinatal management for viral infections in pregnancy

Virus	Family, Subfamily	Transmission	Diagnosis	Clinical Presentation	Treatment	Perinatal Transmission	Congenital Syndrome	Prevention
Cytomegalovirus (DNA)	Herpesviridae, betaherpesvirus	Saliva, urine, blood, and semen	Maternal serology—IgM, IgG, and IgG avidity Amniotic fluid viral culture (PCR) after 20 weeks	90% asymptomatic; Mild febrile illness, nonspecific symptoms (fatigue, headache, arthralgia, myalgia, pharyngitis, rhinitis), rash	Rarely needed, indicated in immunocompromised patients such as renal, liver and bone marrow transplant recipients, AIDS	35%–40% risk with primary infection 3% with recurrent or reinfection	Sensorineural hearing loss, stillbirth, neonatal death, deafness, microcephaly, neurocognitive and motor delay, and seizures	Behavioral risk reduction[a] Treatment with Valaciclovir, CMV immunoglobulin and vaccines under investigation
Ebola virus (RNA)	Filoviridae, Ebola virus	Blood, feces, saliva, semen, sweat, urine; contaminated objects	Maternal viral RT-PCR	Day 1–3: early febrile[b] illness, malaise, fatigue day 3–10: Gastrointestinal complaints (ie, epigastric and abdominal pain, nausea, vomiting, diarrhea) with persistent fevers and onset delirium Day 7–12: hypovolemic shock, oliguria, coma Day 10: GI hemorrhage, seizures, meningoencephalitis. Atypical presentation in pregnancy	Ansuvimab (mAb114) Atoltivimab, maftivimab, and odesivimab-ebg (REGN-EB3).	Case report of 2 pregnant patients with EVD who survived and suffered subsequent fetal demise; placental and fetal blood tests RT-PCR positive for Ebola virus even after maternal tests were negative[c]	Uncertain, stillbirths reported	Infection control precautions[d] RVSV-ZEBOV vaccine

(continued on next page)

Table 1
(continued)

Virus	Family, Subfamily	Transmission	Diagnosis	Clinical Presentation	Treatment	Perinatal Transmission	Congenital Syndrome	Prevention
Hepatitis B (DNA)	Hepadnaviridae, orthohepadnavirus	Blood via parenteral, percutaneous and sexual contact; transplacental	Maternal serology—HBsAg, anti-HBc Ab, HBsAb, HBeAg HBV DNA levels	Acute infection: may be subclinical (70%) right upper quadrant pain, scleral icterus, transaminitis, jaundice, extrahepatic manifestations. Chronic infection: may be asymptomatic, cirrhosis, hepatocellular carcinoma	Tenofovir disoproxil fumarate (TDF) or tenofovir alafenamide (TAF) preferred	90% with acute infection 30%–40% with chronic infection	Chronic hepatitis B, increased risk and earlier manifestation of cirrhosis, hepatocellular carcinoma	Maternal Hepatitis B Vaccine Neonatal HBIG and HBV vaccine and antiviral treatment (risk < 3%)
Herpes Simplex Virus (DNA)	Herpesviridae, alphaherpesvirus	Mucosal contact with active, infectious lesions	Vesicular lesion—PCR viral culture direct fluorescent antigen testing Maternal serology—HSV-1 or HSV-2 IgG or IgM	Primary infection characterized by first occurrence of genital lesion and no preexisting antibodies, often associated with viral prodrome Non-primary first episode characterized by different causative strain in previously seropositive patient. Recurrent characterized by genital lesions in which type specific antibodies are concordant. Ocular manifestations include keratitis, conjunctivitis Cutaneous manifestations	Acyclovir Valacyclovir	40%–45% with primary infection near delivery 25%–30% with nonprimary first episode 1%–3% with recurrent episode	Triad of cutaneous lesions (active lesions, scarring, hypo/hyperpigmentation), neurologic manifestations (microcephaly, intracranial calcifications, hydranencephaly), and ocular manifestations (chorioretinitis, microphthalmia, optic atrophy) with congenital infection	Suppressive therapy at 36 weeks Cesarean delivery for those with active lesions or prodromal symptoms

include erythema multiforme, eczema herpeticum. Severe manifestations include hepatitis, encephalitis, aseptic meningitis

Virus	Family/Genus	Transmission	Testing	Clinical manifestations	Treatment		Sequelae	Prevention
Zika virus (RNA)	Flaviviridae, Flavivirus	Mosquito; semen; transplacental	Symptomatic patients: (1) Serum, dengue and ZIKV RT-PCR (2) Urine ZIKV RT-PCR (3) Serum dengue-IgM[e] Sonographic concern: ZIKV RT-PCR on maternal serum and urine, maternal serum ZIKV IgM, and confirmatory PRNT	Asymptomatic in 50%–80%, low-grade fever, maculopapular pruritic rash, arthralgia, conjunctivitis, Guillain Barre syndrome	Supportive care	Yes	Microcephaly, neurocognitive disorders, seizures, ocular abnormalities (ie, chorioretinal atrophy, optic nerve hypoplasia, coloboma	Prevention of mosquito bite (DEET insect repellent, mosquito nets, cover arms and legs); avoid sexual transmission with infected or at-risk partner Vaccines under investigation
Influenza virus (RNA)	Orthomyxoviridae	Respiratory	Respiratory sample—molecular assays (NAAT, RT-PCR), antigen tests	Uncomplicated illness, complicated illness (pneumonia, CNS, cardiac, and muscular complications, multisystem organ failure)	Supportive care; oseltamivir, treatment of concomitant infection	Rare	—	Influenza vaccine; chemoprophylaxis with oseltamivir

Abbreviation: RT-PCR, reverse transcription polymerase chain reaction.

a Behavioral risk reduction consists of handwashing; avoid direct contact with saliva in children younger than 6 years; do not share toys, food, drinks, and utensils especially with those who work in child care and health care settings.

b Follows the stages of clinical pathophysiology, which include viral replication, cytokine storm, and finally consumptive coagulopathy.

c Baggi FM, Taybi A, Kurth A et al. Management of pregnant women infected with Ebolavirus in a treatment centre in Guinea, June 2014. Euro Surveill. 2014; 19(49): 20983. https://doi.org/10.2807/1560-7917.es2014.19.49.20983.

d Isolation of suspected or confirmed patients, personalized protective equipment, standard, contact, and droplet precautions.

e Testing only recommended for symptomatic patients; PRNT (plaque reduction neutralization test) measure virus specific neutralizing antibody titers.

been extrapolated from their use in nonpregnant adults. Pregnancy-specific data to guide dosing are limited. Further, data regarding effects to the developing fetus are imperfect. Monoclonal antibodies readily cross the placenta, with increasing transfer with advancing gestational age.[6] Postmarketing surveillance has not demonstrated teratogenic potential or serious adverse pregnancy outcomes.[7]

CYTOMEGALOVIRUS
Background

Affecting 0.5% to 2.0% of all live births, maternal human cytomegalovirus (CMV) infection is the most common nongenetic cause of congenital sensorineural hearing loss and neurologic damage and the most frequent congenital infection.[8] In the United States, CMV infects as many as 40,000 infants annually and is associated with stillbirth, neonatal death, deafness, microcephaly, neurocognitive and motor delay, and seizures.[9]

CMV is an ubiquitous virus that can be transmitted through blood, saliva, semen, transplacental, perinatally through cervicovaginal shedding or breastmilk, or following solid organ or stem cell transplant.[10] Infection is categorized into primary, latent with reactivation, or reinfection.[11] Primary infection occurs when an individual with no immunity becomes infected for the first time. Reactivation of latent infection occurs when an endogenous latent virus reactivates. Reinfection occurs following contact with an infectious individual, resulting in superinfection of someone with existing natural immunity. The risk of fetal transmission for primary infection is 30% to 40% in the first and second trimesters and 40% to 70% in the third trimester.[8] The risk of transmission following nonprimary infection is much lower (1%–2%).[8,12] Although transmission is more likely to occur later in gestation, the clinical sequelae and risk of fetal complications are greatest with primary infection during the first trimester. Perinatal acquisition occurs primarily from transplacental transmission but also intrapartum cervicovaginal shedding, as well as through breastmilk, although transplacental acquisition poses the highest risk of infant morbidity.[10]

Therapeutics

Currently approved antivirals target CMV via 2 distinct pathways. Ganciclovir, valganciclovir, cidofovir, and foscarnet inhibit pUL54, a DNA polymerase essential for viral replication.[13] Letermovir inhibits the viral terminase complex that is essential for viral capsid formation.[12,13] Ganciclovir was the first Food and Drug Administration (FDA)-approved treatment of CMV in nonpregnant, immunocompromised patients.[14] It is a synthetic purine nucleoside analogue of guanosine and competitively inhibits viral DNA polymerase. Primary side effects include granulocytopenia, thrombocytopenia, azoospermia, and increased serum creatinine. It is administered intravenously due to poor oral bioavailability. Ganciclovir is not recommended for use in pregnancy because of its teratogenic potential and toxicity. Valganciclovir is a prodrug of ganciclovir with more favorable oral bioavailability and less side effects and, therefore, is the preferred therapy for CMV.[13] Foscarnet and cidofovir are used for strains resistant to ganciclovir but are substantially more toxic. Cidofovir must be administered with probenecid to prevent irreversible renal damage. Letermovir is the preferred agent for primary prevention of CMV infection in seropositive recipients of an allogeneic stem cell transplant, given the myelosuppression associated with ganciclovir.

These treatments have been evaluated in immunocompromised patients, and the clinical utility in immunocompetent patients is unknown. Therefore, CMV treatment in pregnancy for maternal benefit is usually reserved for immunocompromised patients or those with severe illness. Otherwise, the disease is self-limiting, and supportive care is sufficient.[11]

CMV treatment of fetal benefit is an active area of research. Given the toxicity and teratogenic effects of ganciclovir, valacyclovir has been studied for both primary prophylaxis and for the treatment of infected, symptomatic fetuses. A prospective, double-blind trial conducted in Israel randomized participants with evidence of primary infection in the first trimester to either valacyclovir 8 g/d for a minimum of 7 weeks or placebo.[15] Valacyclovir was associated with a 71% reduced incidence of congenital infection (11% in treated group vs 30% in untreated group). However, the trial was limited by high rates of side effect such as nausea (22%), headache (13%), and abdominal pain (4%). As there are currently no guidelines for universal screening in the United States, identifying patients who would benefit from early treatment is also a challenge. However, a phase II open-label randomized trial of high-dose valacyclovir (8 g/d in 4 divided doses) in fetuses with signs of congenital infection demonstrated both a reduction of viral concentration and an increase in the proportion of asymptomatic infants at birth (82% in treated group compared with 43% in historical cohort).[16]

Passive immunization with hyperimmune globulin (HIG) has been studied for the prevention of congenital infection but the data do not clearly indicate clinical benefit. An initial nonrandomized trial showed that treatment was associated with a near 70% reduction in congenital infection; however, 2 follow-up randomized trials have not shown any benefit and further, have suggested an increased risk for worsened obstetric outcomes.[9,17,18] However, the use of HIG remains an area of investigation, especially as recent data has suggested potential benefit when given biweekly in patients with primary infection.[19]

In summary, there is no effective treatment to prevent congenital CMV. Valacyclovir seems promising; however, more data are needed to inform cost-effective screening strategies. Currently, therapeutic interventions during pregnancy should only be administered in the context of a clinical trial.

EBOLA VIRUS
Background

Zaire Ebolavirus is one of the 4 Ebolavirus species that can cause fatal human disease. The virus is not considered endemic anywhere and outbreaks typically occur from new introduction of the virus into community from an animal reservoir, leading to person-to-person transmission.[20] The largest recorded outbreak of Ebola virus disease (EVD) occurred from 2014 to 2016, with 28,616 cases and 11,310 deaths in Guinea, Liberia, and Sierra Leone.[20]

Human to human transmission occurs through direct contact through broken skin or mucous membranes with blood and bodily fluids, such as semen, urine, sweat, feces, and saliva and contaminated objects (ie, clothes, bedding, medical equipment), where it remains active for several hours up to several days. It also persists in areas of the body that are immunologically privileged, such as testes and cerebrospinal fluid.[20]

The initial presentation is a nonspecific febrile illness followed by gastrointestinal symptoms (epigastric pain, anorexia, nausea, vomiting, or diarrhea). Bleeding abnormalities occur in less than half of patients.[21] Common neurologic symptoms include delirium and agitation, which typically precedes severe lethargy. It is fatal in up to 90% of cases, which usually occurs 7 days after symptom onset.[20,21] Those still alive after 2 weeks are 75% likely to recover. The clinical course reflects underlying pathophysiology, which is first characterized by viral replication, followed by cytokine storm and inflammation, and finally consumptive coagulopathy.

Paucity of data limits accurate understanding of the specific impact of EVD during pregnancy. The initial presentation may differ, given that part of the disease severity is immune mediated, and pregnancy is an immunologically privileged status. A case report of a pregnant woman who presented with high plasma viral loads, yet remained asymptomatic for 3 days, until ultimately becoming symptomatic and suffering still-birth and maternal death highlights this issue.[22] Further, it is unclear whether pregnancy presents an independent risk for worse EVD outcome. Initial reports described pregnant patients as particularly vulnerable to death as well as at higher risk for pregnancy loss, stillbirth, and neonatal death.[23] Only two births to Ebola survivors have ever been reported.[24]

Therapeutics

Optimized supportive care involves early and aggressive volume resuscitation, electrolyte repletion, antipyretics, blood products, and respiratory support. Pregnant patients may require 5 to 10 L or more of intravenous or oral fluid per day to maintain circulating volume.[23]

The World Health Organization (WHO) recently updated guidance providing a strong recommendation for 2 monoclonal antibody treatments: ansuvimab (mAb114) and Inmazeb (REGN-EB3).[25] The latter is a combination of 3 separate MAbs and the only FDA-approved treatment of Ebola.[25] The WHO also strongly recommends against the use of remdesivir and ZMapp for the treatment of EVD. This same guidance should be applied for pregnant patients with EVD as well.

HEPATITIS B
Background

Hepatitis B virus (HBV) is the most common blood borne pathogen worldwide. The WHO estimates that approximately 300 million individuals have chronic HBV and that an estimated 1.5 million new infections occur annually.[26] It is transmitted through blood and body fluids, often through sexual and parenteral contact.

The natural history of HBV has been divided into 2 types of infection. Approximately 90% to 95% of acute HBV infections in adults resolve. However, 5% to 10% of adults with acute HBV infection develop chronic infection, characterized by persistent viremia and varying degrees of transaminitis.[27] If untreated, 40% will progress to cirrhosis, of whom 30% will be diagnosed with hepatocellular carcinoma within 10 years.[27]

Perinatal transmission accounts for most cases of chronic HBV infection worldwide. Universal screening for hepatitis B surface antigen (HBsAg) is recommended during every pregnancy.[28] Without immunization, 30% to -40% of infants born to HBV-infected mothers are infected in utero, during delivery, or in infancy due to close contact.[29] The risk of chronic infection following acute infection is inversely related to age at time of exposure: only 5% to 10% of HBV-exposed adults with acute infection will develop chronic infection, whereas 90% of infants with acute infection develop chronic infection.[26] Positive hepatitis B envelop antigen and high HBV DNA viral load confer the highest risk for perinatal transmission, even if postnatal active and passive immunity are provided.[29,30]

Therapeutics

The primary indication for treatment during pregnancy is to reduce the risk of perinatal transmission. Because Since the 1991 adoption of a comprehensive strategy to eliminate HBV transmission in the United States, the prevalence of HBV infection in children younger than 4 years has decreased by 94%.[31] The strategy includes administration of birth dose vaccine within 24 hours to medically stable infants weighing greater than 2000 grams or within 12 hours to HBV-exposed infants (infants born to HBsAg + mothers). Birth dose vaccination is followed by completion of a 3-dose HBV vaccination series. In addition, HBIg should be given within 12 hours of birth to all newborns of HBsAg-positive mothers.

However, this immunoprophylaxis fails in 10% to 30% of infants, especially among those born to mothers with an HBV DNA level of more than 200,000 IU/mL.[32] To improve these outcomes, the WHO, the Society for Maternal Fetal Medicine, and other organizations recommend HBV antiviral therapy for people with an HBV DNA level greater than 200,000 IU/mL ($5.3log_{10}$ IU/mL) beginning at 28 weeks through delivery.[30]

Oral treatments for HBV inhibit the RNA-dependent DNA polymerase reverse transcriptase and include lamivudine, adefovir, entecavir, tenofovir disoproxil (TDF), and tenofovir alafenamide (TAF). All agents are well tolerated, with the most common side effects being fatigue, dizziness, nausea, mild gastrointestinal (GI) disturbance, and headache. Prolonged TDF use is associated with a recoverable reduction in bone mineral density.[33] There is also an association between TDF and renal toxicity.[33] TAF, the prodrug of TDF, has greater plasma stability, resulting in higher intracellular active drug levels with less systemic exposure and reduced renal and bone toxicity.[33]

Tenofovir is currently the recommended first-line agent for the treatment of HBV in pregnancy.[34] In trials including pregnant patients, there was no adverse effect of treatment on fetal development and growth.[34] Further, its high barrier to resistance confers an advantage to women who may need to resume future treatment. TDF, 300 mg, or TAF, 35 mg, is administered orally once daily. Testing for HIV co-infection is imperative before beginning therapy.

Evidence also supports opportunistic hepatitis B immunity screening (HBsAg, anti-HBc, HBsAb) and vaccination during pregnancy. Prabhu and colleagues[35] analyzed the cost-effectiveness of universal hepatitis B immunity screening and vaccination during pregnancy. Assuming 84% adherence to immunity screening, 61% adherence to vaccination, and 90% seroconversion after vaccination, the investigators determined that, "in a theoretical cohort of 3.6 million women, universal HBV immunity screening and vaccination resulted in 1,702 fewer cases of HBV, seven fewer cases of decompensated cirrhosis, four fewer liver transplants, and 11 fewer deaths over the life expectancy of a woman after pregnancy." The preliminary updated guidance from the Centers for Disease Control and Prevention (CDC) recommends persons without documentation of a completed vaccine series should be offered either opportunistic vaccination or screening with the 3-test panel in pregnancy.[36]

INFLUENZA VIRUS
Background

Influenza virus is a respiratory virus that infects the nose, throat, and lungs causing the "flu." Two main types of influenza viruses, types A and B, are responsible for the annual seasonal flu. Some groups of people are at increased risk of adverse outcomes with influenza infection, including young children, the elderly, those with chronic health conditions such as asthma or heart disease, and pregnant persons.

Pregnant people are more likely to have severe illness from influenza than nonpregnant people of reproductive age because of changes in the immune, respiratory, and cardiovascular systems in pregnancy. During the 2009 H1N1 pandemic pregnant women accounted for 5% of all influenza deaths reported to the CDC despite representing only 1% of the general population.[37] Another study in the same time period found that pregnancy was associated with an increased risk of hospital and intensive care unit admissions and death. Also, pregnant persons who received delayed treatment with neuraminidase inhibitors were more likely to develop severe disease.[38] It is rare for infants of mothers with influenza to test positive for infection at birth; however, many neonates require neonatal intensive care unit admission due to the increased risks of prematurity associated with maternal infection.[38]

Therapeutics

Pregnant persons with suspected or confirmed influenza should begin antiviral treatment with the viral neuraminidase inhibitor, oseltamivir (75 mg orally twice daily for 5 days) and acetaminophen if febrile.[39] The alternate antivirals zanamivir and peramivir are also approved for influenza and are not contraindicated in pregnancy.[39]

Given the risk of maternal and neonatal morbidity with influenza infection, the CDC advises consideration of postexposure antiviral chemoprophylaxis for pregnant persons with close contact to someone infected with influenza (oseltamivir, 75 mg, once daily for 7–10 days depending on source of exposure).[39] Although delayed treatment is associated with more severe disease in pregnancy, starting antivirals even 3 to 4 days after symptom onset may still provide benefit.[38] The data regarding fetal exposure are reassuring, with a meta-analysis of 9 studies showing no increased risk of congenital malformations, low Apgar score, or preterm birth compared with unexposed, uninfected patients. Use of oseltamivir was associated with reduced risks of low birth weight (odds ratio [OR] 0.79, 95% confidence interval [CI] 0.68–0.92) and small for gestational age infant (OR 0.78, 95% CI 0.69–0.88), compared with infected, untreated patients.[38]

SIMPLEX VIRUS
Background

Herpes simplex virus types 1 and 2 (HSV-1, HSV-2), similar to other members of the herpes virus family, establish and maintain latency in infected cells and reactivate following cellular stress.

HSV is transmitted through direct mucosal surface contact with an infected person. Infection with HSV-1 generally occurs in the oropharyngeal mucosa with latency established in the trigeminal ganglion. Infection with HSV-2 usually occurs in the genital, perigenital, or anal skin sites with seeding of the sacral ganglia. It has been increasingly common to detect evidence of HSV-1 in the genital tract and HSV-2 in oral infections; however, recurrence at these alternate sites is uncommon. Studies estimate seroprevalence of HSV-1 and HSV-2 in pregnant persons as 59.3% and 21.1%, respectively, with 2% to 3% acquiring new infection during pregnancy.[40]

HSV infection is classified into primary, nonprimary first episode, and recurrent infection. Primary infection indicates first infection in susceptible, seronegative individuals. Nonprimary first episode occurs in individuals with clinically severe apparent primary infection with preexisting antibodies that differ from the causative type. Recurrent HSV is an infectious lesion with the same HSV strain as preexisting antibodies.[41] Approximately 75% of pregnant persons with evidence of prior HSV infection will have at least one recurrence during pregnancy and 14% will have prodromal symptoms or lesions at time of delivery.[42] Recurrence is more likely in persons after a primary infection during pregnancy or a history of 1 to 2 recurrences per year.[41]

The global incidence of perinatal HSV infection is approximately 10 per 100,000 live births, with an annual estimate of 1500 cases in the United States.[43] Transmission to neonates can occur in utero (5%), perinatally (85%), or postnatally (10%). Primary and nonprimary first-episode infections near time of delivery are associated with approximately 40% risk of transmission, whereas recurrent infections are associated with 1% to 3% risk of transmission.[44] However, most mothers of infants with perinatally acquired HSV lack clinical evidence of infection at delivery.[45]

Although antiviral therapies have improved outcomes, neonatal HSV is lifelong and associated with recurrent mucocutaneous and eye lesions, central nervous system, and disseminated disease. Neonates with disseminated disease face up to a 30% mortality within the first year of life as well as risk for seizures and fulminant liver failure.[46]

Therapeutics

At the time of any outbreak, antiviral medication should be offered to reduce the duration and severity of symptoms and viral shedding. Acyclovir, 400 mg, orally, 3 times daily for 7 to 10 days, with treatment beyond 10 days for persistent symptoms is the recommended therapy in pregnancy.[42] Acyclovir, a synthetic purine nucleoside analogue, which stops replication of HSV DNA, is well tolerated and is not associated with increased risk of adverse maternal, fetal, or neonatal outcomes.[42] Acyclovir is dosed 3 times daily in pregnancy, rather than twice daily in the nonpregnant population, due to increased renal clearance.[47] During acyclovir therapy, it is important to monitor for known adverse reactions, such as acute kidney injury, due to acyclovir crystals, neurotoxicity, and thrombotic microangiopathy.[47,48] Patients with complicated HSV infections, such as disseminated infection, central nervous system disease, or end-organ involvement, require hospitalization for intravenous acyclovir for at least 10 days, which is extended up to 21 days for HSV encephalitis.

In 2020, the American College of Obstetricians and Gynecologists (ACOG) changed their recommendation from providing suppressive therapy to anyone with recurrence during pregnancy, to universal suppressive therapy in anyone with known HSV history at or beyond 36 weeks.[42] Although acyclovir has the most data regarding HSV treatment in pregnancy, other options exist (**Table 2**). For instance, valacyclovir, a prodrug of acyclovir with increased bioavailability and thus less frequent dosing, may be used, although it has less safety and efficacy data.[42] Although maternal suppressive therapy has reduced the risk of neonatal acquisition by 30% to 50%, research investigating the therapeutic efficacy of newer antivirals to further reduce neonatal HSV incidence is needed.[46]

ZIKA VIRUS
Background

The Zika virus (ZIKV) is a positive-sense RNA arbovirus, belonging in the family Flaviviridae, which is closely related to dengue, yellow fever, and West Nile. The first human outbreak occurred in 2007 in Micronesia, with reemergence initially in French Polynesia in 2013 to 2014, then in Brazil in February 2015. By March 2016, the virus had spread to 33 countries and territories in the Americas and was declared a Public Health Emergency of International Concern by the WHO. Since the 2016 outbreak, reported Zika cases in the Americas have declined by 30- to 70-fold with the last confirmed case of locally acquired Zika in the continental United States in September 2017.[49]

Mosquito and nonmosquito transmission occurs. The predominant mode of nonmosquito transmission is transplacental, which occurs in approximately 26% of infected pregnant people.[42] Transmission can also occur sexually to partners of

Table 2
Pharmacologic management of viral infections and pregnancy-specific considerations

Drug	Dose[a]	Preferred Agent	Drug Class/Mechanism of Action	Indications for Treatment During Pregnancy[b]	Potential Side Effects	Monitoring & Treatment Considerations	Pregnancy Considerations
CMV – fetal							
Valacyclovir	Oral 8 g/day	N/A	Nucleotide analogue, inhibits viral DNA synthesis	Use outside a clinical trial not currently recommended. In clinical trials, administered to women with primary CMV infection or extracerebral or mild brain abnormalities on US or MRI	Granulocytopenia, anemia, thrombocytopenia, pancytopenia, inhibition of spermatogenesis and female infertility, diarrhea,	Drug reaction with eosinophilia and systemic symptoms (DRESS)	Safety and tolerability of high dose limit use in pregnancy
CMV—maternal							
Ganciclovir or valganciclovir	Varies by indication, intravenous or intravitreal	✔	Nucleotide analogue, inhibits viral DNA synthesis	Most cases of CMV in an immunocompetent host will self-resolve without antiviral therapy. Treatment should be offered to those with immunocompromising conditions (ie, transplant, AIDS) or with severe end-organ disease[c]	Granulocytopenia, anemia, thrombocytopenia, pancytopenia, inhibition of spermatogenesis and female infertility, diarrhea, potential carcinogenic	—	Treatment of maternal infection has not been shown to decrease perinatal transmission Teratogenic (cleft lip/palate, anophthalmia, brachygnathia, others), hydrocephalus, embryo lethality. Intraocular injection preferred over systemic therapy for CMV retinitis, to limit first trimester exposure
Foscarnet	Varies by indication, intravenous or intravitreal	—	Pyrophosphate analogue, inhibits viral DNA synthesis	Ganciclovir-resistant CMV	Renal toxicity, seizures, hypocalcemia, nausea, anemia, genital ulcers	Monitor amniotic fluid volume	High risk of fetal skeletal abnormalities, oligohydramnios
Cidofovir	Varies by indication, intravenous or intravitreal	—	Nucleotide analogue inhibits viral DNA synthesis, chain terminator	Salvage therapy for CMV	Dose-dependent nephrotoxicity, nausea, vomiting, neutropenia	Serum creatinine and urine protein 48 hours after first dose, and before next dose	Embryotoxic

	Dosage		Mechanism	Indication	Adverse effects	Monitoring	Pregnancy
Ebola							
REGN-EB3 (Inmazeb, or Atoltivimab/maftivimab/odesivimab-ebgn)[c]	IV 50 mg/kg of each given as a single dose	✓	Combination of 3 human monoclonal antibodies against *Zaire ebolavirus* glycoprotein mediating viral entry and membrane fusion	*Zaire ebolavirus* infection	Hypersensitivity reaction (fevers, chills, hypotension)	May diminish the effect of Ebola Zaire live vaccine, consider 3-month wait after treatment to administer vaccine	Placental transfer expected to occur; amount depends on maternal serum concentration, gestational age, fetal weight, IgG subclass
mAb114 (Ansuvimab)[c]	IV 50 mg/kg as a single dose	✓	Humanized monoclonal neutralizing antibody (IgG$_1$) targeted against viral glycoprotein	*Zaire ebolavirus* infection, including neonates born to an rtPCR positive mother	Hypersensitivity reaction (fevers, chills, hypotension)	May diminish the effect of Ebola Zaire live vaccine, consider 3-month wait after treatment to administer vaccine	Placental transfer expected to occur; amount depends on maternal serum concentration, gestational age, fetal weight, IgG subclass
Hepatitis B							
Tenofovir disoproxil fumarate (TDF)	Oral 300 mg daily	✓	Nucleotide analogue reverse transcriptase inhibitor, prevents viral DNA chain elongation through inhibition of reverse transcriptase, which is necessary for viral replication	HBsAg positive and HBV DNA level greater than 200,000 IU/mL ($>10^6$ copies/mL). Begin therapy at 28–32 weeks and continue postpartum	Nephropathy, Fanconi syndrome, osteomalacia, lactic acidosis	Creatinine clearance at baseline, consider bone density at baseline, if at risk for renal impairment, Cr Cl, serum phosphate, urine protein at least annually. Test for HIV before treatment initiation	Pharmacokinetics not significantly affected by pregnancy. No concern for mutagenicity, embryofetal lethality, renal or bone toxicity
Tenofovir alafenamide (TAF)	Oral 25 mg daily	✓	Nucleotide analogue reverse transcriptase inhibitor with higher intracellular concentrations and reduced plasma concentrations than TDF	HBsAg positive and HBV DNA level greater than 200,000 IU/mL ($>10^6$ copies/mL). Begin therapy at 28–32 weeks and continue postpartum	Lactic acidosis	Assess creatinine clearance, serum phosphorous, and urine protein before initiating and during therapy. Test for HIV before treatment initiation	Pharmacokinetics not significantly affected by pregnancy. No concern for mutagenicity, embryofetal lethality, renal or bone toxicity
Entecavir	Oral 0.5 mg daily	—	Cyclopentyl guanosine analogue, which inhibits viral hepatitis B, viral polymerase and reverse transcriptase activity to reduce viral DNA synthesis	—	Lactic acidosis in decompensated cirrhosis	Test for HIV before treatment initiation	Teratogenic effects observed in animal data

(continued on next page)

Table 2
(continued)

Drug	Dose[a]	Preferred Agent	Drug Class/Mechanism of Action	Indications for Treatment During Pregnancy[b]	Potential Side Effects	Monitoring & Treatment Considerations	Pregnancy Considerations
Pegylated Interferon-α-2a	Subcutaneous 180 mcg weekly	—	Low-molecular-weight, soluble glycoproteins with antiviral, antiproliferative, and immune-regulating activity	—	Flulike symptoms, fatigue, mood disturbance, cytopenia, anorexia, autoimmune disorders	Complete blood count and TSH every 3 months, clinical monitoring for autoimmune, neuropsychiatric, and infectious complications. Test for HIV before treatment initiation	Theoretical concern for pregnancy loss based on animal data, not reported in human data
Lamivudine	Oral 100 mg daily	—	Cytosine analogue reverse transcriptase inhibitor via viral DNA chain termination	—	Pancreatitis, lactic acidosis	Test for HIV before treatment initiation. If HIV-co-infection, dosing for HIV used rather than for chronic HBV. High rates of resistance	Safe for use in pregnancy, poorly tolerated
Adefovir	Oral 10 mg daily	—	Nucleotide analogue of adenosine monophosphate inhibits HBV viral polymerase	Not preferred therapy for chronic hepatitis B; can be used in HBV with lamivudine resistance	Acute renal failure, Fanconi syndrome, lactic acidosis	Creatinine clearance at baseline, consider bone density at baseline, if at risk for renal impairment, Cr Cl, serum phosphate, urine protein at least annually. Used for the treatment of lamivudine-resistance HBV in combination with another nucleoside analogue	Pregnancy outcome data limited
Telbivudine	Oral 600 mg daily	—	Thymidine nucleotide analogue, inhibits viral DNA polymerase	—	Creatine kinase elevation, myopathy, peripheral neuropathy, lactic acidosis	AST/ALT during therapy and following discontinuation, baseline renal function and serum creatinine kinase, baseline neuromuscular function	Not available in the United States

Herpes Simplex Virus

Drug		Mechanism	Indication	Adverse effects	Monitoring	Comments
Acyclovir	✔	Nucleotide analogue, inhibits viral DNA polymerase and viral replication	*Initial episode:* oral 400 mg 3 times daily for 7–10 days[d] *Recurrent episode:* oral 400 mg 3 times daily for 7–10 days[d] *Suppressive therapy:* oral 400 mg 3 times daily *Severe or disseminated disease:* IV 5–10 mg/kg every 8 hours 14–21 days (may include step-down oral therapy)[e]	Primary or nonprimary first-episode genital infection; recurrent episode; suppressive therapy beginning at 36 weeks until onset of labor	Signs and symptoms of neurotoxicity and nephrotoxicity	None needed Viral culture surveillance not recommended	Safety demonstrated during pregnancy Genital culture monitoring not recommended Increase doses for suppressive therapy given increased renal clearance
Valacyclovir	✔	Acyclovir oral prodrug nucleotide analogue, inhibits viral DNA synthesis	*Initial episode:* oral 1g twice daily for 7–10 days *Recurrent episode:* 500 mg or 1g once daily for 5 days twice daily for 3 days *Suppressive therapy:* 500 mg twice daily or 1g once daily	Primary or nonprimary first-episode genital infection; recurrent episode; suppressive therapy beginning at 36 weeks until onset of labor	Granulocytopenia, anemia, thrombocytopenia, pancytopenia, inhibition of spermatogenesis and female infertility, diarrhea	Drug reaction with eosinophilia and systemic symptoms (DRESS)	3- to 5-fold greater oral bioavailability reduces dosing, may be administered to women to reduce pill burden Genital culture monitoring not recommended Safety and tolerability studied in pregnancy

(continued on next page)

Table 2
(continued)

Drug	Preferred Agent	Dose[a]	Drug Class/Mechanism of Action	Indications for Treatment During Pregnancy[b]	Potential Side Effects	Monitoring & Treatment Considerations	Pregnancy Considerations
Influenza							
Oseltamivir	✓	Treatment: Oral 75 mg twice daily for 6 days Prophylaxis: Oral 75 mg once daily for 7 days Dose adjustment required for impaired renal function	Neuraminidase inhibitor (blocks the release of viral progeny from infected cells)	Initiate as soon as symptom start ideally within 48 hours and at least within 4 days	GI distress (nausea, vomiting) Contraindicated if hypersensitivity	Monitor signs and symptoms of delirium	Safety demonstrated in pregnancy, no increased risk of congenital malformation or increased adverse pregnancy outcomes
Zanamivir	—	Treatment: two oral inhalations (10 mg) twice daily for 5 days Prophylaxis dosing varies by household, institutional, or community exposure	Neuraminidase inhibitor	Initiate within 48 hours of symptom onset For use against influenza A/ H1N1 virus strains that are resistant to oseltamivir	Sore throat, cough Contraindicated in patients with underlying respiratory disease (ie, asthma, chronic obstructive pulmonary disease), patients with severe disease warranting hospitalization, or patients with hypersensitivity	—	Not preferred Observational data with no reported adverse pregnancy outcomes No congenital malformations in animal data
Peramivir	—	600 mg intravenously as a single dose	Neuraminidase inhibitor	For use in patients without severe illness who cannot tolerate oral or inhaled medications	Rash common after administration Neurologic side effects	Baseline BUN, Creatinine	Observational data limited
Baloxavir	—	40 kg to <80 kg: 40 mg orally as a single dose ≥80 kg: 80 mg orally as a single dose No dosage adjustments for renal or hepatic impairment	Endonuclease inhibitor inhibits viral gene transcription and replication	Administered within 48 h of symptom onset Associated with faster time to symptom resolution[f]	Diarrhea, vomiting Minor substrate of CYP3A4 enzyme Should not be used for treatment of severe influenza, in immunocompromised patients, or in pregnancy	Monitor for secondary bacterial infection	Observational data limited No congenital malformations in animal data Should not be used in pregnancy

Abbreviations: IV, intravenous; US, ultrasound.

[a] Dosing for adults with normal renal and liver function. Please note renal and hepatic adjustments not provided.

[b] Treatment indications specifically for pregnancy, which may differ from the nonpregnant adult. Indications for treatment of maternal CMV include those with organ complications (retinitis, severe colitis, pulmonary manifestation, neurologic manifestations including Guillain Barre, encephalitis, transverse myelitis, and seizures, pericarditis, and other cardiac complications), treatment of immunocompromised patients, preemptive treatment in solid organ transplant recipients, and prophylaxis in hematopoietic stem cell transplant recipients.

[c] Not commercially available, only distributed during public health emergencies in the United States.

[d] May extend treatment duration beyond 10 days if lesion has not healed by 10 days.

[e] Step-down oral therapy includes transition from IV to oral administration once clinically improved of acyclovir 400 mg TID to complete a 10-day course.

[f] Ison MG, Portsmouth S, Yoshida Y et al. Early treatment with baloxavir marboxil in high-risk adolescent and adult outpatients with uncomplicated influenza (CAPTSONE2): a randomised, placebo-controlled, phase 3 trial. Lancet Infectious Disease. 2020; 20(1): 1204 – 1214.

infected men, independent of symptoms, as well as with blood transfusion and laboratory.[49] Female to male sexual transmission is less common.

Pregnant people with ZIKV disease are at increased risk for preterm birth and neonatal demise.[50] Congenital neonatal ZIKV syndrome is characterized by severe congenital malformations including microcephaly, neurocognitive disorders, seizures, and ocular abnormalities.[51] The highest risk of adverse perinatal outcomes, especially microcephaly, occurs with first trimester infection.[50]

Therapeutics

Maternal treatment focuses on symptomatic control. There are no currently recommended therapeutic options for the prevention of congenital ZIKV, which is an urgent priority. Current prevention measures include avoiding mosquito bites, reducing sexual transmission, and environmental control of the mosquito vector. Recommendations for persons considering or attempting pregnancy or who are currently pregnant are to avoid unnecessary travel to areas of ongoing ZIKV transmission; avoid unprotected sexual contact with partners at risk for ZIKV infection; use Environmental Protection Agency–approved mosquito repellent containing an active ingredient against mosquitos (eg, DEET); and use permethrin treatment for clothing, bed nets, window screens, and air conditioning as able.

SUMMARY

Viral infections in pregnancy are associated with unique risks, including worsened maternal disease, congenital infection, and adverse perinatal outcomes. Because the prevalence of antiviral use during pregnancy is increasing,[52] the need for well-designed studies that assess the safety, effectiveness, and pharmacology of viral therapeutics in pregnancy is critical.

CLINICS CARE POINTS

- Many viral infections pose unique threats during pregnancy, including heightened risk for worse disease and adverse perinatal outcomes.
- Antiviral medications include a broad and complex arsenal of therapies, most of which can be safely used for primary or secondary chemoprophylaxis, treatment of active disease, or to reduce the risk of perinatal transmission.

REFERENCES

1. Marani M, Katul GG, Pan WK, et al. Intensity and frequency of extreme novel epidemics. PNAS 2021;118(35). e2105482118.
2. Vardanyan R, Hruby V. Antiviral drugs. In: Vardanyan R, Hruby V, editors. Synthesis of best-seller drugs. Elsevier; 2016. p. 687–736. Copyright: © Academic Press 2016. Imprint: Academic Press.
3. Hazenberg P, Navaratnam K, Busuulwa P, et al. Anti-Infective Dosing in Special Populations: Pregnancy. Clin Pharmacol Ther 2021;109(4):977–86.
4. Castelli MS, McGonigle P, Hornby PJ. The pharmacology and therapeutic applications of monoclonal antibodies. Pharmacol Res Perspect 2019;7(6):e00535.
5. Ballow M. Safety of IGIV therapy and infusion-related adverse events. Immunol Res 2007;38(1–3):122–32.

6. Pham-Huy A, Sadarangani M, Huang V, et al. From mother to baby: antenatal exposure to monoclonal antibody biologics. Expert Rev Clin Immunol 2019; 15(3):221–9.

7. Pham-Huy A, Top KA, Constantinescu C, et al. The use and impact of monoclonal antibody biologics during pregnancy. CMAJ 2021;193(29):E1129–36.

8. Leruez-Ville M, Foulon I, Pass R, et al. Cytomegalovirus infection during pregnancy: state of the science. Am J Obstet Gynecol 2020;223(3):330–49.

9. Hughes BL, Clifton RG, Rouse DJ, et al. A Trial of Hyperimmune Globulin to Prevent Congenital Cytomegalovirus Infection. N Engl J Med 2021;385(5):436–44.

10. Fowler K, Mucha J, Neumann M, et al. A systematic literature review of the global seroprevalence of cytomegalovirus: possible implications for treatment, screening, and vaccine development. BMC Public Health 2022;22(1):1659.

11. Griffiths P, Reeves M. Pathogenesis of human cytomegalovirus in the immunocompromised host. Nat Rev Microbiol 2021;19(12):759–73.

12. Royal College of Obstetricians and Gynecologists. Congenital Cytomegalovirus Infection: Update on Treatment. BJOG 2018;125(1):e1–11.

13. Acosta E, Bowlin T, Brooks J, et al. Advances in the development of therapeutics for cytomegalovirus infections. J Infect Dis 2020;221:32–44.

14. Crumpacker CS. Ganciclovir. N Engl J Med 1996;335(10):721–9.

15. Shahar-Nissan K, Pardo J, Peled O, et al. Valaciclovir to prevent vertical transmission of cytomegalovirus after maternal primary infection during pregnancy: a randomised, double-blind, placebo-controlled trial. Lancet 2020;396(10253): 779–85.

16. Leruez-Ville M, Ghout I, Bussières L, et al. In utero treatment of congenital cytomegalovirus infection with valacyclovir in a multicenter, open-label, phase II study. Am J Obstet Gynecol 2016;215(4):462.e1-10.

17. Nigro G, Adler SP, la Torre R, et al. Passive Immunization during Pregnancy for Congenital Cytomegalovirus Infection. N Engl J Med 2005;353(13):1350–62.

18. Revello MG, Lazzarotto T, Guerra B, et al. A Randomized Trial of Hyperimmune Globulin to Prevent Congenital Cytomegalovirus. N Engl J Med 2014;370(14): 1316–26.

19. Kagan KO, Enders M, Schampera MS, et al. Prevention of maternal-fetal transmission of cytomegalovirus after primary maternal infection in the first trimester by biweekly hyperimmunoglobulin administration. Ultrasound Obstet Gynecol 2019;53(3):383–9.

20. Feldmann H, Sprecher A, Geisbert TW. Ebola N Engl J Med 2020;382:1832–42.

21. WHO Ebola Response Team. Ebola Virus Disease in West Africa-The First 9 Months of the Epidemic and Forward Projections. N Engl J Med 2014;371(16): 1481–95.

22. Akerlund E, Prescott J, Tampellini L. Shedding of Ebola Virus in an Asymptomatic Pregnant Woman. N Engl J Med 2015;372(25):2467–9.

23. Jamieson DJ, Uyeki TM, Callaghan WM, et al. What obstetrician-gynecologists should know about ebola: A perspective from the centers for disease control and prevention. Obstet Gynecol 2014;124(5):1005–10.

24. Ratcliffe R. Safe birth of baby born to Ebola survivor hailed as a medical miracle Daughter of Congolese woman treated for Ebola in December becomes only second healthy child born in such circumstances. 2019. https://www.theguardian.com/global-development/2019/jan/11/safe-birth-baby-born-to-ebola-survivor-hailed-as-medical-miracle-democratic-republic-congo. [Accessed 28 July 2022].

25. World Health Organization. Therapeutics for Ebola Virus Disease. 2022. Available at: https://www.who.int/publications/i/item/9789240055742. Accessed September 8, 2022.

26. World Health Organization. Hepatitis B. 2022. https://www.who.int/news-room/fact-sheets/detail/hepatitis-b. [Accessed 28 July 2022].

27. Tang LSY, Covert E, Wilson E, et al. Chronic Hepatitis B infection a review. JAMA - J Am Med Assoc 2018;319(17):1802–13.

28. Owens DK, Davidson KW, Krist AH, et al. Screening for Hepatitis B Virus Infection in Pregnant Women: US Preventive Services Task Force Reaffirmation Recommendation Statement. JAMA 2019;322(4):349–54.

29. Jonas MM. Hepatitis B and pregnancy: An underestimated issue. Liver Int 2009; 29(SUPPL. 1):133–9.

30. Dionne-Odom J, Cozzi GD, Franco RA, et al. Treatment and prevention of viral hepatitis in pregnancy. Am J Obstet Gynecol 2022;226(3):335–46.

31. Shepard C, Finelli L, Bell B, et al. Acute Hepatitis B Among Children and Adolescents—United States, 1990-2002. J Am Med Assoc 2004;292(24):2967–8.

32. Funk AL, Lu Y, Yoshida K, et al. Efficacy and safety of antiviral prophylaxis during pregnancy to prevent mother-to-child transmission of hepatitis B virus: a systematic review and meta-analysis. Lancet Infect Dis 2021;21(1):70–84.

33. Gallant JE, Daar ES, Raffi F, et al. Efficacy and safety of tenofovir alafenamide versus tenofovir disoproxil fumarate given as fixed-dose combinations containing emtricitabine as backbones for treatment of HIV-1 infection in virologically suppressed adults: a randomised, double-blind, active-controlled phase 3 trial. Lancet HIV 2016;3(4):e158–65.

34. Pan CQ, Duan Z, Dai E, et al. Tenofovir to Prevent Hepatitis B Transmission in Mothers with High Viral Load. N Engl J Med 2016;374(24):2324–34.

35. Prabhu M, Susich MK, Packer CH, et al. Universal Hepatitis B Antibody Screening and Vaccination in Pregnancy: A Cost-Effectiveness Analysis. Obstet Gynecol 2022;139(3):357–67.

36. Centers for Disease Control and Prevention. CDC Recommendations for Hepatitis B Testing and Screening - United States, 2022. 2022. Available at: https://www.regulations.gov/document/CDC-2022-0044-0005. Accessed August 21, 2022.

37. Siston AM, Rasmussen SA, Honein MA, et al. Pandemic 2009 Influenza A(H1N1) Virus Illness Among Pregnant Women in the United States. J Am Med Assoc 2010;303(15):1517–25.

38. Mosby LG, Rasmussen SA, Jamieson DJ. 2009 pandemic influenza A (H1N1) in pregnancy: A systematic review of the literature. Am J Obstet Gynecol 2011; 205(1):10–8.

39. Assessment and Treatment of Pregnant Women With Suspected or Confirmed Influenza: ACOG Committee Opinion No. 753. Obstet Gynecol 2018;132(4): e169–73.

40. Patton ME, Bernstein K, Liu G, et al. Seroprevalence of herpes simplex virus types 1 and 2 among pregnant women and sexually active, nonpregnant women in the United States. Clin Infect Dis 2018;67(10):1535–42.

41. Whitley R, Kimberlin DW, Prober CG. In: Arvin A, Campadelli-Fiume G, Mocarski E, editors. Chapter 32 pathogenesis and disease. Human herpesviruses: biology, therapy, and immunoprophylaxis. Cambridge University Press; 2007. Available at: https://www.ncbi.nlm.nih.gov/books/NBK47449/?report=printable.

42. Management of Genital Herpes in Pregnancy: ACOG Practice Bulletin No. 220. Obstet Gynecol 2020;135(5):e193–202.

43. Looker KJ, Magaret AS, May MT, et al. First estimates of the global and regional incidence of neonatal herpes infection. Lancet Glob Health 2017;5(3):e300–9.
44. Brown ZA, Wald A, Morrow MRA, et al. Effect of Serologic Status and Cesarean Delivery on Transmission Rates of Herpes Simplex Virus From Mother to Infant. JAMA 2003;289(2):203–9.
45. Stone K, Brooks C, Guinan M, et al. National surveillance for neonatal herpes simplex virus infections. Sex Transm Dis 1989;16(3):152–6.
46. James SH, Sheffield JS, Kimberlin DW. Mother-to-child transmission of herpes simplex virus. J Pediatr Infect Dis Soc 2014;3(SUPPL1):S19–23.
47. Kimberlin D, Weller S, Whitley R, et al. Pharmacokinetics of oral valacyclovir and acyclovir in late pregnancy. Am J Obstet Gynecol 1998;179(4):846–51.
48. Frenkel L, Brown Z, Bryson Y, et al. Pharmacokinetics of acyclovir in the term human pregnancy and neonate. Am J Obstet Gynecol 1991;164(2):569–76.
49. Musso D, Ko AI, Baud D. Zika Virus Infection — After the Pandemic. N Engl J Med 2019;381(15):1444–57.
50. Mlakar J, Korva M, Tul N, et al. Zika Virus Associated with Microcephaly. N Engl J Med 2016;374(10):951–8.
51. Paixao ES, Cardim LL, Costa MCN, et al. Mortality from Congenital Zika Syndrome — Nationwide Cohort Study in Brazil. N Engl J Med 2022;386(8):757–67.
52. Avalos LA, Chen H, Yang C, et al. The Prevalence and Trends of Antiviral Medication Use During Pregnancy in the US: A Population-Based Study of 664,297 Deliveries in 2001-2007. Matern Child Health J 2014;18:64–72.

Antiretrovirals for Human Immunodeficiency Virus Treatment and Prevention in Pregnancy

Kristina M. Brooks, PharmD[a], Kimberly K. Scarsi, PharmD, MS[b],*,
Mark Mirochnick, MD[c]

KEYWORDS

- HIV • Pharmacokinetics • Pregnant • Obstetric care • Antiretroviral therapy
- Preexposure prophylaxis

KEY POINTS

- Safe and effective antiretroviral medications during pregnancy and postpartum are key to improving human immunodeficiency virus (HIV) treatment and prevention outcomes in persons of child-bearing potential.
- Pharmacokinetics of all HIV drugs need to be studied in pregnant people to inform appropriate drug dosing.
- Many antiretroviral drugs have altered pharmacokinetics in pregnancy, which sometimes dose adjustment, more intensive clinical monitoring of HIV, or avoidance of certain therapies.
- The most updated recommendations for antiretroviral medication use in pregnant people should always be reviewed, as guidelines are regularly updated based on newly available information.

INTRODUCTION

An estimated 1.3 million births occurred worldwide in women with human immuno-deficiency virus (HIV) in 2020.[1] Globally, HIV-related illnesses remain the leading cause of death among women of reproductive age, and approximately 6000 women acquire HIV every week. Collectively, these numbers demonstrate a need to reduce the morbidity and mortality associated with HIV, prevent new infections,

[a] Department of Pharmaceutical Sciences, University of Colorado Anschutz Medical Campus, 12850 East Montview Boulevard, Mail Stop C238, Aurora, CO 80045, USA; [b] Department of Pharmacy Practice and Science, University of Nebraska Medical Center, 986145 Nebraska Medical Center, Room 3021, Omaha, NE 68198, USA; [c] Boston University School of Medicine, 801 Albany Street, Room 2021, Boston, MA 20118, USA
* Corresponding author.
E-mail address: kim.scarsi@unmc.edu

Obstet Gynecol Clin N Am 50 (2023) 205–218
https://doi.org/10.1016/j.ogc.2022.10.013
0889-8545/23/© 2022 Elsevier Inc. All rights reserved.
obgyn.theclinics.com

and improve the health and safety of people of child-bearing potential with, and at risk for, HIV.

Antiretroviral therapy (ART), a combination of at least 2 antiretroviral medications with different mechanisms of action, is indicated for all persons with HIV to reduce morbidity and mortality and prevent transmission by suppressing HIV to an undetectable level in plasma.[2] Among pregnant people with HIV, ART has benefits for both maternal and child health, leading to significant reductions in perinatal HIV transmission from 25% to 30% without treatment to less than 1% in the setting of virologic suppression with ART.[3] Recommended initial ART options in pregnancy generally consist of 2 nucleoside/nucleotide reverse transcriptase inhibitors (NRTI/NtRTI) plus a third agent from a different class, such as an integrase strand transfer inhibitor (INSTI), boosted protease inhibitor (PI), or nonnucleoside reverse transcriptase inhibitor (NNRTI) (**Table 1**). The mechanism of action of each antiretroviral class is described in **Fig. 1**. Antiretroviral medications can also be used as preexposure prophylaxis (PrEP) to prevent HIV acquisition. Pregnancy through early postpartum represents a period of increased HIV acquisition risk due to behavioral (eg, condomless sex) and biological factors (eg, changes in innate and adaptive immunity). Tenofovir disoproxil fumarate (TDF) with emtricitabine is the only recommended PrEP option in pregnancy,[2] although studies are in development or underway with other PrEP medications.

Here the authors provide a historical perspective on studies assessing antiretrovirals, a high-level summary of pharmacokinetic data supporting the current recommended use of antiretrovirals for HIV treatment and prevention in pregnancy, and areas for future research.

HISTORICAL PERSPECTIVE ON ANTIRETROVIRALS IN PREGNANCY

Since the first antiretroviral, zidovudine, was licensed in 1987, there has been a steady introduction of new antiretrovirals with increased potency, decreased toxicity, and more convenient dosing. There are more than 30 licensed drugs available to treat HIV in the United States, as well as several fixed dose combination products that provide one-pill, once-daily ART.[2] The importance of treating HIV during pregnancy was recognized early in the epidemic. However, pregnant women are generally excluded from antiretroviral drug development programs, leading to drug licensure without pregnancy-specific pharmacokinetic and safety data.[4] Clinicians caring for pregnant persons with HIV face the dilemma of denying them treatment with the newest, most potent, and best tolerated antiretrovirals in favor of older, less desirable agents, or treating them with novel agents in the absence of data.

The academic research community responded by establishing postlicensing pharmacokinetic studies in pregnant women receiving antiretrovirals as part of their clinical care, including the IMPAACT (International Maternal Pediatric Adolescent AIDS Clinical Trials) network P1026s study conducted in the United States, Brazil, southern Africa, and Thailand and PANNA (Pharmacokinetics of newly developed ANtiretroviral agents in HIV-infected pregNAnt women) conducted in Europe. The largest of these, the IMPAACT P1026s study, has performed intensive pharmacokinetic sampling on more than 1000 participants for more than 25 antiretrovirals since 1993. This opportunistic approach has resulted in the publication of more pharmacokinetic studies during pregnancy for antiretrovirals than for any other drug class.[5]

However, there remains an average 6-year lag between drug licensure and availability of pregnancy pharmacokinetic and safety data (**Fig. 2**).[6] During this time, many pregnant people receive antiretrovirals in the absence of any pregnancy-specific data. The

Class	Antiretroviral Medication	Recommended Dosing in Pregnancy
Preferred Initial Antiretroviral Therapy Options[a]		
NRTI/NtRTI	Abacavir[b]	600 mg once daily or 300 mg twice daily
	Emtricitabine	200 mg once daily
	Lamivudine	300 mg once daily or 150 mg twice daily
	Tenofovir alafenamide (TAF)	25 mg once daily or 10 mg once daily (if coformulated with cobicistat)
	Tenofovir disoproxil fumarate (TDF)	300 mg once daily
INSTI	Dolutegravir	50 mg once daily
	Raltegravir	400 mg twice daily[c]
Boosted PIs	Atazanavir/ritonavir[d]	300 mg/100 mg once daily (standard) or 400 mg/100 mg once daily (increased)
	Darunavir/ritonavir	600 mg/100 mg twice daily[e]
Preferred Antiretrovirals for Preexposure Prophylaxis		
NRTI/NtRTI	Tenofovir disoproxil fumarate (TDF)	300 mg once daily
	Emtricitabine	200 mg once daily
Alternative Initial Antiretroviral Therapy Options[f]		
NRTI	Zidovudine[g]	300 mg twice daily
NNRTI	Efavirenz[h]	600 mg once daily
	Rilpivirine[i]	25 mg once daily
Not Recommended as Initial Antiretroviral Treatment & Only Used in Special Circumstances in Treatment-Experienced People[j]		
NNRTI	Etravirine	200 mg twice daily after a meal
	Nevirapine	200 mg once daily x 2 wk, then 200 mg twice daily thereafter
Boosted PIs	Lopinavir/ritonavir	400 mg/100 mg twice daily (standard) or 600 mg/150 mg twice daily (increased)
Entry inhibitors	Fostemsavir	600 mg twice daily
	Maraviroc	150 mg twice daily (if coadministered with CYP3A4 inhibitors)
		300 mg twice daily (if coadministered with drugs that are not strong CYP3A4 inhibitors)
		600 mg twice daily (if coadministered with CYP3A4 inducers)
	Enfuvirtide (T-20)	90 mg subcutaneous injection twice daily

Table 1
Recommended antiretroviral medications in pregnancy

Abbreviations: ART, antiretroviral therapy; CYP3A4, cytochrome P450 type 3A4; INSTI, integrase strand transfer inhibitor; NNRTI, nonnucleoside reverse transcriptase inhibitor; NRTI, nucleoside reverse transcriptase inhibitor; PI, protease inhibitor.

[a] Drugs designated as Preferred options based on clinical trial data showing efficacy, durability, acceptable toxicity, ease of use, and pregnancy-specific PK data to guide dosing. Available data must suggest a favorable risk-benefit balance compared with other ART options; risk/benefit assessment should incorporate maternal, pregnancy, fetal, and infant outcomes. All available data should be considered when selecting ART for a pregnant person.

[b] Must be HLA-B*5701 negative; should not be used in persons with pretreatment HIV RNA greater than 100,000 copies/mL if in combination with atazanavir/ritonavir or efavirenz.

[c] Once-daily formulation has not been studied in pregnancy and thus is not recommended.

[d] Atazanavir can cause maternal hyperbilirubinemia through UGT1A1 inhibition; no clinically significant neonatal hyperbilirubinemia or kernicterus reported, but monitoring is recommended;

cannot be administered with proton pump inhibitors and requires specific dose timing when combined with H2 blockers or antacids.

[e] Must be administered twice daily in pregnancy.

[f] Drugs are designated as Alternative options based on clinical trial data showing efficacy and generally favorable, but more limited, data. Concerns with PK, dosing, tolerability, formulation, administration, or interaction more notable than those in the Preferred category, and some regimens are still useful in cases where drug-drug interactions need to be avoided with Preferred medications or are not eligible for Preferred single tablet, once daily regimens.

[g] Requires twice daily administration; associated with hematologic toxicities.

[h] Screening for antenatal and postpartum depression is recommended. Higher rate of adverse events than some Preferred drugs.

[i] Consider monitoring viral load more frequently in pregnancy. Take with food to help increase absorption. Not recommended if pretreatment HIV RNA greater than 100,000 copies/mL or CD4 counts less than 200 cells/mm³. Cannot be administered with proton pump inhibitors and requires specific spacing if receiving H2 blockers or antacids.

[j] Generally not recommended as initial therapy as data about the PKs, safety, and efficacy of these drugs during pregnancy are limited (except lopinavir/ritonavir and nevirapine). Lopinavir/ritonavir is associated with greater risk of nausea and preterm birth in comparison to other options, and nevirapine is associated with toxicities, requires complex lead-in dosing, and has a low barrier to resistance compared with other options. However, certain circumstances may exist in which patients who are ART-experienced may need to initiate or continue these drugs during pregnancy to reach or maintain viral suppression.

Adapted from Panel on Treatment of HIV During Pregnancy and Prevention of Perinatal Transmission. Recommendations for Use of Antiretroviral Drugs in Transmission in the United States. Available at https://clinicalinfo.hiv.gov/sites/default/files/guidelines/documents/Perinatal_GL.pdf. Accessed Oct 9, 2022.

risks involved in this approach are highlighted by the failure of some antiretrovirals to attain sufficient exposure during pregnancy, such as those containing the pharmacoenhancer, cobicistat. Licensure of cobicistat-containing products occurred in 2012 and 2015, but data describing substantially lower exposures during pregnancy did not become available until 2018. These data led to changes in the product labels of all cobicistat-containing antiretrovirals, indicating that they should not be used in pregnancy.[7] Recommendations for how evaluating antiretroviral pharmacokinetics in pregnancy can be optimized to accelerate the availability of data is beyond the scope of this review but is discussed in a 2018 World Health Organization meeting report.[4]

PHARMACOKINETIC DATA DURING PREGNANCY

This review briefly summarizes available pharmacokinetic data for antiretrovirals currently listed as preferred or alternative options (see **Table 1**) and select antiretroviral medications that are not recommended in pregnancy (**Table 2**).[2] Maternal-to-cord blood ratios are summarized in **Table 3**, which are important for characterizing in utero drug exposure and potential protection against perinatal HIV transmission.

Pharmacokinetic Enhancers

Ritonavir and cobicistat are commonly used as pharmacoenhancers to increase plasma drug concentrations of antiretrovirals, including PIs, elvitegravir, and tenofovir alafenamide (TAF), allowing for lower pill burden and less frequent dosing.[8] Both drugs increase plasma antiretroviral exposures by inhibiting specific efflux (eg, P-glycoprotein) and other uptake transporters and CYP enzymes, notably CYP3A4, to increase absorption and decrease the elimination of drugs transported and metabolized through these mechanisms.

Ritonavir

Ritonavir was originally licensed as an antiretroviral given as 600 mg twice daily, but its use was limited by poor tolerability with marked gastrointestinal intolerance and low

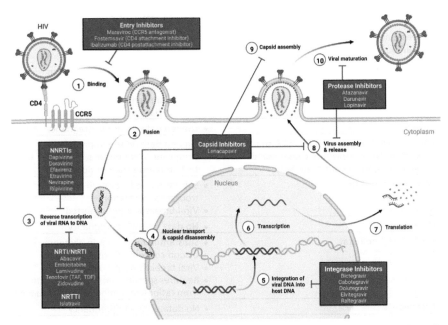

Fig. 1. Antiretroviral mechanisms of action. NNRTI, non-NRTI; NRTI/NtRTI, nucleoside/nucleotide reverse transcriptase inhibitor; NRTTI, nucleoside reverse transcriptase translocation inhibitor. (Created with BioRender.com.)

potency.[8] Ritonavir is now exclusively used at doses of 100 to 200 mg daily. At these doses, ritonavir is subtherapeutic for antiviral activity but remains a potent inhibitor of intestinal and hepatic CYP3A4 and efflux transporters. Ritonavir area under the concentration-time curve (AUC) and minimum concentrations (C_{min}) are reduced by 44% to 86% and 20% to 67%, respectively, during pregnancy compared with postpartum.[9–11] These reductions in plasma ritonavir concentrations likely lead to decreased inhibition of hepatic metabolism and contribute to lower plasma exposures of boosted PIs during pregnancy, as described in the PI section.

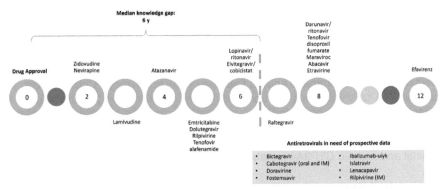

Fig. 2. Delay between regulatory drug approval and availability of pharmacokinetic data. (*Adapted from* Colbers A, Mirochnick M, Schalkwijk S, Penazzato M, Townsend C, Burger D. Importance of Prospective Studies in Pregnant and Breastfeeding Women Living With Human Immunodeficiency Virus. Clin Infect Dis. 2019;69(7):1254-1258.)

Table 2
Antiretroviral medications not currently recommended in the United States perinatal human immunodeficiency virus treatment guideline

Antiretroviral	Rationale Behind Recommendation
Atazanavir/cobicistat	• Substantial reductions in atazanavir trough concentrations • Limited data on use in pregnancy
Bictegravir	• Limited data on use in pregnancy
Cabotegravir (long-acting) for PrEP and cabotegravir + rilpivirine (copackaged long-acting formulation for ART)	• Limited data on use in pregnancy • Drug concentrations may persist for up to 12 mo after the last dose
Darunavir/cobicistat	• Substantial reductions in darunavir trough concentrations • Viral breakthroughs reported
Doravirine	• No data on use in pregnancy
Elvitegravir/cobicistat	• Substantial reductions in elvitegravir trough concentrations • Viral breakthroughs reported • Requires specific spacing of medication from cation-containing prenatal vitamins
Fostemsavir	• No data on use in pregnancy
Ibalizumab	• No data on use in pregnancy
Tenofovir alafenamide/emtricitabine for PrEP	• No efficacy data supporting tenofovir alafenamide/emtricitabine in persons at risk through vaginally receptive sex • No data on use in pregnancy

Adapted from Panel on Treatment of HIV During Pregnancy and Prevention of Perinatal Transmission. Recommendations for Use of Antiretroviral Drugs in Transmission in the United States. Available at https://clinicalinfo.hiv.gov/sites/default/files/guidelines/documents/Perinatal_GL.pdf. Accessed Oct 9, 2022.

Cobicistat

Cobicistat was developed as an alternative pharmacoenhancer to ritonavir with better tolerability, ability to coformulate with other medications, and less potential for complex drug-drug interactions. Because of increased CYP3A4 activity in pregnancy, cobicistat plasma exposures are markedly reduced. Cobicistat AUC and C_{min} are 35% to 63% and 61% to 83% lower during pregnancy compared with postpartum.[12–15] These low exposures likely lead to inadequate inhibition of hepatic CYP3A4 and contribute to lower PI and elvitegravir exposures during pregnancy. In 2018, the Food and Drug Administration product labels for all cobicistat products were updated to recommend against their use during pregnancy.[7] Cobicistat also increases TAF concentrations through inhibition of efflux transporters in the gut.[8] In contrast to the failure of cobicistat to adequately boost PIs and elvitegravir during pregnancy, cobicistat remains an effective booster of TAF, which is likely due to its ability to still inhibit efflux transporters in the intestinal tract before undergoing intestinal and hepatic CYP3A4 metabolism.[16,17]

Protease Inhibitors

Three PIs are currently recommended during pregnancy: atazanavir and darunavir as preferred agents and lopinavir in special circumstances (see **Table 1**).[2] These drugs are predominantly metabolized by CYP3A4 and require administration with a

Table 3
Cord blood-to-maternal transfer ratios of antiretroviral medications

Low (<0.3)	Moderate (0.3–0.6)	High (>0.6)	Unknown
Atazanavir	Efavirenz[a]	Abacavir	Bictegravir
Cobicistat	Etravirine[a]	Dolutegravir	Cabotegravir
Darunavir	Maraviroc	Elvitegravir	Doravirine
Lopinavir	Rilpivirine[a]	Emtricitabine	Fostemsavir
Ritonavir		Lamivudine	Ibalizumab-uiyk
Tenofovir alafenamide		Nevirapine	
		Raltegravir	
		Tenofovir[b]	
		Zidovudine	

[a] Moderate to high transfer.
[b] When administered as either tenofovir alafenamide (TAF) or tenofovir disoproxil fumarate (TDF).
Adapted from Panel on Treatment of HIV During Pregnancy and Prevention of Perinatal Transmission. Recommendations for Use of Antiretroviral Drugs in Transmission in the United States. Available at https://clinicalinfo.hiv.gov/sites/default/files/guidelines/documents/Perinatal_GL.pdf. Accessed Oct 9, 2022.

pharmacoenhancer to increase drug exposures. During pregnancy, the recommended pharmacoenhancer is ritonavir.

Atazanavir

In nonpregnant adults, atazanavir may be given without a pharmacoenhancer; however, in pregnancy, only atazanavir with ritonavir is recommended.[2] Atazanavir AUC and C_{min} are reduced by 6% to 47% in pregnancy with atazanavir, 300 mg/ritonavir, 100 mg, once daily.[10,18] Increasing the dose to atazanavir, 400 mg/ritonavir, 100 mg, during pregnancy results in similar atazanavir exposures to those in nonpregnant adults receiving 300 mg/100 mg.[18,19] Some experts recommend that this increased dose should be used in all pregnant patients receiving atazanavir-ritonavir, whereas the atazanavir label recommends use of the increased dose only in treatment-experienced pregnant women also receiving TDF or an H2-receptor antagonist, both of which can further reduce atazanavir exposures.

Darunavir

Although given once-daily in most people with HIV, only twice-daily darunavir/ritonavir is recommended for pregnant women due to reductions in plasma darunavir exposure during pregnancy.[2] Darunavir C_{min} was decreased by 42% to 50% with once-daily darunavir/ritonavir, 800 mg/100 mg, dosing and 12% to 42% with 600 mg/100 mg twice-daily dosing.[11,20] Increasing the twice-daily dose to 800 mg/100 mg failed to significantly increase darunavir exposure compared with the standard twice-daily dosing.[21] As darunavir is highly protein-bound (95%) and the free drug is ultimately what exerts activity, some studies evaluated unbound concentrations and identified either no change or clinically insignificant decreases between pregnancy and postpartum.[20]

Lopinavir

Similar to darunavir, the recommended dosing for lopinavir/ritonavir during pregnancy is twice daily with either standard or increased dosing; once daily dosing is not recommended.[2] Lopinavir exposures are decreased by 21% to 67% during pregnancy compared with standard twice-daily dosing (400 mg with ritonavir, 100 mg) post-partum. Increasing the twice-daily dose to 600 mg/150 mg resulted in similar exposure to standard-dose lopinavir/ritonavir postpartum.[9,22] Studies of lopinavir protein binding found higher free fractions of lopinavir despite lower total concentrations during pregnancy than in nonpregnant adults, suggesting that dose adjustments during pregnancy might not be necessary.[23–25] Increased dosing should be considered in PI-experienced persons or pregnant persons starting treatment with a detectable viral load.[2]

Nucleoside/Nucleotide Reverse Transcriptase Inhibitors

NRTIs/NtRTIs form the backbone of both ART and HIV PrEP in pregnancy. Plasma abacavir exposures are not lower in pregnancy.[26,27] Although none require dose adjustment during pregnancy, emtricitabine,[28] lamivudine,[29] and tenofovir (in the form of TDF and TAF)[30,31] exposures are decreased by ~20% to 30%, primarily due to increased renal clearance. The magnitude of difference between pregnancy and postpartum for TAF varies based on co-administered antiretrovirals (eg, pharma-coenhancers due to inhibition of intestinal efflux transporters).[16,17] TAF exposure with pharmacoenhancers did not significantly differ between pregnancy and postpartum,[17] but without a pharmacoenhancer, TAF was 33% to 46% lower during pregnancy compared with the same women postpartum.[16] However, exposures during pregnancy were comparable to historical data in nonpregnant adults, so no dose adjustments were deemed necessary. Zidovudine is 1 of 2 antiretrovirals available in an intravenous (IV) formulation and previously was standard of care during delivery. With modern options for maternal ART, IV zidovudine is now recommended at delivery as add-on therapy when HIV viral suppression has not been achieved or is unknown to reduce the risk of perinatal transmission. Zidovudine pharmacokinetic data are more limited in pregnancy,[32] but the oral formulation has been associated with lower exposures and more variable absorption during the delivery period; thus the IV formulation is preferred. Another key consideration with NRTIs/NtRTIs is that the active phosphorylated forms within cells have longer half-lives than the plasma parent form. A strong relationship between intracellular drug concentrations of TDF, TAF, and emtricitabine; adherence; and HIV prevention/treatment outcomes in nonpregnant adults has been demonstrated.[21] However, data describing intracellular concentrations of NRTIs/NtRTIs and their metabolized are very limited in pregnancy,[33] although multiple studies are ongoing.

Nonnucleoside Reverse Transcriptase Inhibitors

Efavirenz and oral rilpivirine are alternative ART options during pregnancy.[2] Studies of efavirenz, 600 mg, daily have either shown slightly lower exposures or no differences between pregnancy and postpartum or nonpregnant adults.[34,35] More recently, efavirenz, 400 mg, daily has become available. A physiologically based pharmacokinetic (PBPK) model suggests extensive CYP2B6 metabolizers may have subtherapeutic exposures during the third trimester in comparison to intermediate and slow metabolizers.[36] Thus, efavirenz, 400 mg, is not recommended in pregnancy until additional data are available.[2] Oral rilpivirine exposures are ~30% to 50% lower in pregnancy, and one study showed the unbound fraction was ~25% lower.[37,38] Given the magnitude of these reductions, more frequent viral load monitoring should be performed during pregnancy.

Etravirine and nevirapine are only recommended in some circumstances and without dose adjustment.[2] Studies have varied regarding whether nevirapine exposures differ during pregnancy, with some showing no effect and others showing

~30% lower exposures.[39,40] Etravirine is generally limited to use in treatment-experienced persons with HIV. In contrast to most other antiretrovirals, etravirine exposures are 30% to 90% higher during pregnancy owing to decreased CYP2C19 activity, and unbound concentrations were unchanged.[41] Newer NNRTI strategies are not recommended in pregnancy due to insufficient data. In 3 women who became pregnant in clinical trials while receiving the long-acting injectable rilpivirine, rilpivirine concentrations were comparable to nonpregnant women. A PBPK model for doravirine suggests exposures may be reduced by 55%,[42] but prospective data are needed.

Integrase Strand Transfer Inhibitors

INSTIs are part of all recommended ART regimens for non-pregnant adults with HIV due to their potency, high barrier to resistance, and tolerability. Both dolutegravir and raltegravir are preferred options during pregnancy. Dolutegravir AUC and C_{min} are 14% to 37% and 20% to 37% lower, respectively, during pregnancy in comparison to postpartum.[43–45] However, because dolutegravir plasma unbound and total concentrations remain greater than the desired threshold for effectiveness, standard dose dolutegravir is recommended throughout pregnancy. Studies of raltegravir, 400 mg, twice daily found that the AUC decreased 24% to 53% during pregnancy, but the C_{min} was not lower, and thus no dose adjustment is necessary.[46] Raltegravir is also approved in nonpregnant adults as 1200 mg once-daily, which results in a lower C_{min} than twice-daily dosing. A population pharmacokinetic model predicted the once-daily dose C_{min} would be 49% lower during pregnancy. Therefore, only raltegravir twice daily is recommended during pregnancy.[2]

Although some INSTIs are preferred in pregnancy, 3 are not recommended during pregnancy. Elvitegravir is only available coformulated with cobicistat, and plasma elvitegravir AUC and C_{min} were 24% to 44% and 77% to 82% lower, respectively, during pregnancy.[12,47] Therefore, elvitegravir should only be considered as continuation of ART in people who become pregnant while receiving elvitegravir, with more frequent HIV viral load monitoring. The 2 newest INSTIs, bictegravir and cabotegravir (oral and injectable formulations), have insufficient data to recommend during pregnancy. Although studies are ongoing, a single case report describes bictegravir use during pregnancy.[48] Pharmacokinetic data from 3 participants who became pregnant during clinical trials of long-acting ART demonstrate cabotegravir exposure persisted throughout pregnancy, despite discontinuing the long-acting injections and switching to oral ART, with similar elimination to nonpregnant participants.

Entry Inhibitors

Entry inhibitors are not commonly used as ART components, except in patients with drug-resistance. Ibalizumab-uiyk, a monoclonal antibody, and fostemsavir, a postattachment inhibitor, are not recommended in pregnancy due to insufficient evidence.[2] Only maraviroc has available data during pregnancy, and similar to other CYP3A4-metabolized antiretrovirals, AUC and C_{min} were 15% to 28% lower during pregnancy, but the C_{min} remained greater than the desired threshold for effectiveness in most participants.[49] Therefore, standard-dose maraviroc should only be used for people who become pregnant while receiving this medication.

PREEXPOSURE PROPHYLAXIS

The only recommended PrEP option for pregnant people at risk for HIV acquisition is TDF 300 mg/emtricitabine 200 mg given once daily.[2] Data supporting TDF/emtricitabine use for PrEP in pregnancy are largely extrapolated from available pharmacokinetic data in pregnant people with HIV on ART and systematic reviews indicating PrEP efficacy and lack of safety concerns in pregnant people using TDF/emtricitabine. People who were assigned male at birth may use less frequent dosing of TDF/emtricitabine for PrEP (eg, "on-demand" PrEP) or daily TAF/emtricitabine as alternative oral PrEP options, but these strategies are not approved for persons at risk through vaginal sex. The only available pharmacokinetic data in pregnant women at risk for HIV showed that intracellular tenofovir-diphosphate (the active form of tenofovir) in dried blood spots were 39% lower during pregnancy in comparison to postpartum, suggesting that daily adherence in pregnancy is critical.[33] The newest PrEP option is injectable long-acting cabotegravir, which is highly effective at preventing HIV in persons at risk through vaginal sex but has not yet been studied in pregnancy. Internationally, a monthly vaginal ring containing dapivirine, an NNRTI, is approved for PrEP.[50] A clinical trial is underway to evaluate this PrEP strategy in pregnant women (NCT03965923). Although the current product is not expected to be approved in the United States, other dapivirine-containing rings, including those coformulated with a hormonal contraceptive, are in development.

THERAPIES ON THE HORIZON

Significant gaps remain in both pharmacokinetic and safety data to support modern ART and PrEP during pregnancy. Notable examples in need of additional data include bictegravir, one of the most commonly used oral antiretrovirals in nonpregnant adults, and the first long-acting ART (cabotegravir/rilpivirine) and PrEP (cabotegravir) that provides effective therapy and prevention with just 6 injection visits per year. Bictegravir and doravirine are both actively under investigation in pregnancy, and a protocol for the long-acting injectable combination of cabotegravir-rilpivirine is in development. Additional data are also expected from the open-label, extension study of long-acting cabotegravir for PrEP in women, which will allow participants who become pregnant to choose if they wish to continue cabotegravir. Medications for treatment-experienced persons, such as fostemsavir and ibalizumab, are also in need of data. Other antiretrovirals are also in various stages of development, notably long-acting therapies (eg, islatravir, lenacapavir), with the promise of reducing the frequency of drug dosing, but plans for prospective assessments in pregnant people are either unclear or nonexistent.

SUMMARY

Pharmacokinetic data in pregnancy are critical for informing the appropriate dosing of antiretroviral medications. However, these data consistently lag studies in nonpregnant adults, which creates challenges when selecting or trying to optimize ART or PrEP in this population. Although a wealth of data has been generated in pregnant people with HIV, there is still much to be learned, and multiple antiretroviral drugs are still in need of prospective data. Pregnant people with, and at risk for, HIV need to be prioritized in research efforts to ensure they receive safe and efficacious therapy at the appropriate dose.

CLINICS CARE POINTS

- All pregnant people with HIV should be treated with ART. All pregnant people at risk for HIV acquisition should be offered PrEP.

- Preferred initial ART regimens in pregnancy include the combination of an NRTI backbone with either an INSTI or boosted PIs.
- Selection of appropriate ART in pregnancy requires consideration of patient-specific factors, evidence supporting use of certain combinations, and minimization of toxicities and drug-drug interactions. Consultation of the most up-to-date versions of the perinatal treatment guidelines and with HIV specialists is advised.
- Multiple antiretroviral drugs have altered pharmacokinetics in pregnancy. But only a few require dose adjustment or are recommended against due to subtherapeutic exposures (eg, cobicistat-containing ART). Dolutegravir, raltegravir, NRTIs/NtRTIs, and NNRTIs do not require dose adjustment.
- All pregnancy outcomes (maternal and infant) in patients receiving antiretrovirals should be prospectively reported to the Antiretroviral Pregnancy Registry: http://www.apregistry.com/.

FUNDING

This work was supported by the National Institute of Allergy and Infectious Diseases, United States (grant number K08AI152942 to KMB). The content is solely the responsibility of the authors and does not necessarily represent the official views of the National Institutes of Health.

DISCLOSURE

K.M. Brooks has received consulting fees from ViiV Healthcare. K.K. Scarsi receives grant support paid to her institution from Organon, Netherlands, LLC. M. Mirochnick receives grant support paid to his institution from Gilead Sciences, United States, ViiV Healthcare and Merck; serves on 2 DSMBs for AstraZeneca; and is a consultant for Merck.

REFERENCES

1. UNAIDS. Start Free, Stay Free, AIDS Free: Final report on 2020 targets. 2021. Available at: https://reliefweb.int/attachments/31ef0276-cc4e-3f3f-830a-033c5b6bcf3e/Start%20Free%2C%20Stay%20Free%2C%20AIDS%20Free%20-%20Final%20Report%20on%202020%20Targets%20-%20July%202021.pdf.
2. Panel on Treatment of Pregnant Women with HIV Infection and Prevention of Perinatal Transmission. Recommendations for the Use of Antiretroviral Drugs in Pregnant Women with HIV Infection and Interventions to Reduce Perinatal HIV Transmission in the United States. Available at: http://aidsinfo.nih.gov/contentfiles/lvguidelines/PerinatalGL.pdf. Accessed October 09 2022.
3. Nesheim SR, FitzHarris LF, Mahle Gray K, et al. Epidemiology of Perinatal HIV Transmission in the United States in the Era of Its Elimination. Pediatr Infect Dis J 2019;38(6):611–6.
4. Abrams EJ, Mofenson LM, Pozniak A, et al. Enhanced and Timely Investigation of ARVs for Use in Pregnant Women. J Acquir Immune Defic Syndr 2021;86(5):607–15.
5. Pariente G, Leibson T, Carls A, et al. Pregnancy-Associated Changes in Pharmacokinetics: A Systematic Review. Plos Med 2016;13(11):e1002160.
6. Colbers A, Mirochnick M, Schalkwijk S, et al. Importance of Prospective Studies in Pregnant and Breastfeeding Women Living With Human Immunodeficiency Virus. Clin Infect Dis 2019;69(7):1254–8.

7. Boyd SD, Sampson MR, Viswanathan P, et al. Cobicistat-containing antiretroviral regimens are not recommended during pregnancy: viewpoint. AIDS 2019;33(6): 1089–93.

8. Eke AC, Mirochnick M. Ritonavir and cobicistat as pharmacokinetic enhancers in pregnant women. Expert Opin Drug Metab Toxicol 2019;15(7):523–5.

9. Best BM, Stek AM, Mirochnick M, et al. Lopinavir tablet pharmacokinetics with an increased dose during pregnancy. J Acquir Immune Defic Syndr 2010;54(4): 381–8.

10. Mirochnick M, Best BM, Stek AM, et al. Atazanavir pharmacokinetics with and without tenofovir during pregnancy. J Acquir Immune Defic Syndr 2011;56(5): 412–9.

11. Stek A, Best BM, Wang J, et al. Pharmacokinetics of Once Versus Twice Daily Darunavir in Pregnant HIV-Infected Women. J Acquir Immune Defic Syndr 2015;70(1):33–41.

12. Momper JD, Best BM, Wang J, et al. Elvitegravir/cobicistat pharmacokinetics in pregnant and postpartum women with HIV. AIDS 2018;32(17):2507–16.

13. Momper JD, Wang J, Stek A, et al. Pharmacokinetics of Atazanavir Boosted With Cobicistat in Pregnant and Postpartum Women With HIV. J Acquir Immune Defic Syndr 2022;89(3):303–9.

14. Momper JD, Wang J, Stek A, et al. Pharmacokinetics of darunavir and cobicistat in pregnant and postpartum women with HIV. AIDS 2021;35(8):1191–9.

15. Crauwels HM, Osiyemi O, Zorrilla C, et al. Reduced exposure to darunavir and cobicistat in HIV-1-infected pregnant women receiving a darunavir/cobicistat-based regimen. HIV Med 2019;20(5):337–43.

16. Brooks KM, Momper JD, Pinilla M, et al. Pharmacokinetics of tenofovir alafenamide with and without cobicistat in pregnant and postpartum women living with HIV. AIDS 2021;35(3):407–17.

17. Brooks KM, Pinilla M, Stek AM, et al. Pharmacokinetics of Tenofovir Alafenamide With Boosted Protease Inhibitors in Pregnant and Postpartum Women Living With HIV: Results From IMPAACT P1026s. J Acquir Immune Defic Syndr 2022;90(3): 343–50.

18. Conradie F, Zorrilla C, Josipovic D, et al. Safety and exposure of once-daily ritonavir-boosted atazanavir in HIV-infected pregnant women. HIV Med 2011;12(9): 570–9.

19. Kreitchmann R, Best BM, Wang J, et al. Pharmacokinetics of an increased atazanavir dose with and without tenofovir during the third trimester of pregnancy. J Acquir Immune Defic Syndr 2013;63(1):59–66.

20. Colbers A, Molto J, Ivanovic J, et al. Pharmacokinetics of total and unbound darunavir in HIV-1-infected pregnant women. J Antimicrob Chemother 2015;70(2): 534–42.

21. Eke AC, Stek AM, Wang J, et al. Darunavir Pharmacokinetics With an Increased Dose During Pregnancy. J Acquir Immune Defic Syndr 2020;83(4):373–80.

22. Santini-Oliveira M, Estrela Rde C, Veloso VG, et al. Randomized clinical trial comparing the pharmacokinetics of standard- and increased-dosage lopinavir-ritonavir coformulation tablets in HIV-positive pregnant women. Antimicrob Agents Chemother 2014;58(5):2884–93.

23. Aweeka FT, Stek A, Best BM, et al. Lopinavir protein binding in HIV-1-infected pregnant women. HIV Med 2010;11(4):232–8.

24. Chen J, Malone S, Prince HM, et al. Model-Based Analysis of Unbound Lopinavir Pharmacokinetics in HIV-Infected Pregnant Women Supports Standard Dosing in the Third Trimester. CPT Pharmacometrics Syst Pharmacol 2016;5(3):147–57.

25. Cressey TR, Urien S, Capparelli EV, et al. Impact of body weight and missed doses on lopinavir concentrations with standard and increased lopinavir/ritonavir doses during late pregnancy. J Antimicrob Chemother 2015;70(1):217–24.

26. Best BM, Mirochnick M, Capparelli EV, et al. Impact of pregnancy on abacavir pharmacokinetics. AIDS 2006;20(4):553–60.

27. Schalkwijk S, Colbers A, Konopnicki D, et al. The pharmacokinetics of abacavir 600 mg once daily in HIV-1-positive pregnant women. AIDS 2016;30(8):1239–44.

28. Stek AM, Best BM, Luo W, et al. Effect of pregnancy on emtricitabine pharmacokinetics. HIV Med 2012;13(4):226–35.

29. Benaboud S, Treluyer JM, Urien S, et al. Pregnancy-related effects on lamivudine pharmacokinetics in a population study with 228 women. Antimicrob Agents Chemother 2012;56(2):776–82.

30. Best BM, Burchett S, Li H, et al. Pharmacokinetics of tenofovir during pregnancy and postpartum. HIV Med 2015;16(8):502–11.

31. Bukkems VE, Necsoi C, Hidalgo Tenorio C, et al. Tenofovir Alafenamide Plasma Concentrations Are Reduced in Pregnant Women Living With Human Immunodeficiency Virus (HIV): Data From the PANNA Network. Clin Infect Dis 2022;75(4):623–9.

32. Moodley J, Moodley D, Pillay K, et al. Pharmacokinetics and antiretroviral activity of lamivudine alone or when coadministered with zidovudine in human immunodeficiency virus type 1-infected pregnant women and their offspring. J Infect Dis 1998;178(5):1327–33.

33. Stranix-Chibanda L, Anderson PL, Kacanek D, et al. Tenofovir Diphosphate Concentrations in Dried Blood Spots From Pregnant and Postpartum Adolescent and Young Women Receiving Daily Observed Pre-exposure Prophylaxis in Sub-Saharan Africa. Clin Infect Dis 2021;73(7):e1893–900.

34. Kreitchmann R, Schalkwijk S, Best B, et al. Efavirenz pharmacokinetics during pregnancy and infant washout. Antivir Ther 2019;24(2):95–103.

35. Lartey M, Kenu E, Lassey A, et al. Pharmacokinetics of Efavirenz 600 mg Once Daily During Pregnancy and Post Partum in Ghanaian Women Living With HIV. Clin Ther 2020;42(9):1818–25.

36. Chetty M, Danckwerts MP, Julsing A. Prediction of the exposure to a 400-mg daily dose of efavirenz in pregnancy: is this dose adequate in extensive metabolisers of CYP2B6? Eur J Clin Pharmacol 2020;76(8):1143–50.

37. Osiyemi O, Yasin S, Zorrilla C, et al. Pharmacokinetics, Antiviral Activity, and Safety of Rilpivirine in Pregnant Women with HIV-1 Infection: Results of a Phase 3b, Multicenter, Open-Label Study. Infect Dis Ther 2018;7(1):147–59.

38. Tran AH, Best BM, Stek A, et al. Pharmacokinetics of Rilpivirine in HIV-Infected Pregnant Women. J Acquir Immune Defic Syndr 2016;72(3):289–96.

39. Capparelli EV, Aweeka F, Hitti J, et al. Chronic administration of nevirapine during pregnancy: impact of pregnancy on pharmacokinetics. HIV Med 2008;9(4):214–20.

40. Lamorde M, Byakika-Kibwika P, Okaba-Kayom V, et al. Suboptimal nevirapine steady-state pharmacokinetics during intrapartum compared with postpartum in HIV-1-seropositive Ugandan women. J Acquir Immune Defic Syndr 2010;55(3):345–50.

41. Mulligan N, Schalkwijk S, Best BM, et al. Etravirine Pharmacokinetics in HIV-Infected Pregnant Women. Front Pharmacol 2016;7:239.

42. Bukkems VE, van Hove H, Roelofsen D, et al. Prediction of Maternal and Fetal Doravirine Exposure by Integrating Physiologically Based Pharmacokinetic

Modeling and Human Placenta Perfusion Experiments. Clin Pharmacokinet 2022; 61(8):1129–41.

43. Bollen P, Freriksen J, Konopnicki D, et al. The Effect of Pregnancy on the Pharmacokinetics of Total and Unbound Dolutegravir and Its Main Metabolite in Women Living With Human Immunodeficiency Virus. Clin Infect Dis 2021;72(1):121–7.

44. Mulligan N, Best BM, Wang J, et al. Dolutegravir pharmacokinetics in pregnant and postpartum women living with HIV. AIDS 2018;32(6):729–37.

45. Waitt C, Orrell C, Walimbwa S, et al. Safety and pharmacokinetics of dolutegravir in pregnant mothers with HIV infection and their neonates: A randomised trial (DolPHIN-1 study). Plos Med 2019;16(9):e1002895.

46. Watts DH, Stek A, Best BM, et al. Raltegravir pharmacokinetics during pregnancy. J Acquir Immune Defic Syndr 2014;67(4):375–81.

47. Bukkems V, Necsoi C, Tenorio CH, et al. Clinically Significant Lower Elvitegravir Exposure During the Third Trimester of Pregnant Patients Living With Human Immunodeficiency Virus: Data From the Pharmacokinetics of ANtiretroviral agents in HIV-infected pregNAnt women (PANNA) Network. Clin Infect Dis 2020;71(10): e714–7.

48. Bukkems VE, Hidalgo-Tenorio C, Garcia C, et al. First pharmacokinetic data of bictegravir in pregnant women living with HIV. AIDS 2021;35(14):2405–6.

49. Colbers A, Best B, Schalkwijk S, et al. Maraviroc Pharmacokinetics in HIV-1-Infected Pregnant Women. Clin Infect Dis 2015;61(10):1582–9.

50. Organization WH. WHO recommends the dapivirine vaginal ring as a new choice for HIV prevention for women at substantial risk of HIV infection. Accessed 08 Oct, 2022. Updated 26 January 2021 Available at:. https://www.who.int/news/item/26-01-2021-who-recommends-the-dapivirine-vaginal-ring-as-a-new-choice-for-hiv-prevention-for-women-at-substantial-risk-of-hiv-infection

A Clinical Review of the Use of Common Psychiatric Medications in Pregnancy
Guidelines for Obstetrical Providers

Shakked Lubotzky-Gete, PhD[a], Lucy C. Barker, MD, FRCPC[b],
Simone N. Vigod, MD, MSc, FRCPC[b],*

KEYWORDS

- Pregnancy • Antidepressant • Benzodiazepine • Hypnotic • Antipsychotic

KEY POINTS

- Psychotropic medications are prescribed in about 10% of pregnancies, with antidepressant medications being the most common type.
- Decisions about the use of psychotropic medication in pregnancy involve weighing the potential benefits of treatment (and risks of nontreatment) against the small but not nonexistent risks of fetal medication exposure.
- In general, the more severe the mental health issue has been, the greater the risks of discontinuing treatment during pregnancy to the pregnant woman or person's mental health and to the health and well-being of the developing fetus, infant, and child.

INTRODUCTION

Psychiatric disorders are common presentations in pregnancy, complicating up to 15% of all pregnancies, and psychotropic medications are prescribed in about 10% of pregnancies in the United States.[1] As such, the issue of how to manage commonly prescribed psychotropic medications around the time of pregnancy is highly relevant to the obstetrical provider. This narrative review focuses on some of the most commonly prescribed psychotropic medications—antidepressants, sedatives and hypnotics, mood stabilizers, and antipsychotic drugs. The aim is neither a complete review of psychiatric disorders in pregnancy nor all possible psychological and pharmacological treatments for mental illness around the time of pregnancy. Rather, the review provides a high-level overview of pharmacological therapeutic considerations for general obstetrical providers. In some cases, general obstetrical providers may be prescribers, or making

[a] Women's College Hospital and Research Institute, 76 Grenville Street, Toronto, Ontario M5S 1B2, Canada; [b] Department of Psychiatry, Women's College Hospital and Research Institute, University of Toronto, 76 Grenville Street, Toronto, Ontario M5S 1B2, Canada
* Corresponding author.
E-mail address: simone.vigod@wchospital.ca

recommendations about prescribing. When individuals have more severe mental illnesses, such as severe depressive disorders, bipolar disorders, and psychotic disorders, specialist psychiatric provider involvement would be strongly recommended. However, even when not prescribing medications for more severe mental health issues, general obstetrical providers care for the pregnant individuals who are taking those medications and will benefit from knowledge of their associated risks and benefits.

ANTIDEPRESSANTS
Clinical Vignette #1

Zara is a 30-year-old woman who takes sertraline for major depressive disorder and is planning her second pregnancy. In her first pregnancy, she stopped sertraline, which resulted in a relapse of depression that continued into the postpartum period and affected her ability to bond with her baby. She is very worried about this happening again. Based on her past experiences, she does not think that therapy alone will be enough to keep her well. After reviewing risks and benefits of sertraline in pregnancy with her family doctor and alternative options, she is reassured by sertraline's safety profile and decides to stay on her medication during this pregnancy to minimize the risk of relapse.

Antidepressant medications are some of the most commonly prescribed medications that need to be addressed around the time of pregnancy. It is estimated that 5% to 10% of individuals are prescribed an antidepressant in the year before conception.[1] Antidepressants are considered first-line medication treatments for major depressive disorder, anxiety disorders such as generalized anxiety disorder and panic disorder, obsessive-compulsive disorders, and posttraumatic stress disorder. They are also used, at times, and with caution, among individuals with bipolar disorders experiencing depressive illnesses nonresponsive to antipsychotic or mood-stabilizing medications.

In this review, we will focus on the most commonly prescribed antidepressants. These include those of the selective serotonin reuptake inhibitor(SSRI) class that includes citalopram, escitalopram, fluoxetine, fluvoxamine, paroxetine, and sertraline, among others and the serotonin norepinephrine reuptake inhibitor (SNRI) class that includes venlafaxine and duloxetine. Bupropion and mirtazapine are frequently prescribed antidepressants as well, used more exclusively for depressive disorders. Most of these antidepressants take effect within 1 to 2 weeks of initiation, with increasing effects for up to 8 to 12 weeks. With partial response, dosages can be titrated upward to the maximum of the dose range. About two-thirds of individuals respond to an initial antidepressant trial, with another 25% to 50% of those not remitted responding to a second or third trial of medication.[2] When this is not effective, individuals may require either augmentation of the antidepressant with another type of psychotropic drug or may be offered a nonmedication somatic treatment given their nonresponse to medications.

There is no evidence that the efficacy of these antidepressant medications is different in pregnancy than at any other time. As outside of pregnancy, individuals should be prescribed the lowest dose that is effective for the remission of their symptoms. The metabolism of many antidepressants, including paroxetine, fluoxetine, sertraline, citalopram, and escitalopram by the liver is increased in the second half of pregnancy, raising the theoretical possibility that dosage increases could be required over the course of a pregnancy to maintain adequate control of depressive symptoms.[3] However, therapeutic drug monitoring is not recommended, and dosages should not be adjusted automatically based on a person's pregnancy status. Instead, decisions about dose increases should be guided by clinical symptomatology. Other potential causes of symptoms (eg, anemia, thyroid dysfunction) should be investigated to ensure that symptom resurgence might not better be addressed by treatment of an underlying condition that can also exacerbate depression or anxiety.

Decisions about whether to start or continue antidepressant medication during pregnancy rest on whether the benefits of the medication outweigh the potential risks of fetal exposure to medication.[4] There is ample evidence that untreated or under-treated depression and anxiety during pregnancy can have negative effects not only on the well-being and quality of life of a pregnant woman or person but also on the developing fetus. Specifically, untreated depression or anxiety is associated with delayed fetal growth and development.[5,6] It is also the strongest risk factor for continued mental illness in the postpartum period,[7] which is strongly linked to problems with the health and development of children across their lifespan.[8] As such, ensuring adequate treatment is of high priority.

For an individual taking antidepressant medication before pregnancy, stopping or reducing the dose of the antidepressant can increase the risk of relapse, with its associated consequences. Although the risk of relapse with medication discontinuation cannot be predicted on an individual level with certainty, the more severe the illness (ie, higher number of episodes, the greater the severity of the episodes) and the more difficult it was to achieve a remission, the greater the risks of relapse and/or the need to reinitiate treatment.[9,10] With new-onset illness in pregnancy, it is reasonable to first attempt a trial of psychological therapy in most cases before initiating antidepressant medication, so as to be able to avoid any concern about fetal medication exposure. However, this is not always possible or advisable.[11] Exceptions would include individuals who have not previously responded to therapy, or who have severe depression requiring more rapid remission.

The safety of antidepressant exposure to the developing fetus has been a subject of intense investigation during the past 30 years. No randomized controlled trials have been conducted, so observational studies comparing exposed and unexposed pregnancies form the basis of the literature in this area. This has presented challenges to interpretation of the literature given that depression and anxiety themselves are associated with adverse fetal outcomes. A summary of the literature suggests, however, that if antidepressants are required for treatment or to maintain remission, the potential risks to the fetus seem to be small.

For the first-line antidepressant medications, the SSRIs and the SNRIs, and to a lesser extent bupropion and mirtazapine, the most well-designed observational studies do not seem to signal that there is a clinically significant increased risk for congenital malformations, preterm birth or low birthweight, or long-term health or developmental problems in the children that is clearly attributable to antidepressant exposure.[12] Some studies have suggested very small absolute risk increases on the order of 1–2/1000 for specific cardiac malformations, and in persistent pulmonary hypertension of the newborn.[13,14] Whether these risk increases are definitively caused by antidepressant exposure remain unclear.

There does seem to be a slightly increased risk for postpartum hemorrhage with exposure close to the time of delivery, which is not surprising due to SSRI impact on platelet-mediated homeostasis and serotonin-mediated myometrial contractility.[15] This does not seem to be of a volume that would be clinically significant to the patient. There is some evidence of an increased risk for neonatal adaptation syndrome in the days to weeks after birth; this is for the most part mild and self-limited, resolving with only supportive care in the first few postnatal weeks.[16] Although lactation is not a focus of this review, the SSRIs, and SNRIs are all considered compatible with breast-feeding; bupropion should be used with more caution given case reports of seizure in exposed infants but is not contraindicated in breastfeeding.[17,18]

SEDATIVES AND HYPNOTICS
Clinical Vignette #2

Taylor is a 26-year-old nonbinary individual who recently found out they are pregnant for the first time. In the past, Taylor has occasionally taken zopiclone for insomnia and asks their family doctor whether this is safe to do in pregnancy. After reviewing the data and discussing alternatives, Taylor decides to start cognitive behavior therapy for insomnia instead of using zopiclone in pregnancy.

Sedative and hypnotic medications include the benzodiazepine class, and the z-drugs, namely zolpidem, zaleplon, and zopiclone/eszopiclone. Benzodiazepines are commonly used for the management of acute anxiety, and for sleep, whereas the z-drugs are used for insomnia. Unlike the antidepressant medications, sedatives and hypnotic medications are intended for short-term use only. In the setting of anxiety, benzodiazepines can sometimes be prescribed for up to 2 weeks while awaiting the effect of an antidepressant drug. Z-drugs may be prescribed for acute insomnia, although it has become clear that nonpharmacological approaches to insomnia, including cognitive behavior therapy for insomnia are highly effective, and should be considered first-line treatment.[19] In practice, many individuals are inappropriately prescribed these medications for long-term use. A systematic review and meta-analysis of 32 studies reporting on 28 countries, found worldwide prevalence of benzodiazepine use during pregnancy was 1.9%. The highest prevalence was found in the third trimester, with lorazepam being the most frequently used benzodiazepine.[20] Considered together, these use profiles suggest that obstetrical providers may be faced with questions about whether and how they can be used in pregnancy.

Historically, investigations into the safety of benzodiazepines and z-drugs have faced the same challenges as the research into antidepressant safety in pregnancy—confounding by indication, that is, is there something about the disease process underlying the indication for the prescription, or factors associated with that disease process, that might explain any observed adverse outcomes associated with their use. Early research suggested that the use of benzodiazepines in the first trimester of pregnancy was associated with an increased risk for cleft lip or palate anomalies; although further research has been less convincing regarding whether this is or is not causally related to the benzodiazepine exposure.[21] There may be an association between benzodiazepine exposure in pregnancy and preterm birth, low birthweight, and small-for-gestational age infants.[22]

High-dose, daily use of benzodiazepines in the third trimester has been associated with neonatal complications, however, including requirement for neonatal intensive care unit (ICU) admissions mainly due to symptoms of hypothermia, lethargy, and respiratory depressions,[22] suggesting that high-dose ongoing use in pregnancy is to be avoided. That being said, periodic use of benzodiazepines, or daily low-dose use, has not been associated with these concerns. There has been less research on the impacts of chronic ongoing use of the z-drugs in nonanimal models, and although, in general, there do not seem to be major long-term developmental impacts, given the low volume of research in this area, caution is advised.[23]

MOOD STABILIZERS
Clinical Vignette #3

Maria was diagnosed with bipolar disorder type 1 at age 22. During her first manic episode, she was hospitalized for 4 weeks and tried multiple antipsychotic medications before finally stabilizing on lithium monotherapy. She was never tried on divalproex because she planned to have a child in the future. At age 25, she has an unplanned pregnancy, and sees her psychiatrist immediately to discuss options. After extensive discussion related to risks of lithium in pregnancy and breastfeeding and risk of relapse if she were to stop lithium, Maria decides to stay on lithium. Her psychiatrist, who has a special interest in perinatal mental health, follows her closely during pregnancy, adjusts her dose as her lithium level changes during pregnancy, and coordinates with her obstetrical team to ensure fetal monitoring for malformations and that adequate supports are in place around delivery for herself and her baby. Maria decides to formula feed, which has the added advantage of allowing her partner to do overnight feeds and minimizes sleep disruption, which could destabilize her mental health.

Mood stabilizers, including lithium and the antiepileptic drugs divalproex (valproate, valpromide, valproic acid, and divalproex sodium), carbamazepine, and lamotrigine are highly effective in the treatment of bipolar disorder. They are used for the treatment of acute mania, and acute depressive episodes, as well as maintenance treatment to prevent relapse. They may be used along with antipsychotic medications, discussed below, or on their own, and sometimes are used in combination with each other.

Pregnant individuals with bipolar disorder are at high risk of relapse with medication discontinuation, with the highest risk on abrupt discontinuation of mood stabilizers.[24] Relapse often results in a depressive episode, and it is estimated that as many as 50% of individuals with bipolar disorder will have a depressive relapse perinatally. There is also a high risk for relapse of mania, and for postpartum psychosis, particularly early in the postpartum period.[24] As such, treatment plans need to be carefully considered to maximize benefit while minimizing exposure to the most high-risk medications.

There are several unique considerations to the use and safety of lithium in pregnancy. Lithium has a narrow therapeutic window, and therapeutic drug monitoring is used to determine dose. Lithium is water-soluble and renally cleared, and so with increased body water in pregnancy and increased renal clearance, levels can drop, increasing the risk for relapse if levels drop lower than the recommended levels for maintenance treatment. As such, in pregnancy, levels need to be monitored more frequently, with weekly monitoring recommended in the third trimester.[25] During labor and delivery, maintaining adequate hydration is important. Given the volume contraction and normalization of glomerular filtration rate that will occur postnatally, levels should be closely followed after delivery with dosage adjustments downward if levels are increasing toward the toxic range. Lithium has been associated with a risk of malformations including cardiac malformations, and in particular Ebstein's anomaly, although these risks are not as high as originally thought.[26] Because of this, high-resolution ultrasound at 20 weeks to check for fetal anomalies is recommended.[25] There is also an increased risk of neonatal admission following lithium exposure, and birth in an appropriately resourced hospital setting is recommended.[25,27] Of note, many individuals taking lithium will choose to not breastfeed due to risks of infant lithium toxicity; in those that continue, infant monitoring is needed.[25]

With respect to the antiepileptic mood stabilizers, divalproex has the most consistently demonstrated risk of teratogenicity and is typically avoided in individuals with childbearing potential and during pregnancy. It is associated with a substantially increased risk of neural tube defects, along with an increased risk of craniofacial, cardiac, and limb defects.[28] In exposed infants, there is also an increased risk of adverse neonatal outcomes including neonatal hypoglycemia and of longer term developmental outcomes including cognitive delay.[28,29] If individuals on divalproex are planning a pregnancy or become pregnant, they should be assessed by a psychiatrist to discuss treatment options. Carbamazepine carries many similar risks to divalproex, and although these are of slightly lower magnitude, individuals should be counselled carefully about its use.[28]

Lamotrigine is another antiepileptic used in bipolar disorder, primarily for the treatment and maintenance of bipolar depression. The metabolism of lamotrigine is substantially increased during pregnancy, so dose adjustments upward may be required. It is advisable to measure therapeutic drug levels before pregnancy or as early as possible after the onset of pregnancy. If individuals begin to have breakthrough symptoms as the pregnancy progresses, the level could be measured again, and if low, the dose could be titrated slowly upward. There is a risk for Stevens-Johnsons Syndrome with lamotrigine, which occurs most often on initiation and rapid titration, so titrations should be slow, and immediate medical attention should be sought if a rash develops. Data on the safety of lamotrigine is more reassuring than for the other antiepileptics.[28,29] There is still some uncertainty including regarding whether it is associated with a slightly increased risk of craniofacial defects but the absolute risk of this outcome seems to be low.[28]

ANTIPSYCHOTICS
Clinical Vignette #4

Victoria is a 32-year-old woman with schizophrenia, currently stable on aripiprazole. She is planning her first pregnancy, so speaks to her family doctor, who refers her to a specialty perinatal psychiatry program. The perinatal psychiatrist lets Victoria know about the risks and benefits of antipsychotic medications in pregnancy, and the substantial risks of relapse with medication discontinuation. Although there are more safety data available for quetiapine than for aripiprazole, Victoria decides to stay on aripiprazole as she previously found quetiapine too sedating and does not want to risk a relapse in the process of a medication switch. She continues to be followed by the perinatal psychiatrist throughout the perinatal period, who works with the obstetrical team to ensure coordinated psychiatric and obstetrical care throughout the perinatal periods.

Antipsychotic medications are less commonly prescribed than antidepressant medications, with estimates of use in about 1% of pregnancies.[1] However, their use—particularly the use of the newer second-generation and third-generation antipsychotics—is increasing in pregnancy (because it is in nonpregnant populations).[30] These medications are first-line treatments for primary psychotic disorders such as schizophrenia, and several second-generation antipsychotics are first-line and second-line treatments for bipolar disorder including for acute mania and depression, and for maintenance treatment. Finally, in recent years, there has been emerging evidence for the use of second-generation antipsychotic medications in augmentation of antidepressant drugs for major depression, anxiety disorders, obsessive-compulsive disorders, and posttraumatic stress disorder.

Similar to the antidepressant medications, there is no reason to suspect that these medications have different efficacy during pregnancy than outside of pregnancy, and there are no specific recommendations for dosing that differ for pregnant populations. For individuals with severe mental illnesses such as schizophrenia and bipolar disorder, the potential for relapse when these medications are stopped is high[31]—with the resultant potential consequences of untreated or undertreated illness to mothers, children, and families. As such, in these cases, the potential risks of discontinuing treatment would almost always outweigh the potential risks of the treatments themselves.

However, it remains important for clinicians and be patients to be aware of the research on their safety. Similar to antidepressant medications, the research is relatively reassuring. Antipsychotic exposure in pregnancy does not seem to be associated with major congenital malformations in the child.[32] One issue that has been examined on several occasions relates to the metabolic effects of the second-generation antipsychotic drugs, including weight gain, diabetes, hypertension, and the metabolic syndrome. Some, but not all, studies found a slightly increased risk for gestational diabetes with antipsychotic exposure in pregnancy but there was no clear evidence of increased risk for exposed infants to be born at the extremes of gestational age.[33–35] Although there is not as high volume a literature as what exists for antidepressant drugs, there are no clear concerns about long-term child health.[36,37]

SUMMARY

Antidepressants, sedatives and hypnotics, antipsychotics, and mood stabilizers are common psychotropic medications prescribed to pregnant people. Decisions about when to use these medications involve a careful weighing of the known benefits of treatment versus the potential risks of maternal and fetal exposure during the pregnancy. In most cases, the benefits of using medication are most clear when the mental illness has been severe, hard to treat, or not responsive to less invasive treatments such as psychological therapy. However, when these medications are required for maternal well-being, it is reassuring that, for most medications, the potential risks to fetal well-being are small.

CLINICS CARE POINTS

- Decisions about when to use psychotropic medication in pregnancy involve a careful weighing of the known benefits of treatment vs. the potential risks of maternal and fetal exposure.

- In many cases, maternal well-being will be at risk if medications are stopped or dosages are reduced, and this should be carefully considered when weighing benefits and risks.

- Divalproex has the most consistently demonstrated risk of teratogenicity, and should be avoided in pregnancy.

DISCLOSURE

Dr S.N. Vigod receives royalties from UpToDate Inc for authorship of materials related to depression and pregnancy. The other authors have no disclosures.

REFERENCES

1. Hanley GE, Mintzes B. Patterns of psychotropic medicine use in pregnancy in the United States from 2006 to 2011 among women with private insurance. BMC Pregnancy Childbirth 2014;14:242.
2. Kennedy SH, Lam RW, McIntyre RS, et al. Canadian Network for Mood and Anxiety Treatments (CANMAT) 2016 Clinical Guidelines for the Management of Adults with Major Depressive Disorder: Section 3. Pharmacological Treatments. Can J Psychiatry 2016;61(9):540–60.
3. Betcher HK, Wisner KL. Psychotropic treatment during pregnancy: research synthesis and clinical care principles. J Womens Health (Larchmt) 2020;29(3):310–8.
4. Walton GD, Ross LE, Stewart DE, et al. Decisional conflict among women considering antidepressant medication use in pregnancy. Arch Womens Ment Health 2014;17(6):493–501.

5. Jarde A, Morais M, Kingston D, et al. Neonatal outcomes in women with untreated antenatal depression compared with women without depression: a systematic review and meta-analysis. JAMA Psychiatry 2016;73(8):826–37.

6. Grigoriadis S, Graves L, Peer M, et al. Maternal anxiety during pregnancy and the association with adverse perinatal outcomes: systematic review and meta-analysis. J Clin Psychiatry 2018;79(5):17r12011.

7. Liu X, Wang S, Wang G. Prevalence and risk factors of postpartum depression in women: a systematic review and meta-analysis. J Clin Nurs 2021.

8. Stein A, Pearson RM, Goodman SH, et al. Effects of perinatal mental disorders on the fetus and child. Lancet 2014;384(9956):1800–19.

9. Wikman A, Skalkidou A, Wikstrom AK, et al. Factors associated with re-initiation of antidepressant treatment following discontinuation during pregnancy: a register-based cohort study. Arch Womens Ment Health 2020;23(5):709–17.

10. Bayrampour H, Kapoor A, Bunka M, et al. The risk of relapse of depression during pregnancy after discontinuation of antidepressants: a systematic review and meta-analysis. J Clin Psychiatry 2020;81(4):19r13134.

11. National Institutes of Clinical Excellence (NICE). Antenatal and postnatal mental health: clinical management and service guidance (CG192). London: NICE; 2014.

12. Uguz F. Neonatal and childhood outcomes in offspring of pregnant women using antidepressant medications: a critical review of current meta-analyses. J Clin Pharmacol 2021;61(2):146–58.

13. De Vries C, Gadzhanova S, Sykes MJ, et al. A systematic review and meta-analysis considering the risk for congenital heart defects of antidepressant classes and individual antidepressants. Drug Saf 2021;44(3):291–312.

14. Masarwa R, Bar-Oz B, Gorelik E, et al. Prenatal exposure to selective serotonin reuptake inhibitors and serotonin norepinephrine reuptake inhibitors and risk for persistent pulmonary hypertension of the newborn: a systematic review, meta-analysis, and network meta-analysis. Am J Obstet Gynecol 2019;220(1): 57 e51–e57 e13.

15. Andrade C. Selective serotonin reuptake inhibitor use in pregnancy and risk of postpartum hemorrhage. J Clin Psychiatry 2022;83(2).

16. Wang J, Cosci F. Neonatal withdrawal syndrome following late in utero exposure to selective serotonin reuptake inhibitors: a systematic review and meta-analysis of observational studies. Psychother Psychosom 2021;90(5):299–307.

17. Chaudron LH, Schoenecker CJ. Bupropion and breastfeeding: a case of a possible infant seizure. J Clin Psychiatry 2004;65(6):881–2.

18. Stewart DE, Vigod S. Postpartum Depression. N Engl J Med 2016;375(22): 2177–86.

19. Xu D, Cardell E, Broadley SA, et al. Efficacy of face-to-face delivered cognitive behavioral therapy in improving health status of patients with insomnia: a meta-analysis. Front Psychiatry 2021;12:798453.

20. Bais B, Munk-Olsen T, Bergink V, et al. Prescription patterns of benzodiazepine and benzodiazepine-related drugs in the peripartum period: A population-based study. Psychiatry Res 2020;288:112993.

21. Grigoriadis S, Graves L, Peer M, et al. Benzodiazepine use during pregnancy alone or in combination with an antidepressant and congenital malformations: systematic review and meta-analysis. J Clin Psychiatry 2019;80(4):18r12412.

22. Grigoriadis S, Graves L, Peer M, et al. Pregnancy and delivery outcomes following benzodiazepine exposure: a systematic review and meta-analysis. Can J Psychiatry 2020;65(12):821–34.

23. Wang X, Zhang T, Ekheden I, et al. Prenatal exposure to benzodiazepines and Z-drugs in humans and risk of adverse neurodevelopmental outcomes in offspring: a systematic review. Neurosci Biobehav Rev 2022;137:104647.
24. Wesseloo R, Kamperman AM, Munk-Olsen T, et al. Risk of postpartum relapse in bipolar disorder and postpartum psychosis: a systematic review and meta-analysis. Am J Psychiatry 2016;173(2):117–27.
25. Poels EMP, Bijma HH, Galbally M, et al. Lithium during pregnancy and after delivery: a review. Int J Bipolar Disord 2018;6(1):26.
26. Patorno E, Huybrechts KF, Bateman BT, et al. Lithium use in pregnancy and the risk of cardiac malformations. N Engl J Med 2017;376(23):2245–54.
27. Munk-Olsen T, Liu X, Viktorin A, et al. Maternal and infant outcomes associated with lithium use in pregnancy: an international collaborative meta-analysis of six cohort studies. Lancet Psychiatry 2018;5(8):644–52.
28. Galbally M, Roberts M, Buist A, et al. Mood stabilizers in pregnancy: a systematic review. Aust N Z J Psychiatry 2010;44(11):967–77.
29. Haskey C, Galbally M. Mood stabilizers in pregnancy and child developmental outcomes: a systematic review. Aust N Z J Psychiatry 2017;51(11):1087–97.
30. Toh S, Li Q, Cheetham TC, et al. Prevalence and trends in the use of antipsychotic medications during pregnancy in the U.S., 2001-2007: a population-based study of 585,615 deliveries. Arch Womens Ment Health 2013;16(2):149–57.
31. Tosato S, Albert U, Tomassi S, et al. A systematized review of atypical antipsychotics in pregnant women: balancing between risks of untreated illness and risks of drug-related adverse effects. J Clin Psychiatry 2017;78(5):e477–89.
32. Andrade C. Major congenital malformations associated with exposure to second-generation antipsychotic drugs during pregnancy. J Clin Psychiatry 2021;82(5):21f14252.
33. Wang Z, Wong ICK, Man KKC, et al. The use of antipsychotic agents during pregnancy and the risk of gestational diabetes mellitus: a systematic review and meta-analysis. Psychol Med 2021;51(6):1028–37.
34. Vigod SN, Gomes T, Wilton AS, et al. Antipsychotic drug use in pregnancy: high dimensional, propensity matched, population based cohort study. BMJ 2015;350:h2298.
35. Wang Z, Man KKC, Ma T, et al. Association between antipsychotic use in pregnancy and the risk of gestational diabetes: Population-based cohort studies from the United Kingdom and Hong Kong and an updated meta-analysis. Schizophr Res 2021;229:55–62.
36. Wang Z, Chan AYL, Coghill D, et al. Association between prenatal exposure to antipsychotics and attention-deficit/hyperactivity disorder, autism spectrum disorder, preterm birth, and small for gestational age. JAMA Intern Med 2021;181(10):1332–40.
37. Halfdanarson O, Cohen JM, Karlstad O, et al. Antipsychotic use in pregnancy and risk of attention/deficit-hyperactivity disorder and autism spectrum disorder: a Nordic cohort study. Evid Based Ment Health 2022;25(2):54–62.

Opioids and Opioid Use Disorder in Pregnancy

Aalok R. Sanjanwala, MD[a], Grace Lim, MD, MSc[b,c], Elizabeth E. Krans, MD, MSc[d,*]

KEYWORDS

- Opioid use disorder • Pregnancy • Postpartum • Methadone • Buprenorphine

KEY POINTS

- Addiction is a treatable, chronic medical disorder involving complex interactions among brain circuits, genetics, the environment, and an individual's life experiences.
- The pathways to the development of a substance use disorder often differ by sex and gender.
- The use of medications for opioid use disorder, such as methadone and buprenorphine, is the recommended treatment of opioid use disorder during pregnancy and is associated with a decrease in the risk of adverse outcomes including overdose and preterm birth.
- A multimodal approach to pain management is often necessary to achieve effective pain control during labor and delivery for patients with opioid use disorder.

INTRODUCTION

From 2010 to 2017, maternal opioid-related diagnoses during pregnancy increased across nearly all states and demographic groups and opioid-related maternal deaths increased by 220%.[1] As a result, drug overdose is a leading cause of pregnancy-associated mortality in the United States.[2] Over the past 20 years, the opioid epidemic has evolved through three distinct but overlapping trends in opioid use: prescription opioid use in the 1990s, heroin use from 2010 to 2017, and synthetic opioid use (eg, fentanyl) starting in 2014 which continues to dominate the opioid market in most regions in the United States (**Fig. 1**).[3,4] In 2021, over two-thirds of the 107,662 drug overdose deaths that occurred in the United States involved a synthetic opioid, which is a 1,040% increase in the rate of overdose since 2013.[5]

[a] Department of Obstetrics, Gynecology & Reproductive Sciences, Division of Maternal-Fetal Medicine, University of Pittsburgh School of Medicine, 300 Halket Street Pittsburgh, PA 15213, USA; [b] Department of Anesthesiology and Perioperative Medicine, University of Pittsburgh School of Medicine, 300 Halket Street, Pittsburgh, PA 15213, USA; [c] Department of Obstetrics, Gynecology & Reproductive Sciences, University of Pittsburgh School of Medicine, 300 Halket Street, Pittsburgh, PA 15213, USA; [d] Department of Obstetrics, Gynecology & Reproductive Sciences, University of Pittsburgh School of Medicine, Magee-Womens Research Institute, 300 Halket Street, Pittsburgh, PA 15213, USA
* Corresponding author. Department of Obstetrics, Gynecology & Reproductive Sciences, University of Pittsburgh School of Medicine, 300 Halket Street, Pittsburgh, PA 15213.
E-mail address: kransee@upmc.edu

Obstet Gynecol Clin N Am 50 (2023) 229–240
https://doi.org/10.1016/j.ogc.2022.10.015
obgyn.theclinics.com

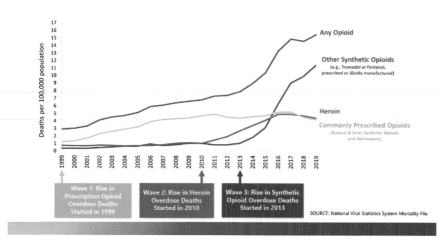

Fig. 1. Three waves of the rise in opioid overdose deaths.

Medications for opioid use disorder (MOUD), such as methadone and buprenorphine, significantly reduce the risk of overdose, recurrent illicit substance use, and infectious disease morbidity.[6,7] In a comparative effectiveness study of different opioid use disorder (OUD) treatment pathways among over 40,000 individuals, MOUD was the only intervention to decrease the risk of overdose compared with non-MOUD treatment approaches.[8] In pregnancy, MOUD use decreases maternal and perinatal morbidity and is associated with a reduced risk of preterm birth and overdose.[9] Further, for each additional week of prenatal MOUD use, the odds of postpartum MOUD continuation nearly doubles which is critical to mitigate the peak in overdose mortality observed during the first year postpartum.[9,10]

To help obstetric providers care for the growing population of patients with OUD, we review the use of methadone and buprenorphine for pregnant patients with OUD, clinical considerations specific to the use of buprenorphine in the setting of fentanyl use, and approaches to analgesia management during the intrapartum and postpartum period.[4] Owing to the rapidly evolving nature of the epidemic, an evidence-based understanding of clinical management approaches for pregnant patients with OUD is necessary to decrease pregnancy-associated mortality from substance use.

OPIOIDS AND OPIOID USE DISORDER

Opioids are a group of natural, semi-synthetic, and synthetic substances that act at the mu, kappa, and delta opioid receptors in the central and peripheral nervous system.[11] Opioids cause euphoria by activating pleasure-reward pathways in the brain and have analgesic and central nervous system depressant effects. Prolonged or chronic opioid use can result in both physical dependence and tolerance. Although opioid dependence can occur after chronic use, such as among patients with chronic pain, physiologic dependence is not synonymous with addiction. Instead, addiction is a chronic, complex, multidimensional disorder characterized by interactions among the brain, genetics, and an individual's life experiences.[12] As a result of these interactions, the symptoms of addiction are characterized by repeated adverse behaviors used to obtain a substance despite negative consequences, in addition to physical dependence.[12]

Sex and Gender Differences

The pathways to the development of a substance use disorder (SUD) often differ by sex and gender.[13,14] Despite higher rates of substance use among men, women progress more quickly to physical dependence, a process referred to as "telescoping."[15] Women may also be more susceptible to effects of substances due to differences in metabolism, body mass, and endocrine-related interactions.[16] Women are more likely to suffer from depression, anxiety, and post-traumatic stress disorder and often report using substances to address untreated mental health symptoms.[17] The majority of women with an SUD have also experienced intimate partner violence (IPV) and are more likely to report the use of substances to cope with a history of trauma or violence.[18,19] Chronic pain disorders are more common among women[20,21] who may also experience higher levels of emotional distress and anxiety when faced with pain compared with men.[22]

Opioid Withdrawal

Patients with a physiologic dependence to opioids will develop withdrawal symptoms once use is discontinued and the desire to relieve or avoid this withdrawal often drives the drug-seeking behaviors that characterize an SUD.[23] The onset and duration of opioid withdrawal can vary widely according to the amount, type and duration of opioid used. Withdrawal symptoms from short-acting opioids such as heroin and opioid analgesic medications (eg, oxycodone) can start to decrease after 4 to 5 days.[24] In contrast, withdrawal from long-acting opioids such as methadone can take up to 10 to 14 days.[24] Although rarely life threatening, opioid withdrawal is extremely uncomfortable as many patients experience drug cravings, anxiety, restlessness, gastrointestinal distress, diaphoresis, and tachycardia. The Clinical Opioid Withdrawal Scale (COWS) is a commonly used clinical assessment tool that can provide an objective measure of withdrawal severity and can help guide the initiation of MOUD and supportive medications.[25]

The association between opioid use during pregnancy and neonatal opioid withdrawal syndrome (NOWS) has fueled an interest in medically supervised opioid withdrawal during pregnancy to prevent NOWS after delivery.[26] However, a consensus of government agencies and professional organizations, including the American College of Obstetricians and Gynecologists, endorse the use of MOUD versus withdrawal.[27] Abstinence-based approaches to substance use treatment during pregnancy are associated with high rates of illicit drug use, which increases the risk of adverse outcomes such as fetal growth restriction, abruption, preterm labor, infectious disease acquisition and overdose.[27]

Medications for opioid use disorder

MOUD is the recommended, evidence-based treatment approach for OUD during pregnancy because it significantly reduces the risk of overdose and opioid-related morbidity and mortality during pregnancy and the postpartum period.[7] Because many people with OUD re-engage or newly engage in health care services during pregnancy, prenatal providers often assume the role of "first responders" and can play a critical role in initiating and linking patients to MOUD. MOUD is most effective when provided through treatment programs that also offer peer recovery services, social services support (eg, housing, transportation), and linkages to counseling, behavioral therapy, and psychiatric services.[28]

Methadone and buprenorphine are the preferred medications for use during pregnancy.[27] Patients should be counseled that there is no known increase in the risk of birth defects or adverse long-term developmental impacts associated with the use of either medication during pregnancy.[28] However, all infants should be observed for NOWS following the use of MOUD during pregnancy although studies have not identified a relationship between the dose of methadone or buprenorphine and the incidence or severity of NOWS.[29,30] Thus, the choice between the use methadone or buprenorphine is highly individualized and should be the result of a shared decision-making process between each patient and their provider. Factors that should be incorporated into the decision-making process include medication availability, medical contraindications, patient preference, and prior treatment experiences (**Table 1**).

Methadone

Methadone was the first medication used for the treatment of OUD in pregnancy and its safety and effectiveness in pregnancy are well established.[27] Methadone is a long-acting, synthetic mu-opioid receptor agonist that can only be dispensed from federally licensed drug and alcohol treatment centers when used for OUD.[7] Methadone treatment programs offer on-site individual and group counseling, case management, education, and job training services for patients. However, patients early in recovery are often required to present each day for supervised medication administration, which can create barriers to treatment engagement due to childcare, employment, and other conflicting responsibilities.[31]

Methadone has a unique pharmacokinetic profile that can be highly variable across patients. The mean half-life is 24 h but can range from 8 to 59 h. During methadone initiation, it can also take up to 5 days after a stable dose is achieved to reach steady-state plasma levels which can result in a deferred toxicity due to the drug's slow release from tissue reservoirs.[32] Thus, providers should "start low and go slow" when titrating methadone to avoid oversedation and respiratory depression.[32] Methadone is also associated with QTc (QT interval corrected for heart rate) prolongation that can increase the risk for ventricular arrhythmias such as Torsades de Pointes.[33] Thus, all patients should have an electrocardiogram performed before the initiation of methadone. If the QTc interval is $\geq$ 500 ms, methadone is generally not recommended and factors such as the concurrent use of medications that can also prolong the QTc and hypokalemia should be addressed.[32]

In pregnancy, methadone initiation often occurs in the inpatient setting to closely observe patients during dose titration. Patients who present in opioid withdrawal can be started on an initial dose of 10 to 30 mg and should be reassessed 2 to 4 h after dosing, when serum levels peak, to monitor for oversedation or withdrawal.[32] After the initial dose, additional doses of 5 to 10 mg can be given every 4 h as needed to treat withdrawal symptoms. Federal regulations limit the initial dose of methadone to a maximum of 30 mg and the total dose on the first day of treatment to 50 mg.[32] If the patient's symptoms are not controlled after the first day, the total dose of methadone administered over the previous 24 h is administered as the new morning dose and 5 to 10 mg are given every 4 h until the patient does not show signs or symptoms of withdrawal. Although dosing should be individualized to the needs of each patient, methadone doses between 80 and 120 mg/day have been associated with improved treatment outcomes during pregnancy.[34,35]

In the outpatient setting, methadone is typically administered as a single daily dose. However, in pregnancy, changes in metabolism, maternal intravascular volume and renal elimination during the second and third trimesters often require dose escalation to avoid withdrawal.[31,36] However, increasing daily doses to account for pregnancy-associated metabolic shifts can suppress fetal movement and breathing.[37,38] Twice-daily dosing or "split dosing" is an alternative approach to controlling patient's symptoms with more consistent plasma levels.[31,37] In 2022, the Substance Abuse and

Table 1
Clinical considerations to guide shared decision-making when selecting a medication for opioid use disorder (MOUD) during pregnancy

Considerations	Buprenorphine	Methadone
Mechanism of action	• Partial mu opioid receptor agonist	• Full mu opioid receptor agonist
Regulations and availability	• Schedule III • Care can be provided in a non-drug and alcohol licensed outpatient setting • Requires DATA-2000 waiver to prescribe	• Schedule II • Can only be prescribed for opioid use disorder through federally licensed drug and alcohol treatment programs
Dispensing	• Can be dispensed from any outpatient pharmacy	• Often requires daily visits to the treatment program for observed daily dosing, especially in the first 90 days
Patient selection	• Patient preference • Patients without prior MOUD treatment experiences • Lack of methadone availability in the patient's geographic area • Limited resources (eg, lack of transportation or unable to remain complaint with daily treatment program visits)	• Patient preference • Lack of buprenorphine effectiveness or compliance with prior use (eg, buprenorphine unable to mitigate opioid craving or withdrawal)
Retention in treatment	• Some evidence shows greater treatment dropout compared with methadone	• Some evidence shows higher rates of treatment retention compared with buprenorphine
Medication interactions	• CYP3A4 enzyme inhibitors • Risk of respiratory depression with CNS depressants including benzodiazepines • Mixed agonist/antagonist medications can precipitate withdrawal	• CYP450 enzyme inhibitors • Risk of respiratory depression with CNS depressants including benzodiazepines • Mixed agonist/antagonist medications can precipitate withdrawal
Starting dose	• 2 to 4 mg • Lose doses (eg, 10 mcg to 0.5 mg) may be necessary in the setting of synthetic opioid use (eg, fentanyl)	• 10 to 30 mg
Average therapeutic dose	• 16 mg	• 80 to 120 mg
Unique pharmacology	• Long elimination half-life (24 to 69 h) due to high binding affinity	• Can take 5 days (ie, 5 half-lives) to reach steady state concentrations
Pregnancy specific dosing considerations	• BID, TID or QID dosing may provide better steady state concentrations	• BID or "split dosing" is preferred during pregnancy
Contraindications	• Allergy	• Prolonged QTc > 500 • Evaluate concurrent medication use, K and Mag deficiencies • Allergy

Adapted from Substance Abuse and Mental Health Services Administration. Clinical Guidance for Treating Pregnant and Parenting Women With Opioid Use Disorder and Their Infants. HHS Publication No. (SMA) 18-5054. Rockville, MD: Substance Abuse and Mental Health Services Administration, 2018.

Mental Health Services Administration issued a statement recommending take-home flexibilities to facilitate split dosing for pregnant women, especially in the third trimester.[39]

Buprenorphine

The use of buprenorphine during pregnancy has significantly increased over the past decade.[40] Expanded use in outpatient and telehealth settings, a low risk of overdose, and evidence from randomized controlled trials demonstrating a shorter treatment duration for NOWS have made buprenorphine a first-line treatment option for many pregnant patients with OUD.[32] Although providers must obtain a DATA-2000 waiver to prescribe buprenorphine for OUD, in 2021, the Department of Health and Human Services exempted providers from training requirements previously necessary to obtain the DATA-2000 waiver to expand access to buprenorphine.

Buprenorphine is a partial agonist at the mu-opioid receptor and has a significantly greater affinity for the receptor compared with most other opioids. This can have a protective effect against overdose as it prevents other opioids with lower affinity (eg, heroin) from binding and its slow dissociation from the receptor prolongs this effect. Owing to changes in metabolism and renal clearance during pregnancy, buprenorphine may also need to be dosed more frequently (eg, three to four times daily) and the total daily dose may need to be increased (eg, 24 to 32 mg), especially in the third trimester, to prevent withdrawal symptoms.[41,42] Importantly, buprenorphine shows a "ceiling effect" at high doses (ie, $\geq$ 32 mg), which further enhances its safety profile and allows for pharmacy-based dispensing in the outpatient setting without the same degree of regulatory oversight compared with methadone.

Buprenorphine is available in a variety of formulations with and without naloxone including a sublingual tablet, a sublingual film, a buccal film, an implant, and an extended-release subcutaneous injection. Naloxone, an antagonist at the mu-opioid receptor, is combined with buprenorphine in transmucosal preparations to prevent medication misuse because it has poor bioavailability when taken as prescribed. However, if crushed or dissolved for intravenous use, naloxone induces opioid withdrawal. Historically, guidelines recommended the use of buprenorphine without naloxone during pregnancy. However, these risks associated with naloxone have proven to be theoretical as naloxone is only detectable at very low levels when taken sublingually and has not been associated with an increased risk of congenital anomalies. Thus, the American Society of Addiction Medicine has revised their national practice guidelines to state that the use buprenorphine-naloxone is safe and effective for pregnant populations.[43]

Buprenorphine Use in the Age of Fentanyl

Caring for pregnant patients with OUD in the "fentanyl age" has prompted the need for revised approaches to the initiation of buprenorphine during pregnancy due to the increased propensity for precipitated withdrawal. Conventional buprenorphine initiation protocols recommend waiting until the patient is in mild to moderate withdrawal and starting a dose of buprenorphine that minimizes withdrawal symptoms (eg, 2 to 4 mg). If withdrawal symptoms remain, the dose is slowly titrated until a therapeutic dose is achieved (eg, 16 mg). However, fentanyl has a much longer elimination half-life than heroin which results in many patients initiating buprenorphine 'too early" during the withdrawal process when fentanyl is still bound to the receptor. In the setting of a full agonist, buprenorphine's partial agonist activity results in an antagonist effect which results in a sudden worsening or "precipitated" withdrawal. In an evaluation of 1,679 individuals seeking treatment of OUD, the odds of precipitated withdrawal significantly increased when taking buprenorphine less than 24 h (OR 5.202) or 48 h (OR 3.352) after fentanyl use.[44] Precipitated withdrawal is also a deterrent to treatment engagement. In an evaluation of 107 patients undergoing buprenorphine induction, those who experienced precipitated withdrawal dropped out of treatment within the first 3 days.[45]

Low-dose buprenorphine initiation protocols have emerged to minimize precipitated withdrawal that often occurs in the setting of fentanyl use. Low-dose buprenorphine initiation or "micro-dosing" is a broad term that encompasses a variety of approaches that start with very small doses of buprenorphine (eg, 10 mcg to 0.5 mg), which are gradually increased over several days. Full opioid agonists (eg, hydromorphone) are often used in low-dose protocols to mitigate withdrawal symptoms during the period when buprenorphine dosing is subtherapeutic.[46] Hydromorphone is a particularly effective agonist because it has a binding affinity similar to buprenorphine.[47] Outcomes associated with low-dose protocols during pregnancy remain limited. In 2021, a case series reported that a 20-mcg transdermal buprenorphine patch was used to transition 8 patients to sublingual buprenorphine without any cases of precipitated withdrawal.[48]

Naltrexone

Currently, there is insufficient evidence to recommend the routine use of naltrexone, a mu-opioid receptor antagonist, during pregnancy although data are rapidly emerging.[49,50] In a retrospective cohort study comparing 6 pregnant patients taking naltrexone and 13 taking buprenorphine, the naltrexone group had less illicit opioid use during pregnancy.[50] Further, no infants in the naltrexone group were diagnosed with NOWS versus 92 in the buprenorphine group.[50] Although one retrospective study of 68 patients found that urogenital anomalies were more frequent in naltrexone-exposed fetuses compared with methadone or buprenorphine, available studies are not adequately powered to detect differences in the congenital anomaly rate.[51]

MANAGEMENT OF ANALGESIA FOR PEOPLE WITH OPIOID USE DISORDER IN LABOR AND POSTPARTUM

The management of analgesia for patients with OUD can be challenging and a multimodal approach to pain management during labor and delivery is warranted. Chronic opioid use increases the risk for opioid-induced hyperalgesia which may necessitate higher doses of analgesic medications to achieve adequate pain control.[28,52] A complex biopsychosocial phenomenon, pain can be exacerbated by anticipatory fear, stress, poor coping mechanisms, and a lack of social support.[53] Poorly controlled pain can also interfere with one's recovery progress serving as a risk factor for relapse. As such, a pain management plan should be developed for all patients with OUD in the prenatal period to address pain-related concerns and OB anesthesia should be consulted as needed. A multidisciplinary team of providers from obstetrics, anesthesia, and nursing should discuss the pain management plan when a patient with OUD is admitted to labor and delivery to ensure consistency in management during the hospitalization.

Methadone or buprenorphine dosing should be continued throughout the intrapartum and postpartum periods and should not be expected to provide pain relief. Increasing the dose of methadone or buprenorphine will also not improve pain control. Instead, neuraxial anesthesia (eg, spinal, epidural) is highly effective for patients with OUD and should be offered as the first-line intervention for labor-related pain. Opioid-sparing approaches may also have utility for this population including transversus abdominis plane blocks, IV acetaminophen, and gabapentin.[54] Partial opioid agonists such as nalbuphine, butorphanol, or pentazocine should not be used in patients with OUD as these medications can precipitate withdrawal.

In the postpartum period, analgesia after vaginal delivery can usually be attained with non-opioid medications such as non-steroidal anti-inflammatory agents, acetaminophen, and non-pharmacologic interventions such as ice packs, analgesic sprays, and sitz baths. However, cesarean delivery is associated with significantly more pain than vaginal birth. Non-opioid medications such as ketorolac and acetaminophen should be scheduled for the first 48 h after delivery and short-acting opioid analgesic agents may be warranted. When opioids are given, their dosing should be individualized and the use of products without acetaminophen should be prioritized to avoid toxicity for patients with hepatic impairment or when IV acetaminophen is also used.[55,56] For patients receiving methadone, short-acting opioids (eg, oxycodone) for pain relief should be administered in addition to patient's daily methadone dose. For patients receiving buprenorphine, adequate analgesia can be more challenging to achieve because of buprenorphine's high affinity for and partial agonist activity at the mu receptor. As a result, full agonists that have a similar affinity for the mu receptor (ie, hydromorphone) should be used to displace buprenorphine, activate the receptor, and induce an analgesic effect.[47] When prescribing opioids for pain for patients with OUD, providers should discuss the potential for "triggering" with the use of short-acting opioids, prescribe very limited quantities, and provide close follow-up to ensure discontinuation after delivery.

SUMMARY

Pregnancy is a unique opportunity to provide highly effective interventions for patients with OUD and improve maternal and neonatal health outcomes for this population. Obstetric providers are uniquely positioned to create trusting and meaningful relationships with patients who can dramatically improve their recovery trajectory. Health care systems, hospitals, and providers should incorporate algorithms and clinical care pathways that address the needs of pregnant patients with OUD to ensure the use of evidence-based practices during pregnancy, labor and delivery, and the postpartum period. Through coordination, collaboration, and consistency in care, health care providers can mitigate adverse outcomes associated with substance use for pregnant patients and their families.

CLINICS CARE POINTS

- COWS can provide an objective measure of withdrawal severity and guide initiation of MOUD and supportive medications.
- Choosing between buprenorophine and methadone should be a shared decision making process based on medication availability, medical contraindications, patient preference, and prior treatment experiences.
- Buprenorphine use during pregnancy is associated with a decreased severity of NOWS in exposed neonates compared to methadone use.
- In patients using synthetic opioids and desiring buprenorphine initiation, a low dose approach should be considered.
- MOUD should be continued throughout the intrapartum and postpartum period with additional pain medication being individualized on the basis of shared decision making, choice of MOUD, and mode of delivery. MOUD should not be used as a substitute for analgesics.

DISCLOSURE

Dr E.E. Krans is an investigator on grants to Magee-Womens Research Institute from the National Institutes of Health, Gilead, and Merck outside of the submitted work. The other authors report no conflicts of interest.

REFERENCES

1. Hirai AH, Ko JY, Owens PL, et al. neonatal abstinence syndrome and maternal opioid-related diagnoses in the US, 2010-2017. JAMA 2021;325(2):146–55.
2. Gemmill A, KIANG MV, Alexander MJ. Trends in pregnancy-associated mortality involving opioids in the United States, 2007-2016. Am J Obstet Gynecol 2019; 220(1):115–6.
3. Ciccarone D. The rise of illicit fentanyls, stimulants and the fourth wave of the opioid overdose crisis. Curr Opin Psychiatry 2021;34(4):344–50.
4. CDC. Three waves of opioid overdose deaths. 2022. Availbale at: https://www.cdc.gov/drugoverdose/epidemic/index.html. Accessed July 10th, 2022.
5. Ahmad FB, Cisewski JA. Provisional drug overdose death counts. Hyattsville (MD): National Center for Health Statistics; 2021.
6. Volkow ND, Frieden TR, Hyde PS, et al. Medication-assisted therapies–tackling the opioid-overdose epidemic. N Engl J Med 2014;370(22):2063–6.
7. American Society of Addiction Medicine (ASAM). national practice guideline for the use of medications in the treatment of addiction involving opioid use. 2015. Available at: https://www.asam.org/docs/default-source/practice-support/guidelines-and-consensus-docs/asam-national-practice-guideline-supplement.pdf. Accessed September, 2022.
8. Wakeman SE, Larochelle MR, Ameli O, et al. comparative effectiveness of different treatment pathways for opioid use disorder. JAMA Netw Open 2020; 3(2):e1920622.
9. Krans EE, Kim JY, Chen Q, et al. Outcomes associated with the use of medications for opioid use disorder during pregnancy. Addiction 2021;116(12):3504–14.
10. Schiff DM, Nielsen T, Terplan M, et al. Fatal and nonfatal overdose among pregnant and postpartum women in massachusetts. Obstet Gynecol 2018;132(2): 466–74.
11. Djurendic-Brenesel M, Piliga V. Opiate receptors and gender and relevance to heroin addiction. In: Peter M, editor. Neuropathology of drug addictions and substance misuse. vol 1. Cambridge, Massachusetts: Academic Press; 2016. p. 922–32.
12. American Society of Addiction Medicine. Public policy statement: definition of addiction. Chevy Chase (MD): American Society of Addiction Medicine; 2011. Available at. http://www.asam.org/docs/publicy-policy-statements/1definition_of_addiction_long_4-11.pdf?sfvrsn=2.
13. McHugh RK, Devito EE, Dodd D, et al. Gender differences in a clinical trial for prescription opioid dependence. J Subst Abuse Treat 2013;45(1):38–43.
14. NIDA. April 13. Sex and gender differences in substance use disorder treatment. 2021. Available at: https://nida.nih.gov/publications/research-reports/substance-use-in-women/sex-gender-differences-in-substance-use-disorder-treatment   on 2022. July 7. Accessed.
15. Lewis B, Hoffman LA, Nixon SJ. Sex differences in drug use among polysubstance users. Drug Alcohol Depend 2014;145:127–33.

16. Liang Y, Goros MW, Turner BJ. Drug overdose: differing risk models for women and men among opioid users with non-cancer pain. Pain Med 2016;17(12): 2268–79.

17. McHugh RK, Votaw VR, Sugarman DE, et al. Sex and gender differences in substance use disorders. Clin Psychol Rev 2018;66:12–23.

18. Engstrom M, El-Bassel N, Gilbert L. Childhood sexual abuse characteristics, intimate partner violence exposure, and psychological distress among women in methadone treatment. J Subst Abuse Treat 2012;43(3):366–76.

19. Pallatino C, Chang JC, Krans EE. The intersection of intimate partner violence and substance use among women with opioid use disorder. Subst Abuse 2019; 42(2):1–8.

20. Tsang A, Von Korff M, Lee S, et al. Common chronic pain conditions in developed and developing countries: gender and age differences and comorbidity with depression-anxiety disorders. J Pain 2008;9(10):883–91.

21. Andersson HI, Ejlertsson G, Leden I, et al. Chronic pain in a geographically defined general population: studies of differences in age, gender, social class, and pain localization. Clin J Pain 1993;9(3):174–82.

22. Sullivan MJ, Tripp DA, Santor D. Gender differences in pain and pain behavior: the role of catastrophizing. Cognit Ther Res 2000;24(1):121–34.

23. Farrell M. Opiate withdrawal. Addiction 1994;89(11):1471–5.

24. Rehni AK, Jaggi AS, Singh N. Opioid withdrawal syndrome: emerging concepts and novel therapeutic targets. CNS Neurol Disord Drug Targets 2013;12(1): 112–25.

25. Tompkins DA, Bigelow GE, Harrison JA, et al. Concurrent validation of the Clinical Opiate Withdrawal Scale (COWS) and single-item indices against the Clinical Institute Narcotic Assessment (CINA) opioid withdrawal instrument. Drug Alcohol Depend 2009;105(1–2):154–9.

26. Caritis SN, Panigrahy A. Opioids affect the fetal brain: reframing the detoxification debate. Am J Obstet Gynecol 2019;221(6):602–8.

27. Mascola MA, Borders AE, Terplan M, et al. Opioid use and opioid use disorder in pregnancy. Obstet Gynecol 2017;130(2):E81–94.

28. Substance Abuse and Mental Health Services Administration. Clinical guidance for treating pregnant and parenting women with opioid use disorder and their infants. Rockville, MD: Substance Abuse and Mental Health Services Administration; 2018. HHS Publication No. (SMA) 18-5054.

29. Pizarro D, Habli M, Grier M, et al. Higher maternal doses of methadone does not increase neonatal abstinence syndrome. J Subst Abuse Treat 2011;40(3):295–8.

30. Cleary BJ, Donnelly J, Strawbridge J, et al. Methadone dose and neonatal abstinence syndrome-systematic review and meta-analysis. Addiction 2010;105(12): 2071–84.

31. McCarthy JJ, Jones HE, Terplan M, et al. Changing outdated methadone regulations that harm pregnant patients. J Addict Med 2021;15(2):93–5.

32. Substance Abuse and Mental Health Services Administration, Medications for Opioid Use Disorder. Treatment Improvement Protocol (TIP) Series 63, Executive Summary. Publication No. PEP21-02-01-003, 2021, Substance Abuse and Mental Health Services Administration; Rockville, MD.

33. Bednar MM, Harrigan EP, Ruskin JN. Torsades de pointes associated with non-antiarrhythmic drugs and observations on gender and QTc. Am J Cardiol 2002; 89(11):1316–9.

34. Wilder C, Lewis D, Winhusen T. Medication assisted treatment discontinuation in pregnant and postpartum women with opioid use disorder. Drug Alcohol Depend 2015;149:225–31.

35. McCarthy JJ, Leamon MH, Parr MS, et al. High-dose methadone maintenance in pregnancy: maternal and neonatal outcomes. Am J Obstet Gynecol 2005;193(3 Pt 1):606–10.

36. Feghali M, Venkataramanan R, Caritis S. Pharmacokinetics of drugs in pregnancy. Semin perinatology 2015;39(7):512–9.

37. Jansson LM, Dipietro JA, Velez M, et al. Maternal methadone dosing schedule and fetal neurobehaviour. J Matern Fetal Neonatal Med 2009;22(1):29–35.

38. Wittmann BK, Segal S. A comparison of the effects of single- and split-dose methadone administration on the fetus: ultrasound evaluation. Int J Addict 1991;26(2):213–8.

39. SAMHSA, Split Dose Guidance SOTAs CSAT Final, Available at: https://www.samhsa.gov/sites/default/files/split-dose-guidance-sotas-csat.pdf. Accessed June 2022.

40. Krans EE, Kim JY, James AE 3rd, et al. Medication-assisted treatment use among pregnant women with opioid use disorder. Obstet Gynecol 2019;133(5):943–51.

41. Bastian JR, Chen H, Zhang H, et al. Dose-adjusted plasma concentrations of sublingual buprenorphine are lower during than after pregnancy. Am J Obstet Gynecol 2017;216(1):64 e1–e64 e7.

42. Caritis SN, Bastian JR, Zhang H, et al. An evidence-based recommendation to increase the dosing frequency of buprenorphine during pregnancy. Am J Obstet Gynecol 2017;217(4):459 e1–e59 e6.

43. The ASAM national practice guideline for the treatment of opioid use disorder: 2020 focused update. J Addict Med 2020;14:1.

44. Varshneya NB, Thakrar AP, Hobelmann JG, et al. Evidence of buprenorphine-precipitated withdrawal in persons who use fentanyl. J Addict Med 2021;16(4):265–8.

45. Whitley SD, Sohler NL, Kunins HV, et al. Factors associated with complicated buprenorphine inductions. J Subst Abuse Treat 2010;39(1):51–7.

46. De Aquino JP, Parida S, Sofuoglu M. The pharmacology of buprenorphine microinduction for opioid use disorder. Clin Drug Investig 2021;41(5):425–36.

47. Volpe DA, McMahon Tobin GA, Mellon RD, et al. Uniform assessment and ranking of opioid mu receptor binding constants for selected opioid drugs. Regul Toxicol Pharmacol 2011;59(3):385–90.

48. Galati BM, Carter EB, Perez M, et al. Buprenorphine patch as a bridge to sublingual treatment of opioid use disorder in pregnancy. Obstet Gynecol 2021;137(4):713–6.

49. Towers CV, Katz E, Weitz B, et al. Use of naltrexone in treating opioid use disorder in pregnancy. Am J Obstet Gynecol 2020;222(1):83 e1–e83 e8.

50. Wachman EM, Saia K, Miller M, et al. Naltrexone Treatment for Pregnant Women With Opioid Use Disorder Compared With Matched Buprenorphine Control Subjects. Clin Ther 2019;41(9):1681–9.

51. Kelty E, Hulse G. A Retrospective Cohort Study of Birth Outcomes in Neonates Exposed to Naltrexone in Utero: A Comparison with Methadone-, Buprenorphine- and Non-opioid-Exposed Neonates. Drugs 2017;77(11):1211–9.

52. Lee M, Silverman SM, Hansen H, et al. A comprehensive review of opioid-induced hyperalgesia. Pain Physician 2011;14(2):145–61.

53. Che X, Cash R, Ng SK, et al. A systematic review of the processes underlying the main and the buffering effect of social support on the experience of pain. Clin J Pain 2018;34(11):1061–76.

54. Mitchell KD, Smith CT, Mechling C, et al. A review of peripheral nerve blocks for cesarean delivery analgesia. Reg Anesth Pain Med 2019. [Epub ahead of print].

55. Meyer M, Paranya G, Keefer Norris A, et al. Intrapartum and postpartum analgesia for women maintained on buprenorphine during pregnancy. Eur J Pain 2010;14(9):939–43.

56. Meyer M, Wagner K, Benvenuto A, et al. Intrapartum and postpartum analgesia for women maintained on methadone during pregnancy. Obstet Gynecol 2007; 110(2 Pt 1):261–6.

Anticoagulation Regimens in Pregnancy

Antonio Saad, MD*, Melody Safarzadeh, MD, MS, Megan Shepherd, MD

KEYWORDS

- Pregnancy • Postpartum • Anticoagulation • Venous thromboembolism
- Thrombophilia • Unfractionated heparin • Low-molecular-weight heparin

KEY POINTS

- The benefits of anticoagulation therapy in preventing venous thromboembolism (VTE) must be weighed against any potential risk to the developing fetus, as well as an increased risk of bleeding during pregnancy and the postpartum period.
- There are several strategies that providers can use to determine whether a patient is an appropriate candidate for anticoagulation during pregnancy, including a screening method based on personal and/or family history of VTE and the presence of low- or high-risk thrombophilia.
- The continuation of pharmacologic thromboprophylaxis is not recommended during labor and delivery; however, patients receiving antepartum anticoagulation will require continuation after delivery and into the postpartum period.

INTRODUCTION

Pregnancy and the postpartum period are associated with a 4- to 5-fold increased risk of venous thromboembolism (VTE) compared with the nonpregnant state.[1,2] VTE is one of the leading causes of maternal mortality globally. Despite the prevalence and severity of this condition among pregnant and postpartum people, universal thromboprophylaxis is not recommended. Prevention of VTE has centered on anticoagulation strategies for those with additional risk factors apart from pregnancy, including a personal history of VTE or a known thrombophilia.[3]

The benefits of anticoagulation therapy in preventing VTE must be weighed against any potential risk to the developing fetus, as well as an increased risk of bleeding during pregnancy and the postpartum period. The most common pharmacologic anticoagulants used in the general population are warfarin and heparins. Warfarin is a vitamin K antagonist that prevents the formation of active vitamin K-dependent clotting factors.[4] Unfractionated heparin (UFH) binds to and increases the activity of antithrombin

Division of Maternal-Fetal Medicine, Department of Obstetrics and Gynecology, The University of Texas Medical Branch at Galveston, 301 University Boulevard, Galveston, TX 77555, USA
* Corresponding author.
E-mail address: afsaad@utmb.edu

Obstet Gynecol Clin N Am 50 (2023) 241–249
https://doi.org/10.1016/j.ogc.2022.10.010
0889-8545/23/© 2022 Elsevier Inc. All rights reserved.

obgyn.theclinics.com

III (AT3), inhibiting thrombin and Factor Xa.[4] Low-molecular-weight heparin (LMWH) also binds to AT3; however, given its smaller molecular size, it ultimately has a proportionally more significant impact on Factor Xa than on thrombin.[4]

Warfarin is a commonly used anticoagulant in the nonpregnant population. However, it crosses the placenta, and exposure during organogenesis is associated with characteristic embryopathy, including midface hypoplasia, stippled chondral calcification, scoliosis, and short proximal limbs.[5] Warfarin administration later in pregnancy is associated with fetal intracranial hemorrhage and schizencephaly.[5] Because of their large molecular size, neither UFH nor LMWH crosses the placenta. Therefore, they are the preferred anticoagulants in pregnancy.[3]

Oral direct thrombin inhibitors (dabigatran) and anti-Factor Xa inhibitors (rivaroxaban, apixaban, edoxaban, betrixaban) should be avoided during pregnancy and lactation, as there is insufficient data regarding their safety in this patient population.[6–8] In cases of severe heparin allergy or heparin-induced thrombocytopenia, consultation with a hematologist is recommended, and fondaparinux, an indirect inhibitor of Factor Xa, may be the preferred method of anticoagulation.[3]

This manuscript reviews current recommendations for anticoagulation therapy in pregnancy, including outpatient antepartum, intrapartum, and postpartum guidelines. The authors also address the challenges of transitioning between LMWH and UFH.

Antepartum

There are several strategies that obstetricians can use to assess whether a patient is an appropriate candidate for anticoagulation during pregnancy. The American College of Obstetricians and Gynecologists (ACOG) uses a screening method based on personal and/or family history of VTE and the presence of low- or high-risk thrombophilia (**Table 1**).[3] Low-risk thrombophilia includes Factor V Leiden heterozygosity, prothrombin G20210A mutation heterozygosity, protein C or protein S deficiency, and antiphospholipid antibody syndrome.[3] High-risk thrombophilia includes Factor V Leiden homozygosity, prothrombin G20210A mutation homozygosity, heterozygosity for both Factor V Leiden and prothrombin G20210A mutation, and AT3 deficiency.[3] In contrast, the Royal College of Obstetricians and Gynecologists (RCOG) uses a different scoring system to stratify patients into low, intermediate, or high risk of developing VTE.[5] Pregnant patients are assigned points for their preexisting, obstetric, and transient risk factors for VTE, and decisions regarding thromboprophylaxis are made based on their total score.[5]

Recommendations for anticoagulation regimens include prophylaxis, intermediate, and therapeutic (or adjusted) dosing (**Table 2**). Prophylactic dosing consists of either LMWH 40 mg administered subcutaneously daily or UFH 5,000 units to 7,500 units administered subcutaneously every twelve hours during the first trimester; 7,500 units to 10,000 units administered subcutaneously every twelve hours during the second trimester; or 10,000 units administered subcutaneously twice daily during the third trimester unless activated partial thromboplastin time (aPTT) is elevated.[3] The aim of prophylaxis is to reduce VTE risk without increasing the risk of bleeding complications. Intermediate dosing consists of LMWH 40 mg given subcutaneously every twelve hours.[6] Although prophylactic and intermediate dosing are prespecified based on the anticoagulant being used, therapeutic (or adjusted) dosing refers to doses that are adjusted based on maternal weight (LMWH) or aPTT (UFH).[6] The therapeutic dosing regimen for LMWH is 1 mg/kg given subcutaneously every twelve hours with a target anti-Factor Xa level in the range of 0.6 to 1.0 units/mL 4 hours after the last injection.[6] The therapeutic dosing regimen for UFH is 10,000 units or more administered

Table 1
Anticoagulation recommendations in pregnancy and the postpartum period

Clinical Scenario	Antepartum Management	Postpartum Management
No thrombophilia with single prior episode of VTE resulting from transient risk factor unrelated to pregnancy or estrogen	Surveillance without anticoagulation	Prophylactic anticoagulation if patient has additional risk factors[a]
No thrombophilia with single prior episode of VTE resulting from transient risk factor related to pregnancy or estrogen or without an identified precipitating risk factor, not on long-term anticoagulation therapy	Prophylactic-dose LMWH or UFH	Prophylactic-, intermediate-, or therapeutic (adjusted)-dose LMWH or UFH for 6 wk
Two or more prior VTE, with or without thrombophilia, not on long-term anticoagulation therapy	Intermediate- or therapeutic (adjusted)-dose LMWH OR prophylactic- or therapeutic (adjusted)-dose UFH	Anticoagulation therapy equal to the selected antepartum regimen for 6 wk
Two or more prior VTE, with or without thrombophilia, on long-term anticoagulation therapy	Therapeutic (adjusted)-dose LMWH or UFH	Resume long-term anticoagulation therapy
Low-risk thrombophilia[b] without personal or family history of VTE	Surveillance without anticoagulation	Prophylactic anticoagulation if patient has additional risk factors[a]
Low-risk thrombophilia[b] with family history of first-degree relative with VTE	Surveillance without anticoagulation	Prophylactic- or intermediate-dose LMWH or UFH
Low-risk thrombophilia[b] with single prior episode of VTE, not on long-term anticoagulation therapy	Prophylactic- or intermediate-dose LMWH or UFH	Prophylactic- or intermediate-dose LMWH or UFH
High-risk thrombophilia[c] without prior VTE	Prophylactic- or intermediate-dose LMWH or UFH	Prophylactic- or intermediate-dose LMWH or UFH
High-risk thrombophilia[c] with single prior episode of VTE or family history of first-degree relative with VTE	Prophylactic-, intermediate-, or therapeutic (adjusted)-dose LMWH or UFH	Anticoagulation therapy equal to the selected antepartum regimen for 6 wk

[a] Major thrombotic risk factors including obesity, cesarean delivery, or prolonged immobility, or first-degree relative with history of thrombotic episode.
[b] Low-risk thrombophilia: Factor V Leiden heterozygosity, prothrombin G20210A mutation heterozygosity, protein C or protein S deficiency, and antiphospholipid antibody syndrome.
[c] High-risk thrombophilia: Factor V Leiden homozygosity, prothrombin G20210A mutation homozygosity, heterozygosity for both Factor V Leiden and prothrombin G20210A mutation, and antithrombin III (AT3) deficiency.

Adapted from American College of Obstetricians and Gynecologists' Committee on Practice Bulletins—Obstetrics. ACOG Practice Bulletin No. 196: Thromboembolism in Pregnancy [published correction appears in Obstet Gynecol. 2018 Oct;132(4):1068]. Obstet Gynecol. 2018;132(1):e1-e17; with permission.

Table 2	
Anticoagulation regimens in pregnancy	
Anticoagulation Regimen	**Dosage**
Prophylactic LMWH	Enoxaparin 40 mg SC daily
Intermediate-dose LMWH	Enoxaparin 40 mg SC every 12 h
Therapeutic (adjusted)-dose LMWH	Enoxaparin 1 mg/kg SC every 12 h Target anti-Factor Xa level in the range of 0.6–1.0 units/mL 4 h after reference injection[a]
Prophylactic UFH	First trimester: UFH 5,000–7,500 units SC every 12 h Second trimester: UFH 7,500–10,000 units SC every 12 h Third trimester: UFH 10,000 units SC every 12 h unless aPTT is elevated
Therapeutic (adjusted)-dose UFH	UFH 10,000 units or more SC every 12 h Target aPTT level between 1.5 and 2.5 times control, 6 h after injection

Abbreviations: aPTT, activated partial thromboplastin time; SC, subcutaneously.

[a] Pregnant individuals with a mechanical heart valve (MHV) may benefit from trough anti-Factor Xa levels (measured immediately before an injection) in addition to peak anti-Factor Xa levels (measured 4 h after the injection) in order to ensure that minimum anti-Factor Xa levels are maintained throughout the dosing interval (for MHV: target trough anti-Factor Xa level >0.6 U/mL and peak anti-Factor Xa level 1.0–1.2 U/mL).[16]

Modified from American College of Obstetricians and Gynecologists' Committee on Practice Bulletins—Obstetrics. ACOG Practice Bulletin No. 196: Thromboembolism in Pregnancy [published correction appears in Obstet Gynecol. 2018 Oct;132(4):1068]. Obstet Gynecol. 2018;132(1):e1-e17; with permission.

subcutaneously every twelve hours with a target aPTT level between 1.5 to 2.5 times control 6 hours after the last injection.[3]

ACOG suggests that pregnant patients with a single prior episode of VTE resulting from a transient risk factor outside of pregnancy do not require antepartum prophylaxis.[3,6] Low-risk patients with a history of a single VTE associated with either pregnancy or estrogen use should receive antepartum prophylaxis.[3,6] Pregnant patients with a history of multiple VTEs should also receive anticoagulation during pregnancy, regardless of the cause.[3,6] Patients already using long-term anticoagulation at the start of pregnancy should be prescribed a therapeutic dose of anticoagulation during the antepartum period.[3,6] Pregnant people with low-risk thrombophilia without a personal or family history of VTE do not require antepartum anticoagulation.[3,6] In contrast, those with high-risk thrombophilia but no VTE history are candidates for prophylactic- or intermediate-dose anticoagulation therapy.[3,6] Finally, patients with a high-risk thrombophilia with a previous episode of VTE or an affected first-degree relative are candidates for either prophylactic, intermediate-dose, or therapeutic anticoagulation therapy (see **Table 1**).[3,6]

For patients who are candidates for antepartum anticoagulation, therapy should be initiated during the first trimester and continued throughout pregnancy. Anticoagulation dose adjustments should be considered if additional risk factors for VTE are identified during pregnancy. Newly diagnosed VTE during pregnancy is treated using therapeutic subcutaneous LMWH.[6] UFH can be used in the initial treatment of pulmonary embolism or in cases where delivery, surgery, or thrombolysis may be necessary.[6] UFH has a shorter half-life than LMWH, can be rapidly assessed using standard laboratory studies (aPTT), and can be pharmacologically reversed using protamine sulfate, all of which are important considerations for neuraxial anesthesia, delivery, and surgical procedures in general.[3] Once the patient is hemodynamically stable, UFH can be switched to LMWH in anticipation of outpatient management.[6] Anticoagulation therapy should continue for at least 6 weeks postpartum (by which time free protein S is approaching baseline levels),[9] with a minimum total duration of treatment of 3 months.[6]

Optimal surveillance of anticoagulation therapy during pregnancy remains controversial. Pregnancy is associated with certain physiologic changes, including increased plasma volume and increased glomerular filtration rate.[10] Because of these changes, LMWH seems to have higher clearance and a larger volume of distribution earlier in gestation compared with the postpartum period.[10] As pregnancy progresses, the maximum concentration achieved further decreases, consistent with an increase in plasma volume.[10] However, renal clearance of LMWH also decreases in late gestation.[10] In addition, the half-life of LMWH ranges from 3 to 6 hours, and its anticoagulant response to weight-adjusted doses is less variable than that of UFH, which allows for its prophylactic administration to be once daily and without laboratory monitoring.[11] The optimal anti-Factor Xa levels for LMWH prophylaxis in pregnancy have also not been determined.[3] Some retrospective studies have proposed anti-Factor Xa monitoring when there is clinical suspicion that prophylactic dosing may be inadequate.[12] With the exception of mechanical heart valves (MHVs), severe renal insufficiency, and morbid obesity (weight > 150 kg), evidence supporting therapeutic (adjusted) dose monitoring remains unclear.[13] Some investigators favor periodic anti-Factor Xa monitoring as maternal weight changes during pregnancy.[14] At the same time, other studies have demonstrated that few people require increased dosing when a weight-based formula is used.[6] A recent systematic review of 33 studies (4 randomized controlled studies and 29 cohort studies) showed that weight-adjusted, fixed-dosed, and anti-Factor Xa–adjusted LMWH thromboprophylaxis were all the same in terms of effectiveness and safety.[15] Weight-dosed LMWH and anti-Factor Xa–adjusted LMWH had similar efficacy and safety profiles in pregnant individuals with VTE or high thromboembolic risk.[15] Despite having mean peak anti-Factor Xa levels within target ranges, individuals with MHVs still experienced both thrombosis and bleeding.[15] The investigators concluded that anti-Factor Xa monitoring is not indicated when using LMWH as thromboprophylaxis or treatment during pregnancy.[15] In the authors' practice, they monitor anti-Factor Xa levels in pregnant individuals with MHV, morbid obesity (weight > 150 kg), and/or chronic kidney disease. They also recommend using peak and trough anti-Factor Xa levels to guide LMWH dosing in those with MHV.[16] If a patient is transitioned from a therapeutic dose of LMWH to UFH, an aPTT level should be drawn to confirm that it is within the therapeutic range.[3]

Intrapartum

There are several challenges to using anticoagulants in pregnancy, including the risk of bleeding at and around the time of delivery and the unpredictable nature of the onset of labor. Another complicating factor is the use of regional anesthesia for labor and the limitations that come secondary to the use of anticoagulation. Two common approaches to managing thromboprophylaxis around the time of delivery include using UFH or LMWH. As discussed previously, an advantage of UFH, especially near term is the short half-life and the ease of reversal. The half-life of UFH is 30 to 90 minutes in healthy adults, whereas the half-life of LMWH is 3 to 6 hours. However, this can vary based on other comorbid conditions. The clinician may individualize their approach to each patient based on the clinical information to include the likelihood of delivery before 39 weeks, the expected mode of delivery, and the desire for regional anesthesia. The continuation of pharmacologic thromboprophylaxis is not recommended during labor and delivery, but those patients receiving antepartum anticoagulation will require continuation after delivery and into the postpartum period.[5]

If desired, the transition from LMWH to UFH should be around 36 to 37 weeks. In addition, the patient should be instructed to discontinue medication with the onset of signs/symptoms of labor. The risk of hemorrhage is not significantly increased if delivery occurs more than 4 hours after the last dose of prophylactic UFH for both vaginal and cesarean delivery.[17] According to The Society of Obstetric Anesthesia and Perinatology (SOAP), for individuals receiving low-dose UFH (5,000 units 2 or 3 times daily), regional anesthesia may be placed 4 to 6 hours after the last dose or after assessing coagulation status. For intermediate doses (7,500 or 10,000 units 2x daily), regional anesthesia may be placed after 12 hours of the last dose in addition to assessing coagulation status. If the patient is on intravenous heparin, it is recommended that the infusion be stopped for 4 to 6 hours and coagulation status be checked before proceeding with regional anesthesia.[18]

If the decision has been made to continue LMWH, the patient should be instructed to discontinue LMWH 12 to 24 hours before the scheduled induction of labor or with signs/symptoms of labor. Spinal anesthesia can be administered 12 hours after the last dose of a prophylactic dose of LMWH and 24 hours after a dose of therapeutic/weight-based dose of LMWH. There is insufficient data to recommend a specific timing interval between 12 and 24 hours in individuals who are receiving intermediate doses of LMWH (>40 mg daily, >30 mg twice daily, and <1 mg/kg every twelve hours or 1.5 mg/kg daily).[18]

Protamine sulfate is used to reverse both UFH and LMWH. One milligram of protamine sulfate given intravenously inactivates 100 units of heparin.[19] To reverse LMWH within 8 hours of administration, 1 mg of protamine is given intravenously for 1 mg of LMWH administered with a maximum dose of 50 mg.[19] If 8 to 12 hours has elapsed since the last dose of LMWH, 0.5 mg of protamine is given intravenously per 1 mg of LMWH.[19] If more than 12 hours has passed after the last dose, LMWH should not be reversed.[19]

Postpartum

Although the risk of a VTE is increased throughout pregnancy, the most significant risk is thought to be in the postpartum period. It is estimated that of VTEs diagnosed in pregnancy and postpartum, 40% to 60% are diagnosed postpartum.[20] Based on a large study in California, it is thought that the highest risk of VTE was in the first 6 weeks after delivery, but the risk was still increased from 7 to 12 weeks postpartum.[21] One proposed reasoning for this is the delayed normalization of clotting factors in certain individuals.[21] Guidelines from the American College of Chest Physicians and ACOG recommend postpartum thromboprophylaxis for all patients with a personal history of a VTE, all patients with a high-risk thrombophilia regardless of history of VTE, and patients with a low-risk thrombophilia with a family history of VTE irrespective of antepartum anticoagulation.[5]

There is considerable variation in the management of thromboprophylaxis after cesarean delivery. In addition to mechanical prophylaxis, which is recommended for all individuals undergoing cesarean section who are not already on pharmacologic thromboprophylaxis, both ACOG and Society for Maternal Fetal Medicine (SMFM) recommend a subset of people who are at high risk of VTE to have a combination of mechanical and pharmacologic thromboprophylaxis.[6,22] This subset of people includes any history of thrombophilia (low-risk or high-risk), body mass index greater than 35 kg/m², or multiple additional risk factors to include postpartum hemorrhage, infection, and blood transfusion. It is essential to recognize that thromboprophylaxis should be individualized according to each patient's risk factors and that institutional protocols are developed where there are no clear and consistent data.[22]

Timing of initiating thromboprophylaxis after delivery depends on the medication used, dose of thromboprophylaxis, and if regional anesthesia was administered. If regional anesthesia was placed, prophylactic doses of LMWH may be started as early as 4 hours after catheter removal but not earlier than 12 hours after anesthesia. Therapeutic doses may be given 4 hours after catheter removal but not earlier than 24 hours after anesthesia. Indwelling catheters can be continued while receiving prophylactic doses of LMWH. Catheter removal can occur 12 hours after LMWH dose with subsequent dosing at least 4 hours after catheter removal. Prophylactic doses of UFH can be started 1 hour after placement and 1 hour after removal of epidural. Indwelling catheters can be continued with low-dose UFH. The catheter may be removed 4 to 6 hours after the last dose of low-dose UFH with a subsequent dose given at least 1 hour after removal.[17]

Anticoagulants used in pregnancy (LMWH and UFH) and post partum (LMHW, UFH, warfarin) do not accumulate in breast milk, thus they are thought to be safe to use during lactation. When a different class of medication is used for anticoagulation, safety during breastfeeding should be evaluated, and shared decision-making between the patient and clinician is suggested.[23]

CLINICS CARE POINTS

- Warfarin is a commonly used anticoagulant in the nonpregnant population; however, it has been shown to cross the placenta, and exposure during organogenesis is associated with characteristic embryopathy.
- Neither UFH nor LMWH crosses the placenta; therefore, they are the preferred anticoagulants in pregnancy.
- Optimal surveillance of anticoagulation therapy during pregnancy remains unclear; however, pregnant patients receiving prophylactic doses generally do not require monitoring.
- Protamine sulfate can be used to reverse both UFH and LMWH.
- Regional anesthesia can be administered at least 4 to 6 hours after the last dose of UFH and at least 12 to 24 hours after the last dose of LMWH.

DISCLOSURE

The authors have nothing to disclose.

REFERENCES

1. Heit JA, Kobbervig CE, James AH, et al. Trends in the incidence of venous thromboembolism during pregnancy or postpartum: a 30-year population-based study. Ann Intern Med 2005;143(10):697–706.
2. Pomp ER, Lenselink AM, Rosendaal FR, et al. Pregnancy, the postpartum period and prothrombotic defects: risk of venous thrombosis in the MEGA study. J Thromb Haemost 2008;6(4):632–7.

3. Bulletins—Obstetrics ACoOaGCoP. ACOG Practice Bulletin No. 196: Thromboembolism in Pregnancy. Obstet Gynecol 2018;132(1):e1–17.

4. Harter K, Levine M, Henderson SO. Anticoagulation drug therapy: a review. West J Emerg Med 2015;16(1):11–7.

5. Kolettis D, Craigo S. Thromboprophylaxis in Pregnancy. Obstet Gynecol Clin North Am 2018;45(2):389–402.

6. Bates SM, Greer IA, Middeldorp S, et al. VTE, thrombophilia, antithrombotic therapy, and pregnancy: Antithrombotic Therapy and Prevention of Thrombosis, 9th ed: American College of Chest Physicians Evidence-Based Clinical Practice Guidelines. Chest 2012;141(2 Suppl):e691S–736S.

7. Cohen H, Arachchillage DR, Beyer-Westendorf J, et al. Direct Oral Anticoagulants and Women. Semin Thromb Hemost 2016;42(7):789–97.

8. Wiesen MH, Blaich C, Müller C, et al. The Direct Factor Xa Inhibitor Rivaroxaban Passes Into Human Breast Milk. Chest 2016;150(1):e1–4.

9. Bremme KA. Haemostatic changes in pregnancy. Best Pract Res Clin Haematol 2003;16(2):153–68.

10. Casele HL, Laifer SA, Woelkers DA, et al. Changes in the pharmacokinetics of the low-molecular-weight heparin enoxaparin sodium during pregnancy. Am J Obstet Gynecol 1999;181(5 Pt 1):1113–7.

11. Iorio A, Agnelli G. Pharmacokinetic optimisation of the treatment of deep vein thrombosis. Clin Pharmacokinet 1997;32(2):145–72.

12. Boban A, Paulus S, Lambert C, et al. The value and impact of anti-Xa activity monitoring for prophylactic dose adjustment of low-molecular-weight heparin during pregnancy: a retrospective study. Blood Coagul Fibrinolysis 2017;28(3):199–204.

13. Nutescu EA, Spinler SA, Wittkowsky A, et al. Low-molecular-weight heparins in renal impairment and obesity: available evidence and clinical practice recommendations across medical and surgical settings. Ann Pharmacother 2009;43(6):1064–83.

14. Crowther MA, Spitzer K, Julian J, et al. Pharmacokinetic profile of a low-molecular weight heparin (reviparin) in pregnant patients. A prospective cohort study. Thromb Res 2000;98(2):133–8.

15. Kjaergaard AB, Fuglsang J, Hvas AM. Anti-Xa monitoring of low-molecular-weight heparin during pregnancy: a systematic review. Semin Thromb Hemost 2021;47(7):824–42.

16. Berresheim M, Wilkie J, Nerenberg KA, et al. A case series of LMWH use in pregnancy: should trough anti-Xa levels guide dosing? Thromb Res 2014;134(6):1234–40.

17. Horlocker TT, Wedel DJ, Rowlingson JC, et al. Regional anesthesia in the patient receiving antithrombotic or thrombolytic therapy: American Society of Regional Anesthesia and Pain Medicine Evidence-Based Guidelines (Third Edition). Reg Anesth Pain Med 2010;35(1):64–101.

18. Leffert L, Butwick A, Carvalho B, et al. The society for obstetric anesthesia and perinatology consensus statement on the anesthetic management of pregnant and postpartum women receiving thromboprophylaxis or higher dose anticoagulants. Anesth Analg 2018;126(3):928–44.

19. Frontera JA, Lewin JJ, Rabinstein AA, et al. Guideline for Reversal of Antithrombotics in Intracranial Hemorrhage: A Statement for Healthcare Professionals from the Neurocritical Care Society and Society of Critical Care Medicine. Neurocrit Care 2016;24(1):6–46.

20. Simpson EL, Lawrenson RA, Nightingale AL, et al. Venous thromboembolism in pregnancy and the puerperium: incidence and additional risk factors from a London perinatal database. BJOG 2001;108(1):56–60.
21. Kamel H, Navi BB, Sriram N, et al. Risk of a thrombotic event after the 6-week postpartum period. N Engl J Med 2014;370(14):1307–15.
22. Pacheco LD, Saade G, Metz TD. pubs@smfm.org SfM-FMSEa. society for maternal-fetal medicine consult series #51: Thromboembolism prophylaxis for cesarean delivery. Am J Obstet Gynecol 2020;223(2):B11–7.
23. Richter C, Sitzmann J, Lang P, et al. Excretion of low molecular weight heparin in human milk. Br J Clin Pharmacol 2001;52(6):708–10.

Antiseizure Medications in Pregnancy

Alexandra C. Moise, MD*, Elizabeth E. Gerard, MD

KEYWORDS

- Pregnancy • Epilepsy • Antiseizure medication • Teratogenesis

KEY POINTS

- When possible, people with epilepsy and gestational capacity should be treated with an antiseizure medication (ASM) with a favorable teratogenic profile.
- It is important to determine the lowest therapeutic ASM dose so that the corresponding prepregnancy plasma concentration can serve as a target throughout pregnancy.
- Pregnancy can lead to changes in plasma concentrations of the majority of ASMs, thus frequent monitoring is recommended with appropriate dosage adjustments.
- Breastfeeding is recommended for patients taking ASMs, as for most ASMs, benefits have been shown to outweigh risks.

INTRODUCTION

Epilepsy is a common chronic medical condition affecting people of reproductive age. There are roughly 1.5 million people with epilepsy and gestational capacity (PWEGC) in the United States and more than 15 million globally.[1] According to a retrospective study looking at data from the Epilepsy Birth Control Registry between 2010 and 2014, up to 65% of PWEGC reported at least one unplanned pregnancy, which emphasizes the need for early patient counseling and medical optimization.[2] It is important to stress that the majority of PWEGC can have normal pregnancies, but both seizures and antiseizure medications (ASMs) have potential implications for pregnancy outcomes. A balance must be struck between effectively treating the epilepsy and mitigating teratogenic risks that can be associated with ASMs.

Risks of Seizures in Pregnancy

Convulsive seizures can cause obstetric trauma including, but not limited to, placental abruption, internal hemorrhage, direct fetal injury, fetal heart rate changes, and lactic acid build-up.[3,4] The impact of nonconvulsive seizures on pregnancy has not been

Department of Neurology, Feinberg School of Medicine, Northwestern University, 710 North Lake Shore Drive, 11th Floor, Abbott Hall, Chicago, IL 60611, USA
* Corresponding author.
E-mail address: Alexandra.moise@nm.org

Obstet Gynecol Clin N Am 50 (2023) 251–261
https://doi.org/10.1016/j.ogc.2022.10.014
0889-8545/23/© 2022 Elsevier Inc. All rights reserved.

obgyn.theclinics.com

Abbreviations	
ASM	Antiseizure Medication
PWEGC	People with Epilepsy and Gestational Capacity
OR	Odds Ratio
FDA	Food and Drug Administration
RR	Relative Risk
NAAPR	North American AED Pregnancy Registry
EURAP	International Registry of Antiepileptic Drugs and Pregnancy
NEAD	Neurodevelopmental Effects of Antiepileptic Drugs
MoBA	Norwegian Mother and Child Cohort
MONEAD	Maternal Outcomes and Neurodevelopmental Effects of Antiepileptic Drugs
SGA	Small for Gestational Age
MCM	Major Congenital Malformation
NTD	Neural Tube Defect
UKIEPR	UK and Ireland Epilepsy and Pregnancy Register
VPA	Valproate
ASD	Autism Spectrum Disorder

well studied, but focal seizures with impaired awareness (FIAS, formerly known as complex partial seizures) have been associated with fetal heart rate decelerations.[5,6] Nonconvulsive seizures that impair awareness (including FIAS and absence seizures) can put the childbearer at risk for accidents and preclude driving. Pregnant and postpartum patients with epilepsy are also at risk for seizure-related deaths and sudden unexpected death in epilepsy, particularly if not appropriately taking ASMs or receiving specialist care.[7,8] A Taiwanese retrospective cross-sectional study found that seizures bringing people to the hospital during their pregnancy were associated with an increased risk of preterm delivery, lower birth weight, and small for gestational age (SGA).[9]

Pregnancy itself does not significantly alter seizure control; the prospective Maternal Outcomes and Neurodevelopmental Effects of Antiepileptic Drugs (MONEAD) study found that there is no meaningful difference between seizure control in the pregnant and nonpregnant state.[10] However, compared with nonpregnant PWEGC, there was a higher frequency of increases in ASM dosage among pregnant PWEGC. This highlights the importance of therapeutic drug monitoring during pregnancy to maintain seizure control due to known pregnancy-induced changes in ASM metabolism.

Antiseizure Medications and Teratogenesis

Currently, there are more than 20 ASMs on the market. Research has shown significant variability in how exposure to these medications can affect a fetus. The majority of information on structural teratogenesis comes from population-based studies of national pregnancy registries (Norway, Sweden, Finland, and Denmark), as well as prospective registries such as the North American AED Pregnancy Registry (NAAPR), the International Registry of Antiepileptic Drugs and Pregnancy (EURAP), the UK/Ireland Epilepsy and Pregnancy Register (UKIEPR), Australian Pregnancy Register of AEDs, and the Kerala registry of Epilepsy and Pregnancy.[11] There have been several other prospective observational studies including the Neurodevelopmental Effects of Antiepileptic Drugs (NEAD) study, the MONEAD study, and Norwegian Mother and Child Cohort (MoBa) Study that examined cognitive outcomes associated with in utero exposure.[11,12]

Structural teratogenesis

The best-studied outcomes related to ASM use in pregnancy are major congenital malformations (MCMs). They include neural tube defects (NTDs), oral clefts, congenital heart anomalies, and hypospadias.[13] MCMs occur during the peak time of organogenesis, between 3 and 10 weeks of gestation. Rates of MCMs in the general population range from 1.6% to 3.2%.[13] Rates of MCM in children exposed to ASMs in utero vary greatly based on the specific medication exposure. **Fig. 1** provides a graphical summary of comparative MCM rates among the best-studied ASMs across 3 prospective pregnancy registries.

There is strong evidence that valproate (VPA) has significant teratogenic potential. Exposure to VPA monotherapy is associated with MCM rates of 6.7% to 10.3%.[14,15] In a pooled analysis, the absolute risks of specific MCMs were 1.8% for NTDs, 1.7% for cardiac malformations, 1.4% for hypospadias, and 0.9% for oral clefts.[16] In contrast, lamotrigine is a broad-spectrum ASM with a low rate of structural teratogenesis (MCM rates 2.3% to 2.9%).[14,17] Levetiracetam is also a broad-spectrum ASM with a low risk of MCM (Rates 1.7%–3%).[18,19]

Carbamazepine is an ASM used for focal seizures. Monotherapy with carbamazepine is associated with MCM rates of 2.65% to 5.9%.[14,17] Absolute risk of specific MCMs from a pooled analysis include 0.3% for NTDs, 0.8% for cardiac malformations, 0.4% for hypospadias and 0.36% for oral clefts.[16] Oxcarbazepine is a structural analog of carbamazepine and is metabolized to 10,11-dihydro-10-hydroxy-carbazepine.[11] Most of the MCM data on oxcarbazepine are from small cohorts. Based on studies from the NAAPR, Denmark, Norway, EURAP, and Finland, the pooled cumulative MCM rate is roughly 2.5%.[11]

Topiramate monotherapy has been associated with MCM rates that range from 3.9% to 4.2% in small cohorts.[17,20] However, topiramate has specifically been associated with an increased risk of oral clefts (OR 5.4 95% CI: 2.0–14.6), leading the Food

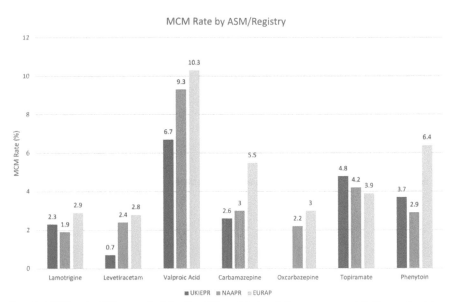

Fig. 1. MCM rate (%) as noted in the UK and Ireland Pregnancy and Epilepsy Registers (UKIEPR),[14] the North American AED Pregnancy Registry (NAAPR),[19] and the International Registry for Antiepileptic Drugs and Pregnancy (EURAP).[18] These were prospective registers that looked at 5206, 7370, and 7555 women, respectively, and for whom outcomes data were available. Some of the variability noted in these rates are due to differing MCM criteria and length of follow-up between the groups.

and Drug Administration to classify it as class D for pregnancy.[20,21] It is also associated low birth weight, and the prevalence of SGA infants was 17.9% (RR 2.4, 95% CI 1.8–3.3).[22]

Phenobarbital is one of the oldest ASMs in use. It is not often used in the United States anymore but is still used internationally due to its affordability and efficacy. MCM rates with phenobarbital monotherapy range from 6% to 7%.[11,23] The most common associated MCMs are cardiac malformations and oral clefts.[16]

Zonisamide, clobazam, and lacosamide are among the newer ASMs that are increasingly prescribed. Not much data regarding their MCM risk exist. Zonisamide has an estimated MCM rate of 3.5% based on data pooled from 142 pregnancies across 5 studies.[17,20,22,24–26] Zonisamide has also been shown to have an increased prevalence of SGA infants (12.2% [RR 1.6, 95% CI 0.90–2.8]).[22] Clobazam has the least MCM data with only 13 monotherapy-exposed pregnancies reported by KREP, with a MCM rate of 21%.[27] However in the same registry, polytherapy including clobazam was associated with a MCM rate of 9.6%, which may be due to lower doses used in polytherapy or a larger sample size.[28] Finally, lacosamide also has very little data with 1 reported MCM in 16 exposed pregnancies.[29] Currently, we have no data on cenobamate, eslicarbazepine, ethosuximide, ezogabine, felbamate, perampanel, rufinamide, and vigabatrin.

ASM-related teratogenesis is associated not only with the specific medication used but also with the dose in early pregnancy. Dose-related teratogenesis has been illustrated for VPA, lamotrigine, and carbamazepine (**Fig. 2**), as well as for phenobarbital.[11,14,23] In the future, studies of ASM levels may be more important than dose given interindividual differences in drug metabolism.

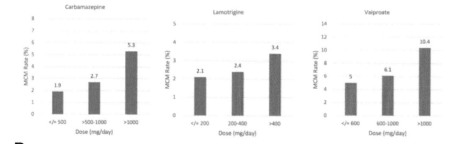

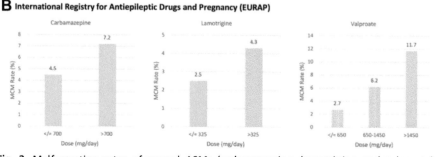

Fig. 2. Malformation rates of several ASMs (carbamazepine, lamotrigine and valproate) show evidence of dose dependence, with higher doses conferring higher rates of MCMs. Panel A shows data as analyzed from the UK/Ireland Pregnancy Registry[14] and panel B shows data as analyzed from the International Registry for Antiepileptic Drugs and Pregnancy.[18]

There is considerable debate about the impact of ASM polytherapy on structural teratogenesis. Polytherapy is often prescribed to patients with more difficult to control epilepsy and may use higher doses of medication. Although older studies suggested polytherapy always conferred higher MCM risk, many of these polytherapy combinations included VPA.[11,30] Polytherapy combinations that include VPA or topiramate are associated with the greatest MCM risk.[31] Within polytherapy combinations, key factors that affect structural teratogenesis include the specific medications within the polytherapy combination and the doses used. In practice, combination therapy for levetiracetam and lamotrigine is often used to avoid VPA.

Behavioral and cognitive teratogenesis

Although the risk of ASM-related structural teratogenesis is important, the risk of cognitive and behavioral teratogenesis is also significant and often overlooked. As with MCMs, VPA has the most data to support a clear association with poorer neurodevelopmental outcomes. Children exposed to VPA in utero have, on average, a 7 to 10-point decrease in IQ compared with children exposed to other ASMs, with higher doses showing greater risk.[32–34] Several studies have also shown that VPA exposure is associated with an increased risk of autism spectrum disorder (ASD),[11,34,35] including a recent study by Bjørk and colleagues,[36] which showed a cumulative 8-year risk of 2.7%. At school-age, children with in utero exposure to VPA or phenobarbital had worse language scores compared with unexposed children from the general population.[37]

At age 6, children with lamotrigine-exposure have similar IQ and verbal abilities compared with controls and better scores when compared with VPA-exposed children.[38,39] In most small prospective cohorts, levetiracetam-exposed children have been found to have cognitive profiles similar to lamotrigine-exposed and control children and superior to VPA-exposed children, with children in some of the studies being followed out to age 9.[40] Small studies of topiramate-exposed children have yielded mixed results on neurodevelopmental outcomes; however, a recent population-based study from 5 Nordic countries has raised concern that topiramate may also have adverse effects on cognitive development.[36] In this study, both VPA and topiramate were associated with significant and dose-related increases in neurodevelopmental disabilities compared with unexposed children. There are limited data on the neurodevelopmental effects of gabapentin, oxcarbazepine, and phenytoin.[39,41] Currently, there is no data on newer medications including, but not limited to, brivaracetam, cenobamate, clobazam, eslicarbazepine, lacosamide, and zonisamide.

In summary, in choosing an appropriate medication for PWEGC, it is important to balance the efficacy of the medication in controlling their epilepsy with the teratogenic profile of that medication. Based on our current data of both structural and cognitive and behavioral teratogenesis, lamotrigine and levetiracetam seem to be among the ASMs with lowest risk in pregnancy. It is our practice that PWEGC with a new diagnosis of epilepsy be started on one of these two medications. If a patient is on a higher risk medication and has not failed levetiracetam or lamotrigine previously, an attempt to transition to one of these two ASMs is recommended, with the caveat that the patient is not currently pregnant and can allow time for the transition to be made and efficacy assessed.

Role of folic acid

Folic acid supplementation has been routinely recommended for PWEGC. Studies in the general population have shown that folic acid supplementation during the periconceptual period is important in preventing NTDs although no clear association with

MCM reduction has been demonstrated in the ASM registries.[42] Folic acid supplementation has been shown to decrease the risk of miscarriage in ASM-exposed pregnancies and, in general, is associated with better cognitive and behavioral outcomes.[32,43] The MoBa study found that periconceptual folic acid supplementation was associated with a lower risk of ASD[44] and severe language delay by age 3.[45] The NEAD study demonstrated that first-trimester folic acid supplementation was associated with a higher IQ in ASM-exposed children.[32] A recently published prospective study found that periconceptual folic acid use was also associated with a lower risk of preterm birth in ASM-exposed pregnancies.[46] However, it is important to note that there is no data on the most beneficial dose of supplementation. A recent publication from the Nordic health databases has shown an association between prescriptions for high-dose (>1 mg/d) folic acid for pregnant patients with epilepsy and an increased risk of cancer in their children.[47] Although this needs further study, it calls into question the common practice of prescribing high-dose folic acid for PWEGC.

Antiseizure Medication Monitoring

ASM plasma concentrations during pregnancy can vary widely based on the medication and the individual patient. Concentrations can decrease during pregnancy due to an increase in the volume of distribution, as well as changes in hepatic metabolism, renal clearance, and protein binding. Studies have shown that a decline in ASM concentrations by greater than 35% from the prepregnancy baseline is associated with decreased seizure control.[48] **Table 1** provides a summary of pregnancy-related changes to dose-normalized concentration of the most commonly used ASM as illustrated in the MONEAD study.

Lamotrigine is 55% protein bound and is metabolized by the hepatic enzyme, uridine 5'-diphospho-glucuronosyltransferase (UGT1A4). During pregnancy, estrogen induces UGT1A4 activity and lamotrigine concentrations can decrease up to 56%.[49,50] Oxcarbazepine is also cleared in part by UGT1A4 and studies have found a 32% decline in total concentrations during pregnancy and a 30.6% decrease in unbound

Table 1	
Many of the commonly used antiseizure medications show decreases in serum concentration during pregnancy	
Antiseizure Medication	**% Max Concentration Decrease From Baseline**
Lamotrigine	56.1
Levetiracetam	36.8
Carbamazepine	17.3
Unbound carbamazepine	No change
Carbamazepine-10,11-epoxide	No change
Oxcarbazepine	32.6
Unbound oxcarbazepin	30.6
Zonisamide	29.8
Lacosamide	39.9

This table shows the maximal percent concentration decrease during pregnancy compared with the nonpregnant state as calculated based on dose-normalized concentration changes seen in the MONEAD study by Pennell et al.[50] It is important to note that these values represent the maximal changes noted and can have significant variation between individuals.

oxcarbazepine.[50] Levetiracetam concentrations can decrease up to 37% during pregnancy, in part due to increased renal clearance although the exact reason for the decline, which can occur early in pregnancy, is not known.[11,50]

In contrast to the above newer ASMs, carbamazepine concentrations seem to be more stable in pregnancy. Carbamazepine is 70% to 80% protein bound and hepatically metabolized by CYP450 3A4 to the active metabolite, known as carbamazepine 10,11-epoxide. Serum concentrations of total carbamazepine can decrease up to 17%; however, unbound carbamazepine and carbamazepine-10,11-epoxide do not change signficantly.[50] Some studies suggest topiramate clearance may increase up to 40% but others have shown no change.[50,51] Phenytoin is 90% protein bound to serum proteins and is hepatically metabolized predominantly by CYP450 2C9 and 2C19. Total drug levels can decrease by up to 60% and free drug levels decrease by 16% to 40% by the third trimester.[13] Finally, VPA is 90% protein bound and cleared by glucuronidation via UGT 1A3 and 2B7 plus other UGTs, as well as several CYP450 enzymes.[11,51] Free levels of VPA remain unchanged during pregnancy.[52]

Considering the relationship between dose-dependent teratogenesis and the concentration changes that occur with many of the ASMs during pregnancy, it is our practice to determine the lowest possible therapeutic dose that controls seizures effectively before pregnancy. Once this dose is determined, a corresponding plasma drug concentration can be used as a goal during pregnancy. For most ASMs, we obtain plasma concentrations monthly. Frequent monitoring may be less important for carbamazepine and VPA because free levels seem to be fairly constant during pregnancy. Medication changes are typically made if ASM concentrations fall below goal and/or if the patient has an increase in seizure frequency.

Postpartum Management

Medication adjustments

For those ASMs that undergo increased clearance during pregnancy, plasma concentrations increase in the first few weeks postpartum. If medication doses were increased during pregnancy, they should be tapered to near the prepregnancy range postpartum. Postpartum clearance changes have been best described for lamotrigine. Lamotrigine concentrations levels increase rapidly in the first few days after delivery and plateau by 3 weeks postpartum.[51,53] For lamotrigine, it is our practice to make dose reductions on postpartum days 3, 7, and 10 to prevent toxicity and recheck concentrations in the third postpartum week. We use a similar plan for other ASMs that were increased in pregnancy. In some cases, doses may be left slightly higher for added protection in the postpartum period when sleep-deprivation is common. However, if seizures are controlled, doses should be returned to baseline doses before the next pregnancy. For any medication, a postpartum weaning plan should be determined at least 1 month before expected delivery date and given to the patient.

Breastfeeding

Breastfeeding has many positive effects for infants in terms of neurodevelopment, decreased risk of infection, and decreased risk of sudden infant death syndrome.[54,55] In general, the known benefits of breastfeeding outweigh largely theoretical concerns about ASM exposure through breastmilk. Reassuringly, the MONEAD study found overall low exposure in breastmilk for several commonly used ASMs, including carbamazepine, lamotrigine, levetiracetam, and oxcarbazepine.[56] An earlier article from the NEAD study found that neurodevelopmental outcomes at age 6 were better in children that were exposed to VPA, carbamazepine, lamotrigine, or phenytoin via breastmilk compared with those of children of PWEGC that were not breastfed.[57] The MoBA study also found no adverse neurodevelopmental outcomes at 36 months in breastfed children exposed to ASMs through breastmilk.[12] The most common ASMs in this cohort were lamotrigine, valproate, and carbamazepine.

SUMMARY

Pregnancy counseling and planning is important for PWEGC and should be offered early and often. Seizures, if poorly controlled, can pose a risk to both the fetus and mother. Each ASM has its own teratogenic risk profile that must be considered, ideally well in advance of pregnancy. Based on current data, lamotrigine and levetiracetam are the ASMs with lowest risks of both structural and cognitive/behavioral teratogenesis. The use of these 2 medications is not always possible, thus shared decision-making is important in each patient's counseling. Once an appropriate medication is selected, the therapeutic dosage and corresponding plasma concentration should be established before pregnancy. This concentration can then serve as a pregnancy target to guide dose adjustments. Monthly levels should be checked for the majority of medications. It is important to note that breakthrough seizures should also prompt a dosage increase and subsequent concentration evaluation. After birth, dosages should be weaned down to prepregnancy ranges during the course of 2 to 3 weeks. A dose-reduction plan should be discussed with the patient 1 month before delivery. It is also important to counsel patients on the benefits of breastfeeding and available information on ASM exposure via breastmilk.

CLINICS CARE POINTS

- It is important to identify a therapeutic ASM regimen with the lowest teratogenic profile for each individual
- Once an appropriate ASM is identified, determine the lowest prepregnancy therapeutic dose and corresponding plasma concentration to serve as a target during pregnancy
- For the majority of ASMs, monthly concentration monitoring is recommended
- Recommend peripartum folic acid supplementation to PWEGC, recognizing that the optimal dose is not known
- Recommend a detailed anatomic ultrasound evaluation between 18 and 22 weeks' gestational age and ultrasonic fetal growth evaluations
- Ensure patient has a postpartum medication reduction plan
- Encourage breastfeeding, stressing the known benefits and low risks related to exposure with several ASMs

DISCLOSURE

E.E. Gerard has served as site PI for clinical trials supported by Stanford University/ Eisai as well as Xenon and Sunovion. She is a site-PI for the MONEAD trial NINDS (U01-NS038455; 2U01-NS038455).

REFERENCES

1. Harden CL, Pennell PB, Koppel BS, et al. Practice Parameter update: management issues for women with epilepsy—Focus on pregnancy (an evidence-based review): Vitamin K, folic acid, blood levels, and breastfeeding. Rep Qual

Stand Subcommittee Ther Technol Assess Subcommittee Am Acad Neurol Am Epilepsy Soc 2009;73(2):142–9.

2. Herzog AG, Mandle HB, Cahill KE, et al. Predictors of unintended pregnancy in women with epilepsy. Neurology 2017;88(8):728–33.

3. Tomson T, Battino D, Bromley R, et al. Management of epilepsy in pregnancy: a report from the International League Against Epilepsy Task Force on Women and Pregnancy. Epileptic Disord 2019;21(6):497–517.

4. Hiilesmaa VK, Teramo KA. Fetal and Maternal Risks with Seizures. In Harden C, Thomas SV, Tomson T, editors. Epilepsy in Women. John Wiley & Sons. p. 115–127.

5. Sahoo S, Klein P. Maternal complex partial seizure associated with fetal distress. Arch Neurol 2005;62(8):1304–5.

6. Nei M, Daly S, Liporace J. A maternal complex partial seizure in labor can affect fetal heart rate. Neurology 1998;51(3):904–6.

7. Edey S, Moran N, Nashef L. SUDEP and epilepsy-related mortality in pregnancy. Epilepsia 2014;55(7):e72–4.

8. Kapoor D, Wallace S. Trends in maternal deaths from epilepsy in the United Kingdom: a 30-year retrospective review. Obstet Med 2014;7(4):160–4.

9. Chen Y-H, Chiou H-Y, Lin H-C, et al. Affect of seizures during gestation on pregnancy outcomes in women with epilepsy. Arch Neurol 2009;66(8):979–84.

10. Pennell PB, French JA, May RC, et al. Changes in seizure frequency and antiepileptic therapy during pregnancy. N Engl J Med 2020;383(26):2547–56.

11. Voinescu PE, Pennell PB. Management of epilepsy during pregnancy. Expert Rev Neurother 2015;15(10):1171–87.

12. Veiby G, Daltveit AK, Schjølberg S, et al. Exposure to antiepileptic drugs in utero and child development: a prospective population-based study. Epilepsia 2013; 54(8):1462–72.

13. Pennell PB. Pregnancy, epilepsy, and women's issues. Continuum (Minneap Minn) 2013;19(3 Epilepsy):697–714.

14. Campbell E, Kennedy F, Russell A, et al. Malformation risks of antiepileptic drug monotherapies in pregnancy: updated results from the UK and Ireland Epilepsy and Pregnancy Registers. J Neurol Neurosurg Psychiatr 2014;85(9):1029–34.

15. Veiby G, Daltveit AK, Engelsen BA, et al. Fetal growth restriction and birth defects with newer and older antiepileptic drugs during pregnancy. J Neurol 2014;261(3): 579–88.

16. Tomson T, Battino D. Teratogenic effects of antiepileptic drugs. Lancet Neurol 2012;11(9):803–13.

17. Tomson T, Battino D, Bonizzoni E, et al. Comparative risk of major congenital malformations with eight different antiepileptic drugs: a prospective cohort study of the EURAP registry. Lancet Neurol 2018;17(6):530–8.

18. Chaudhry SA, Jong G, Koren G. The fetal safety of Levetiracetam: a systematic review. Reprod Toxicol 2014;46:40–5.

19. Scheuerle AE, Holmes LB, Albano JD, et al. Levetiracetam pregnancy registry: final results and a review of the impact of registry methodology and definitions on the prevalence of major congenital malformations. Birth Defects Res 2019; 111(13):872–87.

20. Hernández-Díaz S, Smith CR, Shen A, et al. Comparative safety of antiepileptic drugs during pregnancy. Neurology 2012;78(21):1692–9.

21. Mines D, Tennis P, Curkendall SM, et al. Topiramate use in pregnancy and the birth prevalence of oral clefts. Pharmacoepidemiol Drug Saf 2014;23(10): 1017–25.

22. Hernández-Díaz S, Mittendorf R, Smith CR, et al. Association between topiramate and zonisamide use during pregnancy and low birth weight. Obstet Gynecol 2014;123(1):21–8.

23. Tomson T, Battino D, Bonizzoni E, et al. Dose-dependent risk of malformations with antiepileptic drugs: an analysis of data from the EURAP epilepsy and pregnancy registry. Lancet Neurol 2011;10(7):609–17.

24. McCluskey G, Kinney MO, Russell A, et al. Zonisamide safety in pregnancy: data from the UK and Ireland epilepsy and pregnancy register. Seizure 2021;91: 311–5.

25. Meador KJ, Pennell PB, May RC, et al. Fetal loss and malformations in the MONEAD study of pregnant women with epilepsy. Neurology 2020;94(14):e1502–11.

26. Vajda FJE, Perucca P, O'Brien TJ, et al. Teratogenic effects of zonisamide. Seizure - Eur J Epilepsy 2021;91:490.

27. Thomas SV, Jeemon P, Pillai R, et al. Malformation risk of new anti-epileptic drugs in women with epilepsy; observational data from the Kerala registry of epilepsy and pregnancy (KREP). Seizure 2021;93:127–32.

28. Keni RR, Jose M, Sarma PS, et al. Teratogenicity of antiepileptic dual therapy: dose-dependent, drug-specific, or both? Neurology 2018;90(9):e790–6.

29. Golembesky AK, Cooney MA, Craig JJ, et al. Outcomes following exposure to the antiepileptic drug lacosamide during pregnancy – results from a global safety database (P5.231). Neurology 2017;88.

30. Holmes LB, Mittendorf R, Shen A, et al. Fetal effects of anticonvulsant polytherapies: different risks from different drug combinations. Arch Neurol 2011;68(10): 1275–81.

31. Vajda FJ, O'Brien TJ, Lander CM, et al. Antiepileptic drug combinations not involving valproate and the risk of fetal malformations. Epilepsia 2016;57(7): 1048–52.

32. Meador KJ, Baker GA, Browning N, et al. Fetal antiepileptic drug exposure and cognitive outcomes at age 6 years (NEAD study): a prospective observational study. Lancet Neurol 2013;12(3):244–52.

33. Bromley R, Weston J, Adab N, et al. Treatment for epilepsy in pregnancy: neurodevelopmental outcomes in the child. Cochrane Database Syst Rev 2014; 2014(10):Cd010236.

34. Bromley RL, Mawer GE, Briggs M, et al. The prevalence of neurodevelopmental disorders in children prenatally exposed to antiepileptic drugs. J Neurol Neurosurg Psychiatr 2013;84(6):637–43.

35. Christensen J, Grønborg TK, Sørensen MJ, et al. Prenatal valproate exposure and risk of autism spectrum disorders and childhood autism. JAMA 2013;309(16): 1696–703.

36. Bjørk M-H, Zoega H, Leinonen MK, et al. Association of prenatal exposure to antiseizure medication with risk of autism and intellectual disability. JAMA Neurol 2022;79(7):672–81.

37. Unnikrishnan G, Jacob NS, Salim S, et al. Enduring language deficits in children of women with epilepsy and the potential role of intrauterine exposure to antiepileptic drugs. Epilepsia 2020;61(11):2442–51.

38. Baker GA, Bromley RL, Briggs M, et al. IQ at 6 years after in utero exposure to antiepileptic drugs: a controlled cohort study. Neurology 2015;84(4):382–90.

39. Knight R, Wittkowski A, Bromley RL. Neurodevelopmental outcomes in children exposed to newer antiseizure medications: a systematic review. Epilepsia 2021;62(8):1765–79.

40. Shallcross R, Bromley RL, Cheyne CP, et al. In utero exposure to levetiracetam vs valproate: development and language at 3 years of age. Neurology 2014;82(3): 213–21.

41. Elkjær LS, Bech BH, Sun Y, et al. Association between prenatal valproate exposure and performance on standardized language and mathematics tests in school-aged children. JAMA Neurol 2018;75(6):663–71.

42. Prevention of neural tube defects: results of the Medical Research Council Vitamin Study. MRC Vitamin Study Research Group. Lancet 1991;338(8760): 131–7.

43. Pittschieler S, Brezinka C, Jahn B, et al. Spontaneous abortion and the prophylactic effect of folic acid supplementation in epileptic women undergoing antiepileptic therapy. J Neurol 2008;255(12):1926–31.

44. Surén P, Roth C, Bresnahan M, et al. Association between maternal use of folic acid supplements and risk of autism spectrum disorders in children. JAMA 2013;309(6):570–7.

45. Roth C, Magnus P, Schjølberg S, et al. Folic acid supplements in pregnancy and severe language delay in children. JAMA 2011;306(14):1566–73.

46. Alvestad S, Nilsen Husebye ES, Christensen J, et al. Folic acid and risk of preterm birth, preeclampsia and fetal growth restriction among women with epilepsy: a prospective cohort study. Neurology 2022;99(6):e605–15.

47. Vegrim HM, Dreier JW, Alvestad S, et al. Cancer risk in children of mothers with epilepsy and high-dose folic acid use during pregnancy. JAMA Neurology 2022; 79(11):1130–8.

48. Patel SI, Pennell PB. Management of epilepsy during pregnancy: an update. Ther Adv Neurol Disord 2016;9(2):118–29.

49. Polepally AR, Pennell PB, Brundage RC, et al. Model-Based Lamotrigine Clearance Changes During Pregnancy: Clinical Implication. Ann Clin Transl Neurol 2014;1(2):99–106.

50. Pennell PB, Karanam A, Meador KJ, et al. Antiseizure medication concentrations during pregnancy: results from the maternal outcomes and neurodevelopmental effects of antiepileptic drugs (MONEAD) study. JAMA Neurol 2022;79(4):370–9.

51. Tomson T, Landmark CJ, Battino D. Antiepileptic drug treatment in pregnancy: changes in drug disposition and their clinical implications. Epilepsia 2013; 54(3):405–14.

52. Johannessen SI. Pharmacokinetics of valproate in pregnancy: mother-foetus-newborn. Pharm Weekbl Sci 1992;14(3a):114–7.

53. Pennell PB, Peng L, Newport DJ, et al. Lamotrigine in pregnancy: clearance, therapeutic drug monitoring, and seizure frequency. Neurology 2008;70(22 Pt 2): 2130–6.

54. Thompson JMD, Tanabe K, Moon RY, et al. Duration of breastfeeding and risk of SIDS: an individual participant data meta-analysis. Pediatrics 2017;140(5).

55. Duijts L, Ramadhani MK, Moll HA. Breastfeeding protects against infectious diseases during infancy in industrialized countries. A systematic review. Matern Child Nutr 2009;5(3):199–210.

56. Birnbaum AK, Meador KJ, Karanam A, et al. Antiepileptic drug exposure in infants of breastfeeding mothers with epilepsy. JAMA Neurol 2020;77(4):441–50.

57. Meador KJ, Baker GA, Browning N, et al. Effects of breastfeeding in children of women taking antiepileptic drugs. Neurology 2010;75(22):1954–60.

Moving?

Make sure your subscription moves with you!

To notify us of your new address, find your **Clinics Account Number** (located on your mailing label above your name), and contact customer service at:

Email: journalscustomerservice-usa@elsevier.com

800-654-2452 (subscribers in the U.S. & Canada)
314-447-8871 (subscribers outside of the U.S. & Canada)

Fax number: 314-447-8029

Elsevier Health Sciences Division
Subscription Customer Service
3251 Riverport Lane
Maryland Heights, MO 63043

*To ensure uninterrupted delivery of your subscription, please notify us at least 4 weeks in advance of move.